Optimizing Hemodynamic Support in Severe Sepsis and Septic Shock

Guest Editor

DANE NICHOLS, MD

CRITICAL CARE CLINICS

www.criticalcare.theclinics.com

Consulting Editor
RICHARD W. CARLSON, MD, PhD

April 2010 • Volume 26 • Number 2

SAUNDERS an imprint of ELSEVIER, Inc.

W.B. SAUNDERS COMPANY
A Division of Elsevier Inc.

Elsevier Inc. • 1600 John F. Kennedy Blvd., • Suite 1800 • Philadelphia, Pennsylvania 19103-2899

http://www.theclinics.com

CRITICAL CARE CLINICS Volume 26, Number 2
April 2010 ISSN 0749-0704, ISBN-13: 978-1-4377-1807-2

Editor: Patrick Manley
Developmental Editor: Donald Mumford

Critical Care Clinics (ISSN: 0749-0704) is published quarterly by Elsevier Inc., 360 Park Avenue South, New York, NY 10010-1710. Months of issue are January, April, July, and October. Business and Editorial Offices: 1600 John F. Kennedy Blvd., Suite 1800, Philadelphia, PA 19103-2899. Customer Service Office: 6277 Sea Harbor Drive, Orlando, FL 32887-4800. Periodicals postage paid at New York, NY and additional mailing offices. Subscription prices are $167.00 per year for US individuals, $395.00 per year for US institution, $83.00 per year for US students and residents, $206.00 per year for Canadian individuals, $490.00 per year for Canadian institutions, $240.00 per year for international individuals, $490.00 per year for international institutions and $121.00 per year for Canadian and foreign students/residents. To receive student/resident rate, orders must be accompanied by name of affiliated institution, date of term, and the *signature* of program/residency coordinator on institution letterhead. Orders will be billed at individual rate until proof of status is received. Foreign air speed delivery is included in all *Clinics* subscription prices. All prices are subject to change without notice. POSTMASTER: Send address changes to *Critical Care Clinics*, Elsevier Periodicals Customer Service, 11830 Westline Industrial Drive, St. Louis, MO 63146. **Customer Service: 1-800-654-2452 (US). From outside of the US, call 1-314-447-8871. Fax: 1-314-447-8029. E-mail: journalscustomerservice-usa@elsevier.com (for print support) or journalsonlinesupport-usa@elsevier.com (for online support).**

Reprints. For copies of 100 or more of articles in this publication, please contact the Commercial Reprints Department, Elsevier Inc., 360 Park Avenue South, New York, NY 10010-1710. Tel.: 212-633-3813; Fax: 212-462-1935; E-mail: reprints@elsevier.com.

Critical Care Clinics is also published in Spanish by Editorial Inter-Medica, Junin 917, 1er A, 1113, Buenos Aires, Argentina.

Critical Care Clinics is covered in *MEDLINE/PubMed (Index Medicus), EMBASE/Excerpta Medica, Current Concepts/Clinical Medicine, ISI/BIOMED,* and *Chemical Abstracts.*

Printed and bound in the United Kingdom
Transferred to Digital Print 2011

Contributors

CONSULTING EDITOR

RICHARD W. CARLSON, MD, PhD
Chairman Emeritus, Department of Medicine, Maricopa Medical Center and Director
of Medical Intensive Care Unit; Professor, University of Arizona College of Medicine;
and Professor, Department of Medicine, Mayo Graduate School of Medicine,
Phoenix, Arizona

GUEST EDITOR

DANE NICHOLS, MD
Associate Professor of Medicine, Division of Pulmonary-Critical Care Medicine,
Oregon Health and Sciences University, Portland, Oregon

AUTHORS

LYNN BOSHKOV, MD
Professor of Medicine, Medical Director, Hemostasis and Thrombosis Service, Associate
Director, Transfusion Medicine, Oregon Health and Sciences University, Portland, Oregon

T. MIKO ENOMOTO, MD
Assistant Professor, Division of Critical Care, Department of Anesthesiology and
Perioperative Medicine, Oregon Health and Sciences Univeristy, Portland, Oregon

MATTHEW J. GRIFFEE, MD
Assistant Professor, Department of Anesthesiology and Perioperative Medicine, Oregon
Health and Science University, Portland, Oregon

LOUISE HARDER, MD
Fellow, Department of Critical Care Medicine, Oregon Health and Sciences University,
Portland, Oregon

AKRAM KHAN, MD
Assistant Professor, Division of Pulmonary and Critical Care, Department of Internal
Medicine, Oregon Health and Science University, Portland, Oregon

JENNIFER L. LETOURNEAU, DO, MCR
Assistant Professor, Division of Pulmonary and Critical Care Medicine, Oregon
Health and Science University; Director, Medical Critical Care, Pulmonary Disease
Section, Portland Veterans Affairs Medical Center, Portland, Oregon

LAURIE A. LOIACONO, MD, FCCP, FCCM
Vice Chair, Department of Surgery; Director of Surgical Critical Care; Director of Surgical Education, Associate Professor of Surgery, University of Connecticut School of Medicine, Farmington, Connecticut; Director of Critical Care, Saint Francis Hospital and Medical Center, Department of Surgery; Saint Francis Medical Group, Hartford, Connecticut

LEWIS L. LOW, MD
Clinical Vice President, Medical Specialties Division, Legacy Health, Portland, Oregon

SUPRIYA MADDIRALA, MD
Assistant Professor, Division of Nephrology, Department of Internal Medicine, Oregon Health and Science University, Portland, Oregon

MATTHIAS J. MERKEL, MD, PhD
Assistant Professor, Department of Anesthesiology and Perioperative Medicine, Oregon Health and Science University, Portland, Oregon

IMRAN MOHAMMED, MD
Fellow, Division of Pulmonary and Critical Care, Oregon Health and Science University, Portland, Oregon

RICHARD A. NAHOURAII, MD, FACS
Fellow, Division of Trauma, Critical Care and Acute Care Surgery, Department of Surgery, Oregon Health and Science University, Portland, Oregon

DANE NICHOLS, MD
Associate Professor of Medicine, Division of Pulmonary-Critical Care Medicine, Oregon Health and Sciences University, Portland, Oregon

NATHAN D. NIELSEN, MD, MSc
Assistant Professor of Medicine, Division of Pulmonary-Critical Care, Tulane University, New Orleans, Louisiana

STEPHANIE A. NONAS, MD
Assistant Professor of Medicine, Division of Pulmonary and Critical Care, Oregon Health and Science University, Portland, Oregon

CHARLES PHILLIPS, MD
Division of Pulmonary and Critical Care Medicine, Oregon Health and Science University, Portland, Oregon

SUSAN E. ROWELL, MD, FACS
Assistant Professor, Division of Trauma, Critical Care and Acute Care Surgery, Department of Surgery, Oregon Health and Science University, Portland, Oregon

DAVID S. SHAPIRO, MD
Assistant Professor, Department of Surgery, University of Connecticut School of Medicine, Farmington, Connecticut; Associate Director, Trauma and Surgical Critical Care, Saint Francis Hospital and Medical Center; Saint Francis Medical Group, Hartford, Connecticut

CHRISTOPHER VERNON, DO
Fellow, Critical Care Medicine, Division of Pulmonary and Critical Care Medicine, Oregon Health and Science University, Portland, Oregon

KEVIN S. WEI, MD
Associate Professor, Department of Medicine, Division of Cardiovascular Medicine, Oregon Health and Science University, Portland, Oregon

BRIAN P. YOUNG, MD
Medical Director, Kern Critical Care Unit, Good Samaritan Medical Center, Legacy Health, Portland, Oregon

Contents

Preface   xiii

Dane Nichols

Oxygen Delivery and Consumption: A Macrocirculatory Perspective   239

Dane Nichols and Nathan D. Nielsen

> Severe sepsis is a leading cause of death and resource use throughout the world. This article examines the relationship of oxygen delivery to oxygen use under varying conditions. Topics reviewed include the concept of the critical dissolved oxygen, concerns over shared measurement errors in obtaining estimates of oxygen consumption, seminal articles in this area, and the practice of early goal directed therapy.

Lactic Acidosis: Recognition, Kinetics, and Associated Prognosis   255

Christopher Vernon and Jennifer L. LeTourneau

> Lactic acidosis is a common condition encountered by critical care providers. Elevated lactate and decreased lactate clearance are important for prognostication. Not all lactate in the intensive care unit is due to tissue hypoxia or ischemia and other sources should be evaluated. Lactate, in and of itself, is unlikely to be harmful and is a preferred fuel for many cells. Treatment of lactic acidosis continues to be aimed the underlying source.

Mean Arterial Pressure: Therapeutic Goals and Pharmacologic Support   285

David S. Shapiro and Laurie A. Loiacono

> The Surviving Sepsis Campaign targets central venous pressure, mean arterial pressure, and central venous oxygen saturation as guides for resuscitation. Fluid resuscitation and the use of vasopressors are paramount to the success of the campaign's end points. Although the achievement of supranormal physiologic parameters has been associated with higher mortality in some studies, these slightly higher blood pressures may enable better oxygen delivery, in some observations. This article focuses on the mean arterial pressure goals during sepsis, the measurement of the mean arterial pressure, and the manipulation of this target with volume resuscitation and pharmacologic interventions.

Static Measures of Preload Assessment   295

Richard A. Nahouraii and Susan E. Rowell

> This article focuses on static methods for determining preload, specifically pressure and volumetric indices measured at the bedside. The underlying ventricular function will determine where the patient is located on Frank-Starling ventricular function curve and the patient's response to a fluid

challenge. The proper interpretation and use of such measures, coupled with an understanding of their limitations and knowledge of alternative methods, is necessary to guide properly volume resuscitation in the critically ill.

Dynamic Indices of Preload   307

T. Miko Enomoto and Louise Harder

Hypotension and shock are important issues confronting the intensivist. Volume overload can have dire consequences such as decreased gas exchange and increased myocardial dysfunction. This article explores dynamic means of determining preload responsiveness.

Optimizing Hemodynamic Support in Septic Shock Using Central and Mixed Venous Oxygen Saturation   323

Supriya Maddirala and Akram Khan

Global tissue hypoxia is one of the most important factors in the development of multisystem organ dysfunction. In hemodynamically unstable critically ill patients, central venous oxygen saturation ($Scvo_2$) and mixed venous oxygen saturation (Svo_2) monitoring has been shown to be a better indicator of global tissue hypoxia than vital signs and other clinical parameters alone. Svo_2 is probably more representative of global tissue oxygenation, whereas $Scvo_2$, is less invasive. Svo_2 and $Scvo_2$ monitoring can have diagnostic and therapeutic uses in understanding the efficacy of interventions in treating critically ill, hemodynamically unstable patients.

The Optimal Hematocrit   335

Louise Harder and Lynn Boshkov

Nearly 15 million units of packed red blood cells and whole blood are transfused annually in the United States alone. Until recently, the major risks from blood transfusion were thought to be transmission of viral infections, and overall, blood transfusion was believed by most providers to be safe. A safe hemoglobin threshold above which red cell transfusion is clearly unnecessary has not been established. This article addresses the numerous problems that surround the use and consequences of blood transfusion, such as hemoglobin and hematocrit levels, oxygenation, storage time, immunomodulation, infection, and anemia. The relevant literature is comprehensively reviewed.

Techniques for Determining Cardiac Output in the Intensive Care Unit   355

Imran Mohammed and Charles Phillips

To achieve the goals of resuscitation in critically ill patients, a thorough understanding of the techniques available to measure cardiac output is important. Recently the pulmonary artery catheter has fallen out of favor because of concerns of safety and a lack of efficacy. Newer less invasive techniques since have been developed and are gaining popularity. But is important to remember that the ability of these techniques to improve outcome has yet to be demonstrated, and one should apply caution in how they are used until their use in algorithmic treatment approaches have been shown to improve outcome. This article discusses the invasive and noninvasive techniques to assess cardiac output.

The Role of Echocardiography in Hemodynamic Assessment of Septic Shock   365

Matthew J. Griffee, Matthias J. Merkel, and Kevin S. Wei

Echocardiography is a rapid, noninvasive, comprehensive cardiac assessment option for patients presenting with hemodynamic instability. In patients with septic shock, echocardiography can be used to guide fluid therapy by measuring collapsibility of the inferior vena cava. Sepsis-induced myocardial dysfunction can be diagnosed, and responses to therapy can be monitored with echo. Patients with persistent shock should be evaluated for right heart failure, dynamic left ventricular obstruction, or tamponade if they do not respond to resuscitation and norepinephrine. Unexpected or rare findings that affect management may be revealed using focused echocardiography. This article presents national and international competency statements regarding critical care echocardiography and training resources for intensivists.

Noninvasive Monitoring Cardiac Output Using Partial CO$_2$ Rebreathing   383

Brian P. Young and Lewis L. Low

This article reviews use of partial carbon dioxide rebreathing devices to determine cardiac output and their application for hemodynamic monitoring in the ICU and operating room. The primary focus is on the NICO monitoring device. Compared with conventional cardiac output methods, these techniques are noninvasive, easily automated, and provide real-time and continuous cardiac output monitoring. The advantages and limitations of each technique are different discussed.

Mechanisms, Detection, and Potential Management of Microcirculatory Disturbances in Sepsis   393

Imran Mohammed and Stephanie A. Nonas

Despite improvements in resuscitation and treatment of sepsis, the morbidity and mortality remain unacceptably high. Microvascular dysfunction has been shown to play a significant role in the pathogenesis of sepsis and is a potential new target in the management of sepsis. Clinical studies, aided by new techniques that allow for real-time assessment of the microcirculation, have shown that disturbances in microcirculatory flow are common in sepsis and correlate with worse outcomes. Bedside measurement of microcirculatory perfusion has become simpler and more accessible, and may provide key insights into prognosis in sepsis and guide future therapeutics, much like mean arterial pressure (MAP), lactate, and mixed central oxygen saturation (SvO$_2$) do now. The authors review here the role of microcirculatory dysfunction in sepsis and its potential role as a therapeutic target in sepsis.

Detection of Hypoxia at the Cellular Level   **409**

Laurie A. Loiacono and David S. Shapiro

Organ function is critically linked to the way tissues use available oxygen. In sepsis, tissue-related hypoxic injury is the result of hypoxemia and hypoperfusion and cytokine-mediated mitochondrial dysfunction termed cytopathic hypoxia. Organ dysfunction in sepsis is more likely related to derailment of the metabolic processes of cells to use available oxygen. Cellular dysoxia rather than hypoxia may be the most appropriate way of describing sepsis-related tissue injury. Lactate is a marker of aerobic mitochondrial dysfunction and anaerobic tissue metabolism and in some circumstances is considered the fuel of choice for certain tissues. The concept of cellular metabolic derangement or cytopathic hypoxia as a potential cause for multiorgan system dysfunction in sepsis may direct efforts to optimize outcome in septic patients from the classic targets of CO, tissue perfusion, DVo_2, and Vo_2 toward moderating sepsis-related early cytokine response, maximizing mitochondrial function, and using biomarkers to monitor treatment response.

Index   **423**

FORTHCOMING ISSUES

July 2010
Pharmaconutrition and Nutrition Therapy in Critical Illness
Paul Wischmeyer, MD, *Guest Editor*

October 2010
Critical Care Considerations of the Morbidly Obese
Marilyn T. Haupt, MD, and
Mary Reed, MD, *Guest Editors*

January 2011
Health Economics in Critical Care from a Global Perspective
Donald Chalfin, MD, *Guest Editor*

RECENT ISSUES

January 2010
ICU Management of the Cancer Patient
Stephen Pastores, MD, and
Neil Halpern, MD, *Guest Editor*

October 2009
Sepsis
R. Phillip Dellinger, MD, *Guest Editor*

July 2009
Sedation and Analgesia in the ICU: Pharmacology, Protocolization, and Clinical Consequences
Pratik Pandharipande, MD, and
E. Wesley Ely, MD, *Guest Editors*

RELATED INTEREST

Neurosurgery Clinics Volume 21, Issue 2, April 2010
Aneurysmal Subarachnoid Hemorrhage
P. Nyquist, N.N. Meyer, and R. Tamargo, *Guest Editors*

THE CLINICS ARE NOW AVAILABLE ONLINE!

Access your subscription at:
www.theclinics.com

Preface

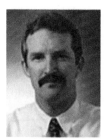

Dane Nichols, MD
Guest Editor

From the early recognition of altered hemodynamics in severe sepsis and septic shock, practitioners have sought new and improved ways to optimize convective oxygen transport, to establish important end points for resuscitation, and to assess the effect of various interventions on organ function and survival. In this regard, investigations of animal models of sepsis have provided unequivocal support for the central role of hemodynamics in determining outcome.[1] Unfortunately, the human experience has been checkered with positive and negative trials, providing clinicians with little certainty about how best to proceed when faced with patients suffering from severe sepsis and septic shock.[2–5] Notwithstanding The Surviving Sepsis Campaign's endorsement of early goal-directed therapy, targets such as mean arterial pressure, central venous pressure, hemoglobin levels, and central venous saturation remain controversial goals and await validation in large, multicentered randomized trials.[6]

Progress in our understanding of the pathophysiology of sepsis and the introduction of new technologies have added to the clinician's dilemma. Which of the available and emerging monitoring devices and techniques offers the best assessment of the state of the circulation? What role does microcirculation play in the development of organ dysfunction? Will changes in the macrocirculation influence microcirculatory blood flow? Does this have any effect on tissue use of oxygen?

In this issue of the *Clinics*, we have attempted to address these and other questions that clinicians routinely face. Articles addressing static and dynamic preload indices, echocardiography, venous blood gas analysis, and the like are meant to provide practitioners with a balanced overview of the topics and seasoned opinions about the current role of these approaches and technologies in the care of patients.

I would like to thank the many contributors for their efforts in reviewing and condensing a large body of work in the area of hemodynamics and oxygen transport.

Crit Care Clin 26 (2010) xiii–xiv
doi:10.1016/j.ccc.2010.02.001
0749-0704/10/$ – see front matter © 2010 Elsevier Inc. All rights reserved.

criticalcare.theclinics.com

In addition, special consideration goes out to Dr Richard Carlson, who has been a sage voice and source of inspiration to me throughout my career.

Dane Nichols, MD
Division of Pulmonary-Critical Care Medicine
Oregon Health & Sciences University
Portland, OR, USA

E-mail address:
nicholda@ohsu.edu

REFERENCES

1. Natason C, Danner RL, Reilly JM, et al. Antibiotics versus cardiovascular support in a canine model of human septic shock. Am J Physiol 1990;259:H1440–7.
2. Bihari D, Smithies M, Gimson A, et al. The effect of vasodilation with prostacyclin on oxygen delivery and uptake in critically ill patients. N Engl J Med 1987;317: 397–403.
3. Hayes MA, Yau EH, Timmins AC, et al. Response of critically ill patients to treatment aimed at achieving supranormal oxygen delivery and consumption: Relationship to outcome. Chest 1993;103(3):886–95.
4. Ronco JJ, Fenwick JC, Tweeddale MG, et al. Identification of the critical oxygen delivery for anaerobic metabolism in critically ill septic and nonseptic humans. JAMA 1993;270:1724–30.
5. Rivers E, Nguyen B, Haystad S, et al. Early goal-directed therapy in the treatment of severe sepsis and septic shock. N Engl J Med 2001;345(19):1368–77.
6. Clinical Trials.Gov. Available at: http://www.clinicaltrial.gov/ct2/results?term= early+goal+directed+therapy. Accessed January 11, 2010.

Oxygen Delivery and Consumption: A Macrocirculatory Perspective

Dane Nichols, MD[a],*, Nathan D. Nielsen, MD, MSc[b]

KEYWORDS

- Oxygen delivery • Oxygen consumption
- Early goal-directed therapy

Despite decades of investigation, severe sepsis continues to be a leading cause of death and resource use throughout the world. Deaths attributable to complications of infection now are thought to be on par with those secondary to acute myocardial infarction. In 2001, Angus and colleagues,[1] using data obtained from all nonfederal hospitals in a seven state area as an estimate of national figures, calculated the number of severe sepsis cases in the United States to be somewhere in the neighborhood of 751,000 cases per annum with an associated mortality of 28.6% or 215,000 deaths overall. This figure was roughly twice that estimated by the Centers for Disease Control (CDC) at the beginning of the 1990s. Moreover, they predicted that the incidence of severe sepsis would continue to increase at an annual rate of 1.5%. This trend was borne out in a longitudinal study using information from a national hospital database representing roughly 20% of nonfederal short-term institutions. Over the period from 1993 to 2003, Dombrovskiy and colleagues[2] reported a doubling in hospitalizations for severe sepsis from 64.7 to 134.6 cases per 100,000 population. In addition, the investigators noted an increase in the percentage of patients developing multiple organ dysfunction during their stay. Whereas acuity of illness and crude severe sepsis rate were clearly increasing, the associated case-fatality rate fell approximately 7% during the decade under study. Not surprisingly, the cases were disproportionately concentrated in the elderly, with patients over the age of 65 accounting for roughly three-fifths of hospitalizations. The expense of caring for patients with this syndrome is staggering. During the calendar year 1995, the cost

[a] Division of Pulmonary & Critical Care Medicine, Oregon Health and Sciences University, OHSU-UHN-67, 3181 SW Sam Jackson Park Road, Portland, OR 97239, USA
[b] Tulane University, SL-9, 1430 Tulane Avenue, New Orleans, LA 70130, USA
* Corresponding author.
E-mail address: nicholda@ohsu.edu

Crit Care Clin 26 (2010) 239–253
doi:10.1016/j.ccc.2009.12.003
0749-0704/10/$ – see front matter © 2010 Elsevier Inc. All rights reserved.

criticalcare.theclinics.com

per case of severe sepsis was estimated to be $22,100, which translated into national expenditures approaching $16.7 billion.[1]

Over the last 5 decades, remarkable advances in our understanding of the pathophysiology of sepsis have occurred. A crucial aspect of the syndrome involves cardiovascular dysfunction that was first appreciated by Waisbren[3] in the 1950s. Early observations suggested that the lactic acidosis and organ dysfunction seen in septic states were occurring in the setting of normal or high oxygen delivery to tissues and, therefore, represented a unique form of shock. Indeed, experimental models revealed that the critical level of oxygen delivery in sepsis was significantly higher than that seen in anemic, stagnant, and hypoxic hypoxia.[4] Another poorly understood phenomenon also seemed to be occurring in septic animals and patients: normal compensatory increases in O_2 extraction to meet tissue demand appeared to be limited, suggesting that the optimal means to meet increased demand would be through an increase in global oxygen delivery.[4,5]

The problem of meeting cellular oxygen needs and maintaining tissue and organ viability in sepsis has become increasingly complex with the modern demonstration of marked microcirculatory disturbances along with early organelle injury and dysfunction. A variety of studies suggest that augmenting convective transport in the macrocirculation often has little impact on the distribution of microcirculatory blood flow or measured oxygen consumption.[6,7] Other studies suggest that oxygen tension within a variety of tissues may be more than adequate for normal cellular respiration implying that as shock progresses treatment strategies based on enhanced convective transport are not likely to be successful.[8,9]

Cellular and organelle injury appears to occur very early on in severe septic conditions. Brealey and colleagues,[10] studying mitochondria obtained from septic patients within the first 24 hours of admission to an ICU, frequently found abnormal activity in electron transport complexes I and IV along with marked alterations in the levels of ATP and the ADP-ATP ratio. Even though initially patients were clinically indistinguishable, nonsurvivors had roughly half the amount of ATP contained within mitochondria than did survivors. Curiously, there also may be important bioenergetic differences in mitochondria from different tissues obtained from patients suffering multiple organ dysfunction and also from patients with different ancestry.[11,12] What does seem clear is that morphologic changes evident on electron microscopy correlate with the organelle's ability to efficiently use oxygen and the cell's ability to function normally. When exposed to lipopolysaccharide, mitochondria undergo changes in size, shape, and density thought secondary to the development of a so-called permeability transition pore. As the process advances, a number of mitochondria may undergo organelle death and subsequent autophagy.[13,14]

Surprisingly, autopsied organs obtained from patients dying of sepsis demonstrate little evidence of ischemic necrosis when assessed by light microscopy. Hotchkiss and colleagues[15] investigating patients within an hour and a half of death found scant amounts of focal necrosis near central veins in hepatic lobules and in organs (heart, kidney, and brain) where infarction had occurred before death. Apoptosis of lymphocytes and endothelial cells was noted on immunohistochemical staining in several organs, but rarely exceeded 5% of the cells examined. These findings, along with a host of other observations in natural and experimental settings, have lead many in the field to develop a new paradigm to explain these discordant findings. Rather than cells undergoing a fatal loss of function secondary to injury or ischemia, cellular processes may be down-regulated in an effort to limit oxidant stress, high-energy phosphate depletion, or other injurious processes as a means to allow for later recovery similar to the hibernation seen in chronically ischemic myocardial tissue.[16]

Although this may prove to be adaptive, at present we do not have the ability to discern the point at which the process becomes maladaptive nor the capability to recover the function of these failing organs.

With this background, the authors examine the relationship of oxygen delivery to oxygen use under varying conditions and review the concept of the critical dissolved oxygen (DO_2crit), the point at which oxygen consumption falls with further decrease in oxygen delivery. In addition, this article addresses the concerns over shared measurement errors in obtaining estimates of oxygen consumption, review the seminal articles in this area, and explore the practice of early goal-directed therapy (EGDT).

CONVECTIVE TRANSPORT AND THE DELIVERED OXYGEN–OXYGEN CONSUMPTION RELATIONSHIP

To sustain aerobic metabolism, cells require a constant supply of oxygen. At the level of the mitochondria, the amount needed seems impossibly small. Under basal conditions, an oxygen partial pressure of $\sim$1mmHg in the vicinity of the mitochondria meets the organelles' metabolic requirements.[17] This supply is maintained through convective and diffusive transport of oxygen and relies heavily on the association properties of hemoglobin (Hgb) for oxygen. Mathematically whole body oxygen delivery (DO_2) is expressed by the following formula:

DO_2 = Arterial oxygen content $\times$ Cardiac Output $\times$ 10

or

$DO_2 = CaO_2 \times CO \times 10$

Where CaO_2= [Hgb x 1.39 mL/gm of Hgb x Saturation of Hgb] + [$PaO_2 \times 0.0031$]. A normal arterial oxygen content is generally between 18 and 20 mL per deciliter of blood. In the setting of a normal cardiac output, total bulk transport in the systemic circulation is then between 900 and 1,100 mL per minute. When indexed to body surface area, a range of 530 to 600 mL/min/m^2 is obtained.

Estimating oxygen consumption (VO_2) can be accomplished in the clinical setting either by expired-gases analysis or through the reverse Fick method. The latter is the more popular approach and uses a mixed venous blood gas obtained from a pulmonary artery catheter to calculate venous oxygen content in the same manner as done on the arterial side of the circulation. Substituting mixed venous central (Cv) and tension (Pv) values into the above equation leads to the following formula: CvO_2 = [Hgb x 1.39 mL/gm of Hgb x saturation of Hgb] + [$PvO_2 \times 0.0031$]. The venous oxygen content under usual conditions runs 13 to 16 mL/dL leading to an arterial-venous (A-V) O_2 content difference of $\sim$3–5 mL/dL. Multiplying the oxygen content difference by the cardiac output obtained from thermodilution measurements then provides a reasonable estimate of total body oxygen consumption. The values obtained are slightly lower than those derived from expired gas analysis that includes O_2 consumption from the alveolar compartment. The reverse Fick equation is expressed mathematically as the following:

VO_2 = A − VO_2 content difference $\times$ CO $\times$ 10

The percentage of oxygen consumed to that delivered is termed the extraction ratio (ER). Normally the ER is around 25%, but can vary significantly depending on the metabolic activities of the tissue and the conditioning of the subject. In well-trained athletes, for example, the extraction ratio near their anaerobic threshold may approach 60%.[18] Extraction ratios can be calculated in one of two ways:

$$ER = VO_2 \div DO_2$$

or

$$ER = (CaO_2 - CvO_2)/CaO_2$$

Intermittent or continuous monitoring of venous oxygen tension in the superior vena cava or pulmonary artery also can often provide important early information with regard to the adequacy of oxygen delivery. By rearranging the following formula and ignoring the small contribution from dissolved oxygen we can demonstrate that when VO_2 is stable venous oxygen saturation (SvO_2) will vary with DO_2.[17,19]

$$\text{Oxygen Delivery } (DO_2) = \text{Oxygen Consumption } (VO_2) +$$
$$[\text{Venous Oxygen Content} \times CO]$$

or

$$SvO_2 = SaO_2 - VO_2/DO_2$$

Originally, it was thought that SvO_2 might serve as an indicator of cardiac output but the correlations in critically ill patients have been disappointing because DO_2 can be influenced by changes in hemoglobin and the partial pressure of oxygen and VO_2 can vary with temperature, activity, nursing interventions, oxygen delivery, and the tissues' ability to extract.[20]

THE ISSUE OF MATHEMATICAL COUPLING

Early studies in the area of DO_2-VO_2 covariance relied on the reverse Fick equation to estimate consumption rather than measuring VO_2 independently through techniques such as indirect calorimetry.[21–23] This methodology led to concerns that systematic or random errors in shared variables such as cardiac output and SaO_2 might force a relationship during regression analysis where in fact none existed. This conclusion was supported by Phang and colleagues[24] in a study of acute respiratory distress syndrome (ARDS) patients. When VO_2 was measured by expired gas analysis during manipulation of oxygen delivery, DO_2 dependence was not apparent, leading to the conclusion that measurement errors in the common elements of the Fick equation were the source of the previously described covariance. This controversy continues to find its way into the literature and can be an ongoing source of confusion for the practitioner. A number of recent papers, however, have provided key insights into the impact of measurement error when common variables are used to establish DO_2-VO_2 dependency and have suggested approaches to mitigate the effect.

Analysis of the problem can be quite complex and is beyond the scope of this article. The interested reader can find in-depth discussions in papers by Squara,[25] De Backer,[26] and Granton and colleagues.[27] The essential elements, however, can be distilled down to (1) the effect of pooled versus individual measurements, (2) the heterogeneity of patient populations, (3) the impact of changing DO_2 in the setting of low cardiac output, and (4) the effect of two versus multiple measurements. Granton and colleagues[27] point out that if the change in DO_2 is large (50–100 mL/min/m²) and multiple measurements are obtained, then the reverse Fick technique and indirect calorimetry approximate each other. Also, if measurement error in cardiac output estimates can be kept to a minimum, then the change in slope of the DO_2-VO_2 relationship attributable to mathematical coupling will be modest and, by itself, inconsistent with supply dependency.[25,27]

It is also important to remember that biologic coupling should not be easily dismissed as a statistical aberration. A number of studies have demonstrated markedly different outcomes across groups depending on the presence or absence of supply-dependency.[28–31] If systematic or random errors were forcing statistical relationships, then one would expect DO_2-VO_2 covariance to be similar between groups and not predictive of patient outcome.

In experimental settings and clinical studies, the slope of the DO_2-VO_2 relationship during supply dependency is quite steep with a range of 30% to 50%. Above DO_2crit, the slope falls to less than 10% but rarely plateaus (**Fig. 1**). The modest slope in oxygen consumption above DO_2crit has been attributed to increased metabolic work necessitated by higher individual organ blood flow, the thermogenic effect of catecholamines, and the conformation of organs to a richer oxygen environment. In light of these observations and the known impact of measurement error, it has been suggested that supply dependency not be diagnosed until the slope of the DO_2-VO_2 relationship is well in excess of 10%.[26]

THE "CRITICAL" DO_2

Normally, changing oxygen needs of the body are easily met through abundant basal flow and a variety of compensatory mechanisms including increased stroke volume and heart rate, vascular redistribution of blood flow, capillary recruitment, and changes in hemoglobin binding affinity. Recently, it has also been shown that the red blood cell itself may be playing an important role in local control of flow through hypoxic regions by generating dilatory nitric oxide from membrane associated nitric oxide synthase.[32] The point at which these compensatory mechanisms fail to meet tissue requirements has been termed the critical DO_2 or anaerobic threshold. At this point, a decrease in oxygen delivery is associated with a fall in oxygen consumption

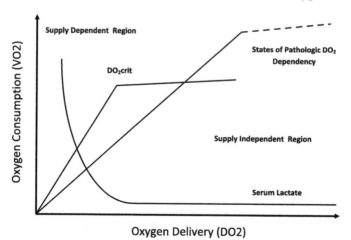

Fig. 1. The classic biphasic DO_2-VO_2 relationship. DO_2crit represents the point at which oxygen consumption falls (becomes dependent on DO_2) with further reduction in oxygen delivery. In states of pathologic DO_2 dependency, the slope of the relationship is altered and covariance is thought to occur over a much wider range of DO_2. Serum lactate arising from anaerobic metabolism will increase when oxygen delivery falls below DO_2crit.

along with an increase in lactate generation. The DO_2-VO_2 relationship is generally biphasic with a supply-dependent and a supply-independent region.[17] The point of transition and the slope of the VO_2-DO_2 relationship will vary depending on the conditions under which measurements are obtained and individual patient characteristics (see **Fig. 1**).

What defines this DO_2crit threshold and whether this threshold changes appreciably based on the physiologic condition of the subject, has long been a subject of study. Initial work in various animal species suggested that the critical DO_2 was in the range of 5 to 10 mL/kg/min depending on study design.[33–35] It was not until the 1980s, however, that systematic investigation of DO_2crit was undertaken in human beings. In the setting of high-risk surgery and ARDS, the values obtained varied widely suggesting that basal conditions could lead to dramatic differences in DO_2crit.[21–23] In an effort to establish minimum delivery requirements, Lieberman and colleagues[36] isovolemically bled normal volunteers down to a Hgb of 5 g/dL then infused esmolol to blunt compensatory tachycardia. None of the participants produced lactate despite an average delivery of 7.3 mL/kg/min establishing that DO_2crit is below this point in normal resting adults. However, mild cognitive and memory changes were described raising the possibility that important individual organ susceptibility may occur and cannot be excluded on the basis of systemic lactate levels or estimated DO_2. Having the subjects breathe high fractional concentrations of oxygen (FiO_2) mitigated the effects of the prior interventions, suggesting that clinically relevant increases in tissue O_2 tension can be achieved in anemic hypoxia by increasing the soluble component of O_2 transport.[37] Shibutani and colleagues,[38] and, later, Komatsu and colleagues,[39] studied patients immediately before coronary artery bypass grafting and then again 15 minutes after coming off bypass. Both studies demonstrated a VO_2 plateau in the majority of patients as DO_2 exceeded 300 to 330 mL/min/m^2. Post-bypass, however, there was a subset of patients who for unclear reasons demonstrated a proportional increase in VO_2 over the range of DO_2 studied suggesting that within this group a higher critical DO_2 existed. The most extreme example of critical DO_2, however, comes from hemodynamic measurements obtained from an 84-year-old patient who for religious beliefs refused blood products in the perioperative period. At the end of the operation, hemoglobin had fallen to 2.6 g with a measured DO_2 of 146 mL/min/$m.^2$ The patient went on to die 8 hours postoperatively with a preterminal DO_2 of 78 mL/min/$m.^2$ Utilizing best-fit regression lines the investigators estimated the DO_2crit to be ~184 mL/min/m^2 (4.9mL/kg/min) while fully ventilated and undergoing sedation and muscle relaxation.[40]

In the situations described above, one would expect compensatory mechanisms to be fully active and that oxygen consumption would proceed normally. Indeed, in the latter case, the extraction ratio was found to be 60% before death.[40] The situation with sepsis has always been considered to be more complex with a much higher range needed to achieve supply independency.[4,5,21–23]

Studies of critically ill patients in the 1980s demonstrated supply dependent VO_2 at much higher levels of DO_2 than previously thought necessary. Mohsenifar and colleagues,[22] using data pooled from patients suffering from ARDS, calculated the critical DO_2 to be 21 mL/kg/min. Later, experimental studies and observations in septic patients suggested that the altered slope of the VO_2-DO_2 relationship and higher DO_2crit represented a new type of "pathologic DO_2 dependency" resulting from altered vasomotor activity, O_2 conformity, and metabolic demands of tissue.[41] Based on observational studies, "supranormal" oxygen delivery was recommended as a strategy to avoid incurring oxygen debt and secondary organ dysfunction. The early suggested targets for supranormal delivery were a cardiac index of 4.5 L/ min/m^2, oxygen delivery in excess of 600 mL/min/m,[2] and an oxygen consumption of greater than 170 mL/min/m[2].[42]

Systematically studying DO_2-VO_2 dependency is now rarely done in critically ill septic patients. Much of the contemporary approach is based upon achieving hemodynamic goals such as mean arterial pressure (MAP), stabilizing organ function, reducing lactate, and increasing SvO_2. In a landmark paper, Ronco and colleagues[43] set out to determine individual anaerobic thresholds in a variety of critically ill patients who were having support withdrawn. Oxygen delivery and consumption were measured repeatedly by independent means to avoid shared measurement errors in the calculation of DO_2 and VO_2. All patients demonstrated the classic biphasic curve as delivery declined. When comparing DO_2crit between septic and nonseptic patients, no significant difference was noted. In these heavily sedated patients, the anaerobic threshold averaged 3.8 ± 1.5 and 4.5 ± 1.3 mL/min/kg respectively. Extraction ratios were also similar and approached those seen in exercising athletes and patients with other forms of shock. The investigators also noted elevated lactate in patients whose baseline oxygen delivery exceeded the measured DO_2crit by as much as threefold. As consumption began to fall in response to declining delivery, lactate levels rose in all patients, suggesting that hyperlactemia may develop from two independent processes—one tied to deranged cellular metabolism and the other to convective O_2 transport. The investigators went on to conclude that DO_2crit is not increased in the terminal phases of septic shock and that oxygen extraction proceeds normally as well. These findings are difficult to reconcile with numerous clinical and experimental studies demonstrating abnormal supply dependency but may reflect important changes in metabolic activity over the course of illness or particular responses to acute bacteremia and endotoxemia. Resting metabolic rate has been shown to vary considerably over the course of illness. In one study, patients were classified on a daily basis as having sepsis, severe sepsis, or septic shock. The lowest metabolic activity was shown to occur when patients met criteria for septic shock. In one striking example, resting metabolic rate moved in a direction opposite to serum endotoxin levels.[44]

TRIALS OF DO_2-VO_2–GUIDED THERAPY

The appreciation of this altered VO_2-DO_2 relationship and elevated DO_2crit led to the proposition that organ damage in critically ill patients could result from an inadequate DO_2, even in settings where DO_2 was normal or modestly elevated. This inadequate DO_2 would, in turn, result in a reduction in VO_2 and consequent tissue hypoxia, injury, and, eventually, organ failure. In landmark observational studies on high-risk surgical patients, Shoemaker and colleagues[23,42] observed that patients who were able to generate a high cardiac output, DO_2, and VO_2 had a significantly higher survival rate than those who did not. This led to the proposition that therapies designed to induce such a "supraphysiologic" state could be life preserving. Based upon median values of survivors noted by Shoemaker and colleagues,[42] the initial targets for these supranormal therapies were a cardiac index of 4.5 L/min/m,[2] DO_2 greater than or equal to 600 mL/min/m,[2] and a VO_2 greater than or equal to 170 mL/min/m,[2] and several studies were undertaken to assess the potential benefit of DO_2-VO_2–guided therapies in the critically ill, particularly among those in severe sepsis and septic shock.[45]

Bihari and colleagues[28] were some of the first investigators to study the impact of increased oxygen delivery on oxygen consumption in a largely septic ARDS population. To augment DO_2, vasodilation of the systemic circulation was produced with a fixed dose of prostacyclin (5ng/kg/min[−1]). The change in DO_2 was 23% higher in survivors and 12% in nonsurvivors. Nonsurvivors, however, demonstrated a 19% increase in VO_2 at the end of the 30-minute infusion period compared with 5% in the surviving population. The extraction ratio increased 11% in nonsurvivors with no apparent change in SvO_2. This was in contrast to survivors in whom the ER fell 17% in association with an increase in SvO_2. The investigators understood this to mean that a large oxygen debt was present in those who went on to die and that this debt could be unmasked by increasing global supply or nonspecifically dilating regional vascular beds. Interpretation of the findings, however, is limited by the baseline differences in severity of illness and base deficit, and an incomplete understanding of the cause of death in the nonsurviving population.

In the only randomized, controlled trial limited to septic shock patients of supranormal DO_2 therapy (CI targeted to >6 L/min/m^2), Tuchschmidt and colleagues[46] found a higher mortality rate in the supranormal DO_2 group compared with the normal DO_2 group (72% vs 50%), though this difference was not statistically significant. However, in a subgroup analysis, treatment group patients who were able to achieve the more modest elevations in CI (>4.5 L/min/m^2) had a survival advantage over control group patients who were not hyperdynamic (CI<4.5 L/min/m^2). This latter finding would seem to suggest that an elevated hemodynamic state confers a survival advantage in septic shock, with or without external intervention. Further, it strongly implies that the inability to achieve a hyperdynamic state in response to septic shock carries a grim prognosis.

Hayes and colleagues[29] conducted a similar trial in a heterogeneous group of critically ill patients with more modest CI goals (>4.5 L/min/m^2), though also using targeted DO_2 (>600 mL/min/m^2) and VO_2 (>170 mL/min/m^2). This study was actually terminated early due to significantly higher in-hospital mortality rates in the treatment group (54%) than in the control group (34%), with mortality differences attributed to multiple organ failure. In the subgroup of patients with septic shock, in-hospital mortality was 52% in the control group as compared with 71% in the treatment group. Whereas nearly all treatment group patients were able to achieve the specified supranormal CI and DO_2 targets, few were able to achieve the targeted oxygen consumption.[47] This points to the conclusion that either VO_2 is not in fact wholly dependent on DO_2 or, less likely, that even higher ranges of DO_2 would be required to normalize VO_2. In a smaller study using only a DO_2 target (>600 mL/min/m^2), Yu and colleagues[48] also failed to identify a therapeutic benefit of a supranormal DO_2 strategy over conventional management, though they also noted that there was a significant survival benefit for patients who were able to reach supranormal DO_2 whether self-generated or from treatment (14% vs 56%).

In the largest randomized, controlled trial of supranormal DO_2 in critically ill patients, Gattinoni and colleagues[49] attempted to assess the effect of raising cardiac indices to supranormal levels (CI>4.5 L/min/m^2) and normalizing mixed venous oxygen saturations ($SmvO_2 \geq 70\%$) as compared with controls. Neither intervention group experienced a reduction in morbidity or mortality (48% in control group, 49% in cardiac index group, 52% in oxygen saturation group). As experienced in prior studies, a large proportion of treatment-arm patients were unable to reach their hemodynamic targets. In this case, only 45% of the cardiac index group and 67% of the mixed venous oxygen saturation group obtained the targeted hemodynamic indices.

Taken collectively, these studies support two conclusions. The first is that supranormal DO_2-based therapeutic strategies are ineffective and potentially harmful. The second is that, although the prognosis for septic patients who can achieve higher than normal oxygen delivery and extraction levels is very good, the prognosis for the substantial number of patients who are unable to increase oxygen consumption despite aggressive inotropic support to increase oxygen delivery is very poor.[50]

However, the premise of directing resuscitation efforts to achieve clearly delineated hemodynamic goals remains an appealing one, though a reorientation of such goals away from achieving supranormal DO_2 levels with inotropes is indicated. The fact that in their studies of high-risk surgical patients, Shoemaker and colleagues[42] were successful in achieving their hemodynamic goals with fluid resuscitation alone in two-thirds of their patients, points to an alternative strategy for the resuscitation of septic patients. Further, as observed by Hayes and colleagues,[29] inotropic support was frequently not started until the patient had been admitted to the ICU, by which time boosting oxygen delivery may not be able to improve the outcome. This distinction is a crucial one and is highlighted below in the discussion of EGDT.

DOBUTAMINE AND DO_2-VO_2

Whereas intentionally raising DO_2 with dobutamine to achieve certain delivery goals has not been shown to improve outcome outside of the early hours of resuscitation, the associated changes in oxygen consumption have been correlated with survival in critically ill and severely septic populations. When Hayes and colleagues[47] reviewed their experience with high dose dobutamine, they noted that patients who did not to achieve all three specified supranormal targets (CI>4.5 L/ min/m,^{2} DO_2>600 mL/ min/m,^{2} and VO_2>170 mL/min/m^2) failed to do so on the basis of inadequate VO_2 response 65% of the time. In this group of inadequate responders, lactate levels remained elevated while SvO_2 increased in association with very high mortality rates.

Vallet and colleagues[31] were one of the first groups of investigators to employ short-term infusions of dobutamine in septic patients to identify important physiologic responses and tie these changes to outcome. Their original study population consisted of normolactemic patients with severe sepsis. Baseline hemodynamics and oxygen transport and use measurements were performed before and 1 hour after an infusion of dobutamine. A less than 15% increase in VO_2 was considered a positive response based on receiver operating characteristic curves. In the responder group, the average increase in oxygen delivery and oxygen consumption approached 40% while nonresponders had a modest 13% increase in DO_2 and no change in VO_2. The behavior of lactate was curious, rising ∼25% in the nonresponder group despite stable VO_2 levels. Among responders the mortality rate was 8.7% while in the nonresponder group mortality was 44.4%.

This approach was later applied by Rhodes and colleagues[30] in a severely septic population that included patients with shock. The groups were characterized based on the VO_2 response to 10 mcg/kg/min of dobutamine given over 1 hour's time. The patients who went on to demonstrate minimal increases in VO_2 tended to be older; had higher APACHE (acute physiology and chronic health evaluation) III scores; and required, on average, higher infusion rates of epinephrine and dopexamine at baseline. Hemodynamics, however, were similar in both groups before the initiation of dobutamine. Responders had a brisk increase in cardiac index that came from both chronotropic and inotropic responses, which may have important clinical implications. The nonresponders had varying effects from dobutamine in terms of CI and DO_2 but, on average, failed to demonstrate a meaningful increase in either of these parameters. The mortality difference was striking. At 28 days, 86% of the responders were alive compared with just 9% of the nonresponders.

The hemodynamic response to graded amounts of dobutamine also appears to have important prognostic implications. In a recent study performed during the first 48 hours of severe sepsis or septic shock, survivors demonstrated an increase in stroke volume index (SVI) of greater than or equal to 8.5 mL/m^2 as dobutamine was infused up to 15 mcg/kg/min. Although both survivors and nonsurvivors demonstrated a chronotropic response to dobutamine, only the former group seemed capable of improving other aspects of cardiac performance. Left ventricular ejection fraction increased ~12% in survivors, but remained essentially unchanged in nonsurvivors. Right ventricular ejection fraction was affected very little by dobutamine, though indices of lusitropy were shown to improve in the survivor group.[51] These findings recapitulate earlier work demonstrating differing hemodynamic responses to septic shock between survivors and nonsurvivors—with the former having, on average, lower heart rates, higher end-diastolic volumes, and better peak systolic pressure to end-systolic volume ratios.[52–54] Whether this represents a critical physiologic reserve or an epiphenomenon of generalized organ dysfunction remains a debated question.

EGDT

The management of severe sepsis and septic shock changed dramatically with the recognition of the "golden hours"—the critical period of time in which recognition and treatment provide maximal benefit. Lundberg and colleagues[55] showed that septic patients on the general wards had a substantial delay in the receipt of intravenous fluids and vasoactive medications in comparison to those in the ICU, with a trend toward decreased survival. In their study of the management of the critically ill in the emergency department, Nguyen and colleagues[56] demonstrated that emergency department management (on average 6 hours in duration) was capable of reducing APACHE II scores and reducing down-stream morbidity and mortality. A possible explanation for the failure of the studies led by Tuchschmidt,[46] Hayes,[29] and Gattinoni[49] was not that the theory behind them was unsound, but that they took too long from the onset of illness (and presumably hemodynamic insult) to initiate therapy as all of their studies initiated treatment upon admission to the ICU (and some allowed enrollment up to 72 hours after admission). These delays in the initiation of treatment may have caused any therapeutic strategy to become ineffective.

In 2001, Rivers and colleagues[57] published a landmark article in which aggressive EGDT was employed from the outset of the recognition of severe sepsis and septic shock, often before admission to the ICU. Specific goals were set to for the first 6 hours of resuscitation and included the following targets: MAP of 65 to 90, a central venous pressure (CVP) of 8 to 12, and a ScvO2 of $\geq$70%. The investigators based this approach on the premise that critical underperfusion was poorly recognized in the early hours of sepsis and that this period of inadequate delivery set the stage for later development of life-threatening organ dysfunction.

In the treatment and standard therapy arms, a high percentage of patients had coexisting conditions such as congestive heart failure, diabetes, hypertension, and liver disease. At the time of enrollment, serum lactates averaged 6.9 ± 4.5 to 7.7 ± 4.7, respectively; with greater than 50% of patients having septic shock. By the end of the first 6 hours of treatment, all subjects had achieved a MAP greater than 65 mmHg. Other conventional targets (CVP, urine output) were met by 86.1% of the standard therapy group and 99.2% of the EGDT group. The greatest difference between the groups was found in measures of saturation of superior vena caval blood (ScvO$_2$). The group receiving conventional treatment met or exceeded the ScvO$_2$ target in 60% of cases compared with 95% of cases in the EGDT group. To achieve the ScvO$_2$ goal in the EGDT group, 60% of patients required red cell transfusions and 14% dobutamine. At 6 hours, the EGDT group had received on average 1.5L of additional fluids over the standard therapy group. This translated into a roughly two-point difference in CVP at the end of the resuscitation period. After intervention, the reported MAPs were exceptionally high for patients with severe sepsis and septic shock. In the EGDT group, MAPs at 6 hours averaged 95 ± 19 mmHg compared with 81 ± 18 mmHg in the standard arm. Despite the high MAP values in both groups, a significant difference in pH, base deficit, lactate, and organ failure scores was found at the end of 6 hours, which persisted into the 7- to 72-hour observation period despite more aggressive fluid and red cell replacement in the standard therapy group during the later period. When mortality was analyzed, the risk of death was reduced at both the 28- and 60-day mark with all subgroups of sepsis benefiting. The benefit afforded by this approach, however, was limited to a reduction in deaths secondary to "sudden cardiovascular collapse." Improvement in outcome related to multiple organ dysfunction syndrome did not achieve statistical significance.

In a subanalysis of the trial, Donnino and colleagues[58] advanced the concept of "cryptic septic shock" as an explanation for some of these findings. Post hoc, the group identified a subset of patients who met the criteria for systemic inflammatory response syndrome, or SIRS, and had lactic acidosis, but in whom early blood pressures were in excess of 100 mmHg (mean ~ 116 mmHg) while $ScvO_2$s were in the mid-40%. A markedly lower mortality rate (20% vs 60.9%) was seen in the patients receiving EGDT. If one makes some assumptions (SVR of 1000 dyne/s·cm⁵) and use average values from the trial, the estimated cardiac output for this group would be in the range of 8 L/min, which is difficult to reconcile with the $ScvO_2$ data. More likely, this group represented a severely hypertensive subset with very limited cardiac reserve. Still, this may be an important group to identify, as aggressive early intervention seems to have lead to a much better outcome.

While the Rivers study has been subject to much analysis and critique in the years since its publication,[59] the fact remains that a resuscitation strategy involving the normalization of hemodynamic parameters beyond that of cardiac output and oxygen delivery remains the most effective management strategy for severe sepsis and septic shock. As such, EGDT was quickly and widely embraced, and became one of the cornerstone of the Surviving Sepsis Campaign and its published guidelines.[60]

Currently a number of studies are underway to assess the value of EGDTs. The questions being addressed include the utility of protocolized care, the value of minimally invasive cardiac assessment, the potential of lactate directed resuscitation, and finally, the benefits of different resuscitation fluids and vasopressors.[61]

SURVIVING SEPSIS CAMPAIGN GUIDELINES

Though a hemodynamic management strategy based primarily on supranormal oxygen delivery has largely been dismissed, the principles behind maintaining normal or even elevated DO_2 in the setting of severe sepsis or septic shock to maintain tissue oxygenation remain sound. In the most recent iteration of the evidence-based guidelines for the management of severe sepsis and septic shock, the Surviving Sepsis Campaign incorporated some of the principles of DO_2 normalization.[60]

Along with CVP, MAP, and urine output goals, initial resuscitation recommendations include maintaining a central or mixed venous O_2 saturation of greater than or equal to 70%, or greater than or equal to 65%, respectively, as a less-invasive measure of adequate oxygen delivery. If the venous O_2 saturation goal is not achieved with fluid resuscitation and vasopressors (norepinephrine or dopamine), then red cell transfusion should be considered if the hematocrit is less than 30%. The use of red blood cell transfusions as a means to increase DO_2 outside of the early phase of severe sepsis remains controversial, however, as other studies have shown a survival benefit with more conservative transfusion strategies in general ICU populations.[62] The current recommendations are to transfuse for hemoglobin below 7 g/dL, although a higher hemoglobin could be required in special circumstances such as myocardial ischemia, severe hypoxemia or acute hemorrhage. If $ScvO_2$ remains below 70% after the above interventions, cardiac output is presumed to be low, and the use of dobutamine to increase delivery is recommended.[60]

SUMMARY

As understanding of the pathophysiology of sepsis has developed so has appreciation of the limited role that supranormal oxygen delivery plays in resuscitation strategies. The window of opportunity to improve outcome through manipulation of convective transport is probably quite narrow and must be exploited at the onset of severe sepsis. EGDT currently offers the best approach to improving outcome. With the completion of a number of ongoing studies, the authors hope that early strategies can be optimized and better endpoints of resuscitation identified. Once cellular injury is well established, increasing delivery of oxygen to the tissues should not be expected to improve oxygen consumption, lactate production and clearance, or outcome.

REFERENCES

1. Angus DC, Linde-Zwirble WT, Lidicker J, et al. Epidemiology of severe sepsis in the United States: analysis of incidence, outcome, and associated costs of care. Crit Care Med 2001;29:1303–10.
2. Dombrovskiy VY, Martin AA, Sunderram J, et al. Rapid increase in hospitalization and mortality rates for severe sepsis in the United States: a trend analysis from 1993 to 2003. Crit Care Med 2007;35:1244–50.
3. Waisbren BA. Bacteremia due to gram-negative bacilli other than the Salmonella: a clinical and therapeutic study. Arch Intern Med 1951;88:467–88.
4. Cain SM, Curtis SE. Experimental models of pathologic oxygen supply dependency. Crit Care Med 1991;19:603–11.
5. Edwards JD. Oxygen transport in cardiogenic and septic shock. Crit Care Med 1991;19:658–63.
6. Krejci V, Hiltebrand LB, Sigurdsson GH. Effects of epinephrine, norepinephrine, and phenylephrine on microcirculatory blood flow in the gastrointestinal tract in sepsis. Crit Care Med 2006;34:1456–63.
7. De Backer D, Creteur J, Dubois M-J. The effects of dobutamine on microcirculatory alterations in patients with septic shock are independent of its systemic effects. Crit Care Med 2006;34:403–8.
8. Sair M, Etherington PJ, Winlove CP, et al. Tissue oxygenation and perfusion in patients with systemic sepsis. Crit Care Med 2001;29:1343–9.
9. Massimo-Girardis M, Rinaldi L, Busani S, et al. Muscle perfusion and oxygen consumption by near-infrared spectroscopy in septic-shock and non-septic-shock patients. Intensive Care Med 2003;29:1173–6.
10. Brealey D, Brand M, Hargreaves I, et al. Association between mitochondrial dysfunction and severity and outcome of septic shock. Lancet 2002;360:219–23.
11. Fredriksson K, Hammarqvist F, Strigård K, et al. Derangements in mitochondrial metabolism in intercostal and leg muscle of critically ill patients with sepsis-induced multiple organ failure. Am J Physiol Endocrinol Metab 2006;291: E1044–50.
12. Baudouin SV, Saunders D, Tiangyou W, et al. Mitochondrial DNA and survival after sepsis: a prospective study. Lancet 2005;366(9503):2118–21.

13. Crouser ED, Julian MW, Dorinsky PM. Ileal VO_2-DO_2 alterations induced by endotoxin correlate with severity of mitochondrial injury. Am J Respir Crit Care Med 1999;160:1347–53.
14. Watts JA, Kline JA, Thornton LR, et al. Metabolic dysfunction and depletion of mitochondria in hearts of septic rats. J Mol Cell Cardiol 2004;36:141–50.
15. Hotchkiss RS, Swanson PE, Freeman BD, et al. Apoptotic cell death in patients with sepsis, shock, and multiple organ dysfunction. Crit Care Med 1999;27:1230–51.
16. Mongardon N, Dyson A, Singer M. Is MOF an outcome parameter or a transient, adaptive state in critical illness? Curr Opin Crit Care 2009;15:431–6.
17. Leach RM, Treacher DF. The pulmonary physician in critical care: oxygen delivery and consumption in the critically ill. Thorax 2002;57:170–7.
18. Dantzker D, Foresman B, Gutierrez G. Oxygen supply and utilization relationships. Am Rev Respir Dis 1991;143:675–9.
19. Guzman JA. Monitoring oxygen transport. In: Kruse JA, Fink MP, Carlson RW, editors. Saunders manual of critical care. p. 781–3, chapter 216.
20. Mahutte CK, Jaffe MB, Sasse SA, et al. Relationship of thermodilution cardiac output to metabolic measurements and mixed venous oxygen saturation. Chest 1993;104:1236–42.
21. Danek SJ, Lynch JP, Weg JG, et al. The dependence of oxygen uptake on oxygen delivery in the adult respiratory distress syndrome. Am Rev Respir Dis 1980; 122(3):387–95.
22. Mohsenifar Z, Goldbach P, Tashkin DP, et al. Relationship between oxygen consumption and oxygen delivery in adult respiratory distress syndrome. Chest 1983;84:267–71.
23. Shoemaker WC, Chang PC, Czer LSC, et al. Cardiorespiratory monitoring in postoperative patients: prediction of outcome and severity of illness. Crit Care Med 1979;7:237–42.
24. Phang PT, Cunningham KF, Ronco JJ, et al. Mathematical coupling explains dependence of oxygen consumption on oxygen delivery in ARDS. Am J Respir Crit Care Med 1994;150:318–23.
25. Squara P. Matching total body oxygen consumption and delivery: a crucial objective? Intensive Care Med 2004;30:2170–9.
26. De Backer D. VO2/DO2 relationship: how to get rid of the methodological pitfalls? Intensive Care Med 2000;26:1719–22.
27. Granton JT, Walley KR, Phang PT, et al. Assessment of three methods to reduce the influence of mathematical coupling on oxygen consumption and delivery relationships. Chest 1998;113:1347–55.
28. Bihari D, Smithies M, Gimson A, et al. The effect of vasodilation with prostacyclin on oxygen delivery and uptake in critically ill patients. N Engl J Med 1987;317: 397–403.
29. Hayes MA, Yau EH, Timmins AC, et al. Response of critically ill patients to treatment aimed at achieving supranormal oxygen delivery and consumption: relationship to outcome. Chest 1993;103(3):886–95.
30. Rhodes A, Lamb F, Malago I, et al. A prospective study of the use of a dobutamine stress test to identify outcome in patients with sepsis, severe sepsis, or septic shock. Crit Care Med 1999;27(11):2361–6.
31. Vallet B, Chopin C, Curtis SE, et al. Prognostic value of the dobutamine test in patients with sepsis syndrome and normal lactate values: a prospective, multicenter study. Crit Care Med 1993;21:1868–75.
32. Gladwin MT, Patel RP. The role of red blood cells and hemoglobin–nitric oxide interactions on blood flow. Am J Respir Cell Mol Biol 2008;38:125–6.

33. Cain SM. Oxygen delivery and uptake in dogs during anemic and hypoxic hypoxia. J Appl Phys 1977;42:228–34.
34. Gutierrez G, Warley AR, Dantzker DR. Oxygen delivery and utilization in hypothermic dogs. J Appl Phys 1986;63:1487–92.
35. Nelson DP, Beyer C, Samsel RW, et al. Pathological supply dependence of O2 uptake during bacteremia in dogs. J Appl Phys 1987;63:1487–92.
36. Lieberman JA, Weiskopf RB, Kelley S, et al. Critical oxygen delivery in conscious humans is less than 7.3 ml O_2 kg^{-1}.min^{-1}. Anesthesiology 2000;92:407–13.
37. Weiskopf RB, Feiner J, Hopf HW, et al. Oxygen reverses deficits of cognitive function and memory and increased heart rate induced by acute severe isovolemic anemia. Anesthesiology 2002;96:871–7.
38. Shibutani K, Komatsu T, Kubal K, et al. Critical level of oxygen delivery in anesthetized man. Crit Care Med 1983;11(8):640–3.
39. Komatsu T, Shibutani K, Okamoto K, et al. Critical level of oxygen delivery after cardiopulmonary bypass. Crit Care Med 1987;15(3):194–7.
40. Van Woerkens EC, Trouwborst A, van Lanschot JJB. Profound hemodilution: what is the critical level of hemodilution at which oxygen delivery-dependent oxygen consumption starts in an anesthetized human? Anesth Analg 1992;75: 818–21.
41. Weg JG. Oxygen transport in adult respiratory distress syndrome and other acute circulatory problems: relationship of oxygen delivery and oxygen consumption. Crit Care Med 1991;19:650–67.
42. Shoemaker WC, Appel PL, Kram HB, et al. Prospective trial of supranormal values of survivors as therapeutic goals in high-risk surgical patients. Chest 1988;94:1176–86.
43. Ronco JJ, Fenwick JC, Tweeddale MG, et al. Identification of the critical oxygen delivery for anaerobic metabolism in critically ill septic and nonseptic humans. JAMA 1993;270:1724–30.
44. Kreymann G, Grosser S, Buggisch P, et al. Oxygen consumption and resting metabolic rate in sepsis, sepsis syndrome, and septic shock. Crit Care Med 1992;21:1012–9.
45. Shoemaker WC, Appel PL, Bland R. Use of physiologic monitoring to predict outcome and to assist in clinical decisions in critically ill postoperative patients. Am J Surg 1983;146:43–50.
46. Tuchschmidt J, Fried J, Astiz M, et al. Elevation of cardiac output and oxygen delivery improves outcome in septic shock. Chest 1992;102:216–20.
47. Hayes MA, Timmins AC, Yau EH. Oxygen transport patterns in patients with sepsis syndrome or septic shock: influence of treatment and relationship to outcome. Crit Care Med 1997;25(6):926–36.
48. Yu M, Levy M, Smith P, et al. Effect of maximizing oxygen delivery on morbidity and mortality rates in critically ill patients: a prospective, randomized, controlled study. Crit Care Med 1993;21(6):830–8.
49. Gattinoni L, Brazzi L, Pelosi P, et al. A trial of goal-oriented hemodynamic therapy in critically ill patients. N Engl J Med 1995;333:1025–32.
50. Vinay K, Sharma VK, Dellinger RP. The International Sepsis Forum's Frontiers in Sepsis: high cardiac output should not be maintained in severe sepsis. Crit Care 2003;7:272–5.
51. Kumar A, Schupp E, Bunnell E, et al. Cardiovascular response to dobutamine stress predicts outcome in severe sepsis and septic shock. Crit Care 2008;12: R35.

52. Parker MM, Shelhamer JH, Natanson C, et al. Serial cardiovascular variables in survivors and non-survivors of human septic shock: heart rate as an early indicator of prognosis. Crit Care Med 1987;10:923–9.
53. Ognibene FP, Parker MM, Natanson C, et al. Depressed left ventricular performance: response to volume infusion in patients with sepsis and septic shock. Chest 1988;93(5):903–10.
54. Parker MM, Ognibene FP, Parrillo JE. Peak systolic pressure/end-systolic volume ratio, a load-independent measure of ventricular function, is reversibly decreased in human septic shock. Crit Care Med 1994;22(12):1955–9.
55. Lundberg JS, Perl TM, Wiblin T, et al. Septic shock: an analysis of outcomes for patients with onset on hospital wards versus intensive care units. Crit Care Med 1998;26:1020–4.
56. Nguyen HB, Rivers EP, Haystad S, et al. Critical care in the emergency department: a physiologic assessment and outcome evaluation. Acad Emerg Med 2000;7(12):1354–61.
57. Rivers E, Nguyen B, Haystad S, et al. Early goal-directed therapy in the treatment of severe sepsis and septic shock. N Engl J Med 2001;345(19):1368–77.
58. Donnino MW, Nguyen B, Jacobsen G, et al. Cryptic septic shock: a sub-analysis of early, goal-directed therapy. Chest 2003;124:90S.
59. Burton T. The Wall Street Journal. Available at: http://online.wsj.com/article/SB121867179036438865.html. Accessed August 14, 2008.
60. Dellinger RP, Levy MM, Carlet JM, et al. Surviving Sepsis Campaign: international guidelines for management of severe sepsis and septic shock. Intensive Care Med 2008;34(1):17–60.
61. Clinical Trials Gov. Available at: http://www.clinicaltrial.gov/ct2/results?term=early+goal+directed+therapy. Accessed December 1, 2009.
62. Hebert PC, Wells G, Blajchman MA, et al. A multicenter, randomized, controlled clinical trial of transfusion requirements in critical care. N Engl J Med 1999;340:409–17.

Lactic Acidosis: Recognition, Kinetics, and Associated Prognosis

Christopher Vernon, DO[a], Jennifer L. LeTourneau, DO, MCR[a,b],*

KEYWORDS

- Lactic acidosis • Mitochondria • Prognosis
- Critical care • Shock • Metabolic diseases

LACTATE HISTORY

Lactic acidosis in the setting of severe illness has a history dating back into the 1800s when Johann Joseph Scherer first measured lactic acid levels in postmortem blood from two women dying of puerperal fever. Subsequently, Folwarczny in 1858 described elevated lactate levels in a living patient with leukemia[1] and was later followed by Salomon in 1878, who observed increased lactate levels in patients with chronic obstructive pulmonary disease, pneumonia, solid tumors, and congestive heart failure.[1] Several years later, Fletcher described how lactic acid was produced by skeletal muscle under anaerobic conditions, noting that when oxygen was readily available, it "either restrains by some guidance of chemical event the yield of acid in the muscle, or is able to remove it after its production."[2] These observations made more than 100 years ago represent the groundwork laid in understanding of lactic acid in the disease states of critically ill patients.

In the late 1950s, Huckabee[3–6] performed a series of important physiologic experiments, summarizing the relationship of blood lactate and pyruvate levels to various oxygen-deficient states, including extreme exercise, breathing of low oxygen tension gases, and impaired cardiac output. He went on to demonstrate elevated levels from patients in various stages of shock.[7] Nearly 2 decades later, Woods and Cohen[8] created a classification scheme of lactic acidosis based on Huckabee's original work, designating type A as that arising from decreased perfusion or oxygenation

[a] Division of Pulmonary and Critical Care Medicine, Oregon Health & Science University, 3181 SW Sam Jackson Park Road, UHN 67, Portland, OR 97239, USA
[b] Pulmonary Disease Section, Portland Veterans Affairs Medical Center, 3710 SW US Veterans Hospital Road, Mailcode P3PULM, Portland, OR 97239, USA
* Corresponding author. Pulmonary Disease Section, Portland Veterans Affairs Medical Center, 3710 SW US Veterans Hospital Road, Mailcode P3PULM, Portland, OR 97239.
E-mail address: Jennifer.Letourneau@va.gov

Crit Care Clin 26 (2010) 255–283
doi:10.1016/j.ccc.2009.12.007
0749-0704/10/$ – see front matter. Published by Elsevier Inc.

criticalcare.theclinics.com

and type B stemming from underlying diseases, medication/intoxication, or inborn error of metabolism. This scheme continues to be used to this day as a means of classifying and understanding the origins of elevated lactate. Further study on lactate metabolism expanded views of lactate use in the body. In the 1980s, the idea of lactate shuttles and lactate itself as a source of energy was first postulated.[9] Lactate was no longer thought of as a dead-end byproduct of metabolism but a normal and at times a preferred source of metabolic fuel.

LACTATE METABOLISM

Lactate is formed from the reduction of pyruvate via the enzyme lactate dehydrogenase:

Pyruvate + NADH $\leftrightarrow$ lactate + NAD$^+$

This process produces two molecules of ATP, making formation of lactate a source of cellular energy during anaerobic metabolism. The reaction occurs within the cytosol as the final step of glycolysis.[10] At a basal physiologic state, the reaction favors lactate formation from pyruvate in an approximately 10:1 ratio.[6] The reduction of pyruvate is the only known pathway for lactate production, making this a unique way of monitoring anaerobic metabolic processes (**Fig. 1**).

Lactate levels in the blood result from the balance between production and clearance, a source of significant scientific interest over the past few decades. Normally, blood lactate levels are less than 2 mmol/L.[11] In normal physiologic conditions, approximately 1500 mmol of lactate are produced daily primarily from skeletal muscle, skin, brain, intestine, and red blood cells.[11] In severe illness, lactate production occurs in many other tissues. The lungs, for example, can be a significant source of lactate during acute lung injury despite the absence of tissue hypoxia.[12] Leukocytes may also produce large amounts of lactate during phagocytosis[13] or when activated in sepsis.[14] The splanchnic organs, such as the liver and intestines, are another potential source of lactate production and may be particularly vulnerable to disproportionate vasoconstriction in low perfusion states. Whether or not this mechanism contributes to elevated gut lactate in sepsis remains a matter of debate.[15] De Backer and colleagues[15] showed, using hepatic venous oximetry, that only 6 of 90 patients with severe sepsis had splanchnic lactate production, even in those with severely elevated serum lactate levels.

Lactate clearance occurs principally in the liver (60%) with important contributions from the kidney (30%) and to a lesser extent other organs (heart and skeletal muscle).[16] Utilization occurs via the Cori cycle where lactate is converted back to pyruvate and eventually to glucose through gluconeogensis.[17] It has been shown that in patients with chronic liver disease (usually grade III or IV encephalopathy),[18] lactate clearance is diminished, thus also contributing to elevated blood levels.[14] In addition to metabolic clearance mechanisms, lactate can be excreted by the kidney once the renal threshold is exceeded (approximately 5 mmol/L).[11] Thus, hepatic and renal impairment can alter lactate clearance.

Lactic acidosis is typically present in shock states in which tissue oxygen delivery (DO_2) is insufficient to meet cellular demand. In this classic type A lactic acidosis, flux through the glycolytic pathway increases, leading to an accumulation of pyruvate. In a low oxygen tension state, pyruvate does not enter the mitochondria for oxidative phosphorylation. Hypoxia has been known to inhibit pyruvate dehydrogenase (PDH) complex[19] involved in aerobic breakdown of pyruvate to acetyl coenzyme A (CoA) for entry into the Krebs cycle. It also is known to inhibit pyruvate carboxylase, which

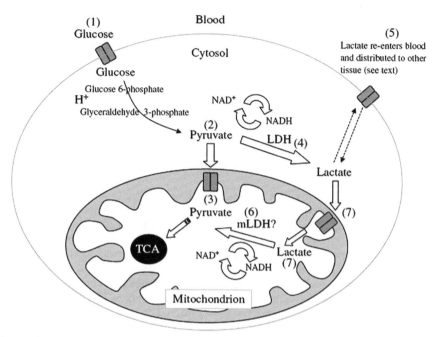

Fig. 1. The processes involved in the lactate shuttle hypothesis (Brooks, 1986[218]). The pathway proposes that (1) glucose enters the cell, where it is sequentially broken down to pyruvate; (2) pyruvate enters the mitochondrion, allowing respiration to continue in the tricarboxylic acid (TCA) cycle; (3) lactate is subsequently formed via the lactate dehydrogenase (LDH) reaction (4) and is then exported from the cytosolic compartment via monocarboxylate transporter (MCT) transport (5), where it is redistributed to a variety of functional sites. Note the suggested presence of mitochondrial lactate dehydrogenase (mLDH) (6), which forms the construct of the intracellular shuttle system (7). (*Reproduced from* Philp A, Macdonald AL, Watt PW. Lactate—a signal coordinating cell and systemic function. J Exp Biol 2005;208(Pt 24):4561–75; with permission. Available at jeb.biologists.org doi:10.1242/jeb.01961.)

converts pyruvate into oxaloacetate early in the process of gluconeogenesis. This causes rapid accumulation of pyruvate, and pyruvate metabolism is subsequently shifted almost in entirety toward lactate formation. Subsequently, intracellular lactate concentration rapidly increases, leading to excretion into the bloodstream. Clinically significant formation of lactate from low perfusion was most notably shown in a group of cardiogenic shock patients by Levy and colleagues[20] where lactate:pyruvate ratios were calculated at 40:1 as compared with controls (10:1). Further evidence for increased lactate production during shock states came from Revelly and colleagues,[21] who compared seven patients with cardiogenic shock and seven patients with septic shock to seven healthy controls. By infusing ^{13}C-radiolabeled lactate and ^{2}H-labeled glucose continuously, they showed that hyperlactatemia resulted from overproduction of lactate and that clearance was similar in all three groups.

Excess lactate production may not be the only contributor to hyperlactatemia in critically ill patients. Levraut and colleagues[16] showed that in patients with hemodynamically stable sepsis, elevated lactate levels are more related to altered clearance than to overproduction. The overall metabolism of lactate in critical illness is, therefore, a highly complex process with many factors influencing blood lactate levels. Lactate itself is probably not harmful and is shuttled to tissues during stress states as a carbon backbone energy fuel. When lactate levels are elevated in the blood, it may be more of an indicator of an underlying stress state and not necessarily the direct cause of the pathogenesis.

ROLE AS A PROGNOSTIC MARKER IN CRITICALLY ILL PATIENTS

Whether or not blood lactate levels are elevated due to increased production or decreased clearance, monitoring levels may prove valuable as a biomarker of an underlying critically ill state, such as shock. Lactate is one of many markers used for prognosis in critically ill patients and a value greater than 4 mmol/L is recommended by the surviving sepsis campaign[22] as suggestive of severe sepsis requiring aggressive resuscitation.

Huckabee performed the first analyses of elevated lactate levels in patients of varying degrees of shock.[7] He reported a case series of nine patients with lactic acidosis complaining of hyperpnea and dyspnea. The clinical syndrome progressed to weakness, stupor, and death during various stages of other severe illnesses (ie, postgastrectomy, poliomyelitis, pneumonia, and bacterial endocarditis). He found a wide range of lactate levels (3–26 mmol/L) at various days into their illness. He noted elevated lactate levels indicative of widespread tissue hypoxia but no apparent cause of the hypoxia. In his article, he states, "the chemical syndrome could be reproduced in animals only by gradual peripheral circulatory failure and this syndrome could not be ruled out in the patients."

By the 1970s, Weil and Afifi[23] and Cady and colleagues[24] expanded on Huckabee's experiments showing prospectively that lactate was a strong predictor for death in critically ill patients. Death occurred in two-thirds of patients with lactate levels above 3.8 mmol/L[24] and approached 90% as levels neared 8 mmol/L.[23] Later, in 1994, Stacpoole and colleagues[25] reported on the natural history of elevated lactate in critically ill medical and surgical patients, demonstrating that elevated lactate levels (>5 mmol/L) predicted death over time. Survival was 59%, 41%, and 17% at 1, 3, and 30 days, respectively, for patients with persistently abnormal lactate levels. Median survival overall in this group was 2 days.

More recently, in 2007, Trzeciak and colleagues[26] observed initial serum lactate levels in more than 1100 patients seen in an emergency department (ED), an intensive care unit (ICU), and general hospital wards. Lactate levels were divided into low (0–2 mmol/L), intermediate (2.1–3.9 mmol/L), and high (>4.0 mmol/L). They found a lactate level of greater than 4 mmol/L to be highly specific (89%–99%) for predicting acute phase of death and in-hospital death in all three groups (**Fig. 2**). They concluded that initial lactate levels (on suspicion of clinical sepsis) could be used to augment but not replace bedside mortality assessment no matter the location of the patient (ED, ward, or ICU).

Shapiro and colleagues[27] took patients with suspected infection in an ED and hypothesized that initial serum lactate levels would predict hospital mortality. Again, lactate levels were stratified into low (<2.5 mmol/L), intermediate (2.5–4 mmol/L), and high (>4 mmol/L). They showed an increasing likelihood of mortality (4%, 9%, and 28.4%, respectively) for each group and calculated 92% specificity for death. Later, in 2007, Shapiro's group[28] enrolled normotensive and hypotensive patients presenting to an ED with suspected infection. They showed an odds ratio of death of 2.2 for those patients with intermediate lactate levels and an odds ratio of 7.1 for high lactate levels. These values were independent of hypotension (**Fig. 3**). Mortality in the normotensive patients with lactate levels greater than 4 mmol/L was similar to normolactatemic patients who had systolic blood pressures less than 70 mm Hg.

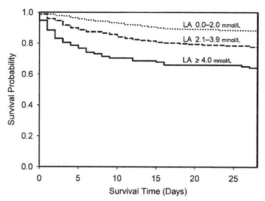

Fig. 2. Kaplan-Meier survival curves. Kaplan-Meier survival curves (truncated at 28 days) for the three a priori defined groups of initial lactate values: low, 0.0–2.0 mmol/L (n = 827); intermediate, 2.1–3.9 mmol/L (n = 238); and high, 4.0 mmol/L or above (n = 112). Time 0 represents the day of lactate measurement. LA, lactic acid. (*From* Springer Science+Business Media. Trzeciak S, Dellinger RP, Chansky ME, et al. Serum lactate as a predictor of mortality in patients with infection. Intensive Care Med 2007;33(6):970–7; with permission.)

The question remains: Is initial lactate level a true risk stratification biomarker or just a manifestation of organ dysfunction? Mikkelsen and colleagues[29] performed a recent single-center cohort of 830 patients with severe sepsis admitted through an ED. They looked at shock and nonshock patients with low (<2.5 mmol/L), intermediate (2.5–4 mmol/L), and high (>4 mmol/L) levels of lactate. They found that initial serum lactate level predicted mortality in both groups and found mortality to be 15.4%, 37%, and 46.9% in the low, medium, and high lactate groups with septic shock, respectively. They also found mortality of 8.7%, 16.4%, and 31.8% in the nonshock groups, respectively. These values were calculated after correction for organ dysfunction with Acute Physiology and Chronic Health Evaluation (APACHE) II scores, showing the predictive power of initial lactate level uniquely as a biomarker. Relatively high mortality was seen in nonshock septic patients with relatively intermediate levels of lactate (2.5–4 mmol/L). Shapiro and Mikkelsen demonstrated predicted mortalities in these patients of approximately 15%. Normotensive patients with presumed sepsis and intermediately high lactate levels likely represent an at-risk subgroup of patients in whom early and aggressive resuscitation may improve mortality. The surviving sepsis campaign recommends early goal directed therapy in individuals with severe sepsis or septic shock, particularly if lactate level is greater than 4 mmol/L. Jansen and colleagues[30] showed that blood lactate levels were strongly associated with Sequential Organ Failure Assessment scores, especially early in the ICU stay. They found that initial lactate levels between 2 and 3 mmol/L corresponded to 60% mortality. Perhaps the initiation of early goal directed therapy as recommended by the surviving sepsis campaign should be expanded to include those patients with presumed sepsis and intermediate lactate levels (2–4 mmol/L). Serum lactate levels as a predictive biomarker may prove most useful in this population.

LACTATE:PYRUVATE RATIOS

Lactate:pyruvate ratios have been employed in prognostication and to distinguish type A from type B hyperlactatemia. Pyruvate assays are not always available, however, and can be inaccurate if the specimen is hemolyzed, stored incorrectly, or

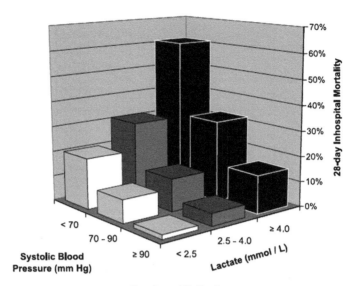

Number of Patients
In Each Lactate/Blood Pressure Group

		Systolic Blood Pressure (mm Hg)		
		< 70	70 - 90	≥ 90
Lactate (mmol / L)	< 2.5	20	99	819
	2.5 - 4.0	13	31	202
	≥ 4.0	18	25	60

Fig. 3. 28-Day in-hospital mortality risk stratified by blood pressure and serum lactate level. (*From* Springer Science+Business Media. Howell MD, Donnino M, Clardy P, et al. Occult hypoperfusion and mortality in patients with suspected infection. Intensive Care Med 2007;33(11):1892–9; with permission.)

not processed within the first 3 hours.[31] An example of their utility can be found in a study by Levy and colleagues[20] in which elevated lactate levels were present in association with increased lactate:pyruvate ratios in nonsurvivors (37:1) relative to survivors (20:1) in patients with septic shock. Suistomaa and colleagues[32] also measured lactate levels and lactate:pyruvate ratios for the first 24 hours of critically ill medical surgical patients. Elevated initial lactate level, continued elevation of lactate, and lactate:pyruvate ratio all predicted mortality. In patients with severe sepsis, lactate elevation was associated with normal lactate:pyruvate ratios whereas in circulatory failure, both were elevated. This gives some support to theories that elevated lactate:-pyruvate ratios support a hypoxic mechanism of lactate production. Normal ratios of lactate to pyruvate in the setting of elevated lactate levels may signify a nonhypoxic mechanism. Further studies are necessary. With the many difficulties in obtaining accurate pyruvate levels, it is doubtful that measuring lactate:pyruvate ratio adds any additional prognostic value for shock resuscitation.

LACTATE CLEARANCE

Single serum lactate measurements may have limitations and perhaps serial measurements improve prognostic ability. Lactate clearance over time was shown to be superior to oxygen-derived variables (DO_2 and oxygen consumption [VO_2]) in septic shock patients.[33] Initial and final phase lactate levels were lower in survivors whereas DO_2 and VO_2 were not different. Bakker and colleagues[34] showed that lactime, or duration of elevated serum lactate levels, most accurately corresponded to organ failure and death and did so better than initial lactate levels, DO_2, and VO_2. Abramson and colleagues[35] demonstrated that all trauma patients who normalized their serum lactate levels by 24 hours survived and that those who cleared by 48 hours had a 75% chance of survival. The ability to normalize lactate to a value of less than 2 mmol/L predicted survival ($P<.0001$) whereas DO_2 and VO_2 did not.

These findings were corroborated by McNelis and colleagues,[36] who demonstrated 100% mortality in surgical ICU patients who had persistently elevated lactate levels. Those who cleared their lactate (lactate level <2 mmol/L) in the first 24 hours had a mortality of 3.9%. Patients who had delayed lactate clearance (>48 hours to lactate level <2 mmol/L) had a mortality of 42.5%. Husain and colleagues[37] furthered the importance of lactate clearance in critically ill surgical ICU patients when he risk-stratified 95 trauma and nontrauma patients into four groups based on their ability to clear lactate: (1) clearance in the first 24 hours, (2) clearance in 24 to 48 hours, (3) greater than 48 hours to normalize, or (4) never normalized. Predicted mortality was calculated as 10%, 20%, 23%, and 67%, respectively, in the four groups. Initial and serial lactate measurements predicted survival with statistical significance.

In a different patient population, Nguyen and colleagues[38] quantified lactate clearance in 111 patients with severe sepsis and septic shock. Survivors had a lactate clearance of 38% versus 12% of nonsurvivors. Low lactate clearance (<10%) within the first 6 hours predicted death two-thirds of the time. It is not clear that any intervention helps improve lactate clearance, but perhaps serial lactate measurements could be used as markers of progress in shock resuscitation.

For many years, it was felt that the lactate itself was harmful and contributed to the worsening acidosis. This has since been shown to likely not be true. In an effort to actively lower lactate levels, however, Stacpoole and colleagues[39] performed a series of experiments with dichloroacetate (DCA). DCA stimulates the PDH complex by binding to and inhibiting PDH kinase, which inactivates the PDH enzyme. Increasing flux through the PDH enzymatic pathway seemed an ideal way to reduce lactate levels and has been studied in a variety of patient populations: children with congenital lactic acidosis,[40] patients with myocardial ischemia,[41] and critically ill patients with shock.[42,43] All studies have shown that DCA safely lowers circulating lactate levels in the blood. The only controlled trial of DCA, however, by Stacpoole and colleagues, for the treatment of lactic acidosis showed a lowering of lactate levels but no change in any significant hemodynamic measurements or survival. Many patients were enrolled with significantly elevated lactate levels and many were enrolled late into their shock states well into developing multiorgan system failure. Nonetheless, DCA has never proved useful in treating critically ill patients with elevated lactate levels.

ARTERIAL VERSUS VENOUS LACTATE

To compare arterial and venous lactate, a series of 74 ED adult patients had arterial and venous lactate drawn within 5 minutes of the other.[44] The correlation between arterial and venous lactate was 0.94 (95% CI, 0.91–0.96). There was a mean venous minus arterial lactate difference of 0.22 mmol/L (95% CI, 0.04–0.41), which ranged from −1.3 to 1.7 mmol/L in individual patients. Of the sample patients, 30% had arterial lactate levels less than 1.6.

In a study of trauma patients, arterial and venous lactate measurements were taken, drawn within 2 minutes of each other in 221 patients.[45] The levels correlated with a correlation of 0.94 (95% CI, 0.94–0.96; P = .0001). The equation for the difference in the values was expressed as arterial lactate = 0.0706 + 0.889 (venous lactate). The difference between arterial and venous values was not statistically significant.

LACTATED RINGER SOLUTION

Some providers have expressed concern about the use of lactated Ringer solution in the setting of lactic acidosis, theorizing that it could make the lactic acidosis worse. One liter of lactated Ringer solution contains 130 mEq sodium, 4 mEq potassium, 3 mEq calcium, 109 mEq chloride, and 28 mEq lactate mixed in sterile water. The electrolyte content is isotonic (273 mOsm/L, calculated) in relation to the extracellular fluid (approximately 280 mOsm/L). The sterile water is acidic (pH 5 to 7) as a result of interactions with air and the plastic bag. The addition of sodium lactate increases pH to approximately 6.6 (range 6.0–7.5). Hence, the lactate acts as a base and as such cannot cause acidosis.[46] Often, due to the diagnosis of lactic acidosis, physicians choose saline for resuscitation fluids. In a study of sixty patients with severe sepsis or septic shock, hyperchloremic metabolic acidosis due to saline infusion was the predominant cause of metabolic acidosis.[47] Furthermore, to determine if lactated Ringer solution increased circulating lactate concentrations, healthy adult volunteers were given 1-L infusions of lactated Ringer solution or 5% dextrose over 1 hour.[48] Lactate concentrations were not significantly different between the two groups. Therefore, elevated blood lactate levels in the setting of lactated Ringer solution infusion are an unexpected finding and should not be attributed to the infusion.

To summarize, the understanding of type A lactate acidosis, initial serum lactate, serial lactate measurements, and lactate clearance may be useful in the management of critically ill patients. Elevated lactate levels are likely related to increased production and decreased clearance depending on the complex metabolic factors of individual patients. Venous lactate levels are easy to obtain, inexpensive, and can provide valuable information in the prognostication of medical and surgical patients with shock.

TYPE B LACTIC ACIDOSIS

Often during the course of critical illness, patients have continued elevations in lactate level without ongoing evidence of cellular hypoxia or ischemia (**Fig. 4**). In these cases it is important to consider what Woods and Cohen labeled type B lactic acidosis.[8] **Box 1** lists causes of type B lactic acidosis. Type B lactic acidosis is divided into type B1 (related to underlying diseases), type B2 (related to the effect of drugs and toxins), and type B3 (associated with inborn errors of metabolism.)

TYPE B UNDERLYING DISEASES
Malignancy-Associated Lactic Acidosis

In the 1920s, Warburg[49] measured VO_2 and lactate production in tumor cells in aerobic and anaerobic conditions. He found that tumor cells had high glucose consumption and lactate production in the presence of oxygen. He believed that this "aerobic glycolysis" was due to abnormal function of mitochondria and was the root of malignant transformation. One factor contributing to the high rate of glycolysis is the overexpression of glycolytic enzymes, such as hexokinase. In contrast with Warburg's hypothesis, the literature supports that, except for a few cancers,[50,51] the mitochondrial impairment in tumors is a result of tumor-related metabolic shifts and not the

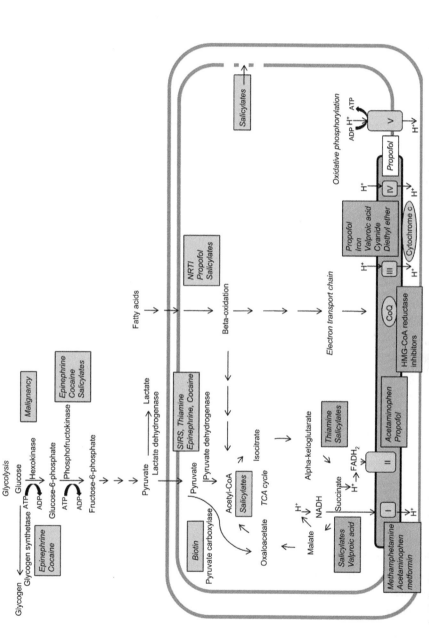

Fig. 4. Proposed etiologies of type B lactic acidosis. Selected pathways in glycolysis, citric acid cycle, and oxidative phosphorylation and the proposed effect of various conditions and medications on those pathways leading to lactic acidosis. ADP, adenosine diphosphate; CoQ, coenzyme Q; $FADH_2$, reduced flavin adenine dinucleotide; H^+ hydrogen ion; NAHD, reduced nicotinamide adenine dinucleotide; TCA, tricarboxylic acid; I, complex I; II, complex II; III, complex III; IV, complex IV; V, complex V.

Box 1
Causes of type B lactic acidosis

Type B1—underlying diseases

Renal failure

Hepatic failure

Diabetes mellitus

Malignancy

Systemic inflammatory response syndrome

Human immunodeficiency virus

Type B2—drugs and toxins

Acetaminophen

Alcohols—ethanol, methanol, diethylene glycol, isopropanol, and propylene glycol

Antiretroviral nucleoside analogs—zidovudine, didanosine, and lamivudine

β-Adrenergic agonists—epinephrine, ritodrine, and terbutaline

Biguanides—phenformin and metformin

Cocaine, methamphetamine

Cyanogenic compounds—cyanide, aliphatic nitriles, and nitroprusside

Diethyl ether

Fluorouracil

Halothane

Iron

Isoniazid

Linezolid

Nalidixic acid

Niacin

Propopol

Salicylates

Strychnine

Sugars and sugar alcohols—fructose, sorbitol, and xylitol

Sulfasalazine

Total parenteral nutrition

Valproic acid

Vitamin deficiencies—thiamine and biotin

Type B3—inborn errors of metabolism

Glucose-6-phosphatase deficiency (von Gierke disease)

Fructose-1,6-diphosphatase deficiency

Pyruvate carboxylase deficiency

PDH deficiency

Methylmalonic aciduria

Kearns-Sayre syndrome

Pearson syndrome

Mitochondrial encephalomyopathy, lactic acidosis, and stroke-like episodes (MELAS)

Myclonic epilepsy with ragged red fibers (MERRF)

etiology of malignancy. Furthermore, not all tumors use glycolysis as the preferred form of energy production.[52] Nonetheless, lactic acidosis has been most frequently reported in hematologic malignancies, such as leukemias and lymphomas,[53] and also reported in melanoma,[54] small cell lung cancer,[55] multiple myeloma,[56,57] sarcoma,[58] breast cancer,[59] oat cell carcinoma,[60] undifferentiated carcinoma,[61] cholangiocarcinoma,[62] and pheochromocytoma (although this is likely due to the high circulating catecholamines [discussed later]).[63] In one review of lactic acidosis in hematologic malignancy, reported lactate levels ranged from 5 to 38 mmol/L with reported mortality of 93% to 96%.[64] Management of the hyperlactemia relies on treating the underlying malignancy. Approaches to acute management of the lactic acidosis in these cases include using intravenous insulin to increase conversion of pyruvate to acetyl CoA, thereby facilitating oxidation of lactate to pyruvate[65] and bicarbonate therapy to buffer the extreme acidosis. Bicarbonate has been shown to increase lactate production in patients with malignancy associated chronic lactic acidosis, however.[66]

Systemic Inflammatory Response Syndrome

Systemic inflammatory response syndrome is typically associated with type A lactic acidosis due to the presumption that the hemodynamic instability leads to inadequate DO_2.[67] Although this is likely at least a partial contributor, there is evidence that increased production of pyruvate,[68] decreased activity of PDH (in part due to increased PDH kinase[69]), lactate production by the lung,[70] and decreased lactate clearance[71] are contributors to lactic acidosis in systemic inflammatory response syndrome.

Hepatic Failure

In critically ill patients with cirrhosis, lactic acidosis portends a grim prognosis with a 7.64 (95% CI, 3.01–19.34) odds ratio for ICU mortality.[72] Individuals with the combination of cirrhosis, acidemia, lactic acidosis, and acute renal failure had 86% ICU mortality and 94% hospital mortality. Liver failure is associated with decreased lactate clearance, which is further exacerbated in sepsis.[16] In cases of severe liver failure, the liver can be a source of lactate production.[73] When lactate measurements were added to King's College Hospital criteria for determining outcome after paracetamol intoxication, an early lactate of greater than 3.5 mmol/L or a postresuscitation lactate of greater than 3.0 mmol/L increased sensitivity for predicting death to 95% whereas specificity was relatively unchanged at greater than 90%.[74]

TYPE B2—DRUGS AND TOXINS
Acetaminophen

Acetaminophen and its toxic metabolite, N-acetyl-p-benzoquinonimine, interferes with mitochondrial oxidative phosphorylation by inhibiting cellular respiration at NADH-linked substrates (energy coupling site I) and at succinate stimulated sites (energy coupling site II).[75–77] In an animal model, the inhibition of mitochondrial respiration preceded overt hepatic necrosis and was completely prevented by treatment with N-acetyl-L-cysteine.[76] Inhibition of oxidative phosphorylation eventually results in a shift toward lactate production. This suggests that the earlier treatment with N-acetyl-L-cysteine is initiated, the better the outcome.

Toxic Alcohols

Toxic alcohol ingestions of ethanol, methanol, ethylene glycol, and diethylene glycol can cause hyperosmolality and lactic acidosis. Propylene glycol intoxication is the most common alcohol intoxication in ICUs.[78] Propylene glycol is the vehicle carrier for several intravenous medications used in ICUs, including lorazepam, diazepam, digoxin, hydralazine, pentobarbital, phenobarbital, nitroglycerin, etomidate, phenytoin, multivitamins, esmolol, and trimethoprim-sulfamethoxazole (**Box 2**). Propylene glycol is oxidized by alcohol dehydrogenase in the liver to lactate and pyruvate.[79] There are many case reports of propylene glycol toxicity, manifested as unexplained anion gap, unexplained metabolic acidosis, elevated lactate, and hyperosmolality.[80–82] The majority of case reports have involved the use of lorazepam, likely due to the relatively higher concentration of propylene glycol in the solution. A 2-mg/mL standard solution of lorazepam contains 830 mg/mL of propylene glycol.[83] A daily dose of propylene glycol of 25 mg/kg of body weight is considered safe.[83] In patients who require greater than 1 mg/kg/day of intravenous lorazepam, following the osmolar gap may help identify those individuals at risk for the development of lactic acidosis, with values greater than 12 mg/dL, suggesting increased risk for propylene glycol toxicity.[84] Treatment includes discontinuation of the agent and in severe cases removal via hemodialysis.[85] Theoretically, fomepizole, which inhibits alcohol dehydrogenase and slows the breakdown of alcohols to their toxic metabolites, might have some utility but its efficacy in propylene glycol intoxication is unclear.[86]

Nucleoside/Tide Reverse Transcriptase Inhibitors

Nucleoside/tide reverse transcriptase inhibitors (NRTIs) have revolutionized treatment of HIV and AIDS (**Table 1**). A typical regimen of highly active antiretroviral therapy consists of two NRTIs and a protease inhibitor or a non-NRTI.[87] Toxicities due to NRTIs are likely due to mitochrondrial toxicity. NRTIs may inhibit DNA polymerase-γ, which interferes with mitochondrial DNA synthesis and can lead to abnormal transcription and translation.[88] Although there is no clinical correlation at present, studies demonstrate that zalcitabine has the greatest inhibition of DNA polymerase γ and lamivudine, abacavir, and tenofovir have the least.[89] Long-chain–fatty-acid oxidation is also impaired by NRTIs. One of the most serious outcomes of the mitochondrial toxicity is lactic acidosis.[90] Elevations in lactic acid is common in individuals treated with NRTIs, affecting approximately 9% individuals in one study.[91] In this group,

Box 2
Commonly used medications in propylene glycol vehicle
Diazepam
Esmolol
Hydralazine
Multivitamins
Pentobarbital
Phenytoin
Digoxin
Etomidate
Lorazepam
Nitroglycerin
Phenobarbital
Trimethoprim-sulfamethoxazole

Table 1	
Currently available nucleoside/tide reverse transcriptase inhibitors	
Generic Name	**Abbreviation**
Abacavir	ABC
Didanosine	ddI EC
Emtricitabine	FTC
Lamivudine	3TC
Stavudine	d4T
Tenofovir	TDF
Zalcitabine	ddC
Zidovudine	AZT, ZDV

among those with elevated lactate, a little over one-third had symptoms possibly consistent with hyperlactatemia, including myalgias, fatigue, and vomiting. Lactic acidosis may occur in single or combination NRTI regimens.[88,91] Risk factors include exposure to didanosine, stavudine, or a combination of the two; female gender; age over 40 years; advanced immunosuppression (lower CD4 counts); and shorter duration of therapy (<12 months), suggesting an idiosyncratic reaction.[92] In patients with symptoms of unexplained nausea, vomiting, abdominal pain, hepatic steatosis, or transaminemia, it may be beneficial to check lactate levels.[88] The lactic acidosis typically resolves with cessation of the NRTI and supportive therapy, although some investigators have suggested supplementation with riboflavin, thiamine, carnitine, and coenzyme Q-10.[93] One study using polymerase chain assay to compare mitochondrial to nuclear DNA in non–HIV-infected controls, HIV-infected individuals not on NRTIs, and HIV-infected individuals on NRTIs with elevated lactate demonstrated that HIV alone can affect the mitochondrial–to–nuclear DNA ratio and, therefore, HIV alone could result in lactic acidosis.[94]

Metformin

The biguanides, metformin and phenformin, have been used to treat diabetes mellitus since the 1950s. Phenformin was pulled off the US market in 1976 due to more than 300 reports of lactic acidosis.[95] Metformin, available since 1995, has a much lower risk of lactic acidosis than its predecessor, phenformin. Metformin inhibits gluconeogenesis from lactate in the liver in a time- and concentration-dependent manner.

In overdose, metformin binds to mitochondrial membranes, specifically complex I, resulting in inhibition of the electron transport system, resulting in a shift toward anaerobic metabolism.[96] Most cases of metformin-related lactic acidosis have been in cases of intentional overdose[97] or in individuals with underlying conditions, such as renal failure, congestive heart failure,[98] hepatic failure, sepsis, and shock.[99] The risk of death in these patients correlates better with organ dysfunction than lactate level or metformin level.[100] There is low mortality in intentional metformin overdose with early recognition, hemodynamic and respiratory support, and hemodialysis. With hemodialysis, approximately 12% per hour of the drug is eliminated in the first 2 hours. After 15 hours of hemodialysis the elimination is approximately 1.5% per hour.[100]

Propofol

Propofol infusion syndrome is a rare, life-threatening complication of propofol infusion. Characterized by metabolic acidosis, rhabdomyolysis of skeletal and cardiac muscle, arrhythmias, myocardial failure, renal failure, hepatomegaly, and death, it has sudden onset usually resulting in death.[101] The majority of case reports have been in individuals receiving relatively higher doses (>4 mg/kg/h) for a prolonged period of time (>48 hours),[102] but it also has been described in low-dose infusion (1.4–2.6 mg/kg/h).[103] Propofol can alter the mitochondrial respiratory chain in multiple ways. Reduction in cytochrome-c oxidase activity and decreased complex IV activity[104] and impaired fatty-acid oxidation with secondary impairment in complex II activity has been described in propofol infusion syndrome.[105] New metabolic acidosis in a patient on propofol infusion should raise suspicion for propofol infusion syndrome. Discontinuation of propofol, resuscitation and cardiocirculatory stabilization, and hemodialysis to eliminate propofol is recommended[106]; however, the syndrome is often rapidly fatal and patients are unresponsive to pressors and inotropes.

Linezolid

Linezolid-related lactic acidosis was not reported during phase III clinical trials,[107] but many case reports and case series have emerged since those.[108–110] Most cases occur after a prolonged duration of therapy,[111] but there are reports with duration of therapy as short as 7 days,[110] In most cases, discontinuation of the linezolid results in resolution of the lactic acidosis.[111] Linezolid kills bacteria by binding to the 23S ribosomal RNA (rRNA) of the bacteria.[112] In mammals, the 16S RNA large ribosomal subunit is homologous to the bacterial 23S rRNA. In two patients with linezolid-related lactic acidosis, polymorphisms were identified in the mitochondrial 16S rRNA, specifically in the region structurally similar to the linezolid binding site located at the bacterial 23S rRNA.[113] Caution should be used when administering linezolid with selective serotonin reuptake inhibitors as they block p-glycoprotein activity and may raise linezolid levels.[114] Serotonin syndrome has been reported with concomitant use of linezolid and selective serotonin reuptake inhibitors.[115]

β_2-Adrenergic Agents—Epinephrine, Ritodrine, Terbutaline, Salbumatol, and Dobutamine

β-Agonists cause lactic acidosis in several ways. First, β_2-adrenergic–mediated stimulation of muscle and hepatic phosphorylase and inhibition of glycogen synthetase stimulates glycolysis and, thereby, an increase in pyruvate production.[116] In skeletal muscle, β-agonists stimulate Na^+-K^+-ATPase via upregulation of cyclic AMP.[117] This increases generation of ADP and then phosphofructokinase, which accelerates glycolysis.[118] Then, the β-agonists inhibit PDH, which leads to decreased oxidation of pyruvate to acetyl CoA and, thereby, increased reduction of the pyruvate to lactate.[119]

Salicylates

Salicylate overdose is characterized by an early respiratory alkalosis and a late metabolic acidosis, mostly due to lactic acidosis.[120] Respiratory acidosis occurs late and is typically a terminal event.[121] The toxicity of salicylates is due to multiple mechanisms, including inhibition of β-oxidation of fatty acids,[122] decreasing the availability of CoA,[123] inhibition of succinate dehydrogenase and α-ketoglutarate dehydrogenase,[124] and increasing permeability of the inner mitochondrial membrane.[125] Furthermore, the early respiratory alkalosis stimulates an increase in 2,3-diphosphoglycerate level, with subsequent increase in phosphofructose kinase activity resulting in accelerated glycolysis.[126] Management consists of administering glucose to keep ward off central nervous system hypoglycemia and keeping the pH 7.45 to 7.5 to decrease central nervous system salicylate concentration and augment renal salicylate excretion. Hemodialysis is indicated in severe intoxications.[127]

Sulfasalazine

Sulfasalazine is broken down in the colon to sulfapyridine and 5-aminosalicylic acid (ASA). The sulfapyridine is absorbed and is mostly acetylated in the liver with the remainder undergoing glucuronidation or hydroxylation before being excreted in the urine. Approximately one-quarter of the 5-ASA is absorbed, which is then acetylated to N-acetyl-5-ASA.[128] In one case report, lactic acidosis with coingestion of paracetamol resulted in lactate levels of approximately 20 mmol/L with survival of the patient despite late administration of N-acetylcysteine.[129]

Other Medications Causing Hyperlactatemia

Case reports of lactic acidosis due to isoniazid (INH),[130] simvastatin,[131] atorvastatin,[132] niacin,[133] and nalidixic acid[134] have been published. It is unclear whether or not the hyperlactatemia is due to hepatic impairment that occurs with these drugs or if there is additional inhibition of cellular respiration. INH inhibits mycobacterial pyridoxal (the oxidized form of pyridoxine) to block bacterial growth and metabolism. Elevated levels of INH could affect human diphosphopyridine nucleotides[135] and decrease metabolism of lactate to pyruvate. Simvastatin and atorvastatin are in a class of drugs known to reduce serum coenzyme Q10, a central cofactor of the mitochondrial respiratory chain.[136] Lactulose has been a mainstay of treatment of hepatic encephalopathy for decades. Colonic bacteria break down lactulose into lactic, acetic, and formic acids. In a case where a cirrhotic patient received treatment with lactulose, severe lactic acidosis occurred, theoretically due to the formation of lactate in the colon, which diffused back across the gut wall, facilitated by intestinal hypomotility.[137]

Thiamine, Biotin, and Iron

Thiamine deficiency resulting in lactic acidosis is most often described in patients with alcoholism,[138] patients receiving total parenteral nutrition,[139] foreign workers whose nutritional habits have changed,[140] and infants receiving a defective soy-based formula.[141] Lactate levels up to 20 mmol/L were recorded in one study.[142] Thiamine, a water-soluble, B-complex vitamin that mammals are unable to synthesize, is an essential cofactor for enzymes in the cytosol and the mitochondria,[143] including keto-lase, PDH, and α-ketoglutarate dehydrogenase.[144] Losses in the activity of PDH and α-ketoglutarate dehydrogenase are thought to lead to reduced pyruvate entry into the TCA cycle[145] and increased lactate production. Lack of transketolase leads to reduction of the pentose phosphate pathway and subsequent reduction in NADH,[146] stimulating anaerobic glycolysis and further lactate production. Administration of glucose stimulates excess lactate production.[147]

Biotin is a cofactor in multiple carboxylation reactions,[148] including pyruvate carboxylation to form oxaloacetate.[149] Deficiency of biotin was demonstrated in humans by feeding them a diet of raw egg whites.[150] Raw egg whites have a glycoprotein called avidin, which binds biotin. Cooking the whites denatures avidin and destroys its affinity for biotin.[151] In individuals fed an egg white diet, symptoms of dermatitis, pallor, changes in mental status, myalgias, anorexia, anemia, and EKG changes consistent with coronary ischemia were seen. Administration of injectable biotin resolved all symptoms within 3 to 5 days. Biotin deficiency has also been described in individuals receiving total parenteral nutrition without biotin[152]; with prolonged use of some anticonvulsants, such as phenytoin, carbamazepine, phenobarbital, and primidone; and in genetic mutation.[153] Theoretically, prolonged antibiotic use could lower biotin levels as biotin is generated by bacteria living in the intestine, and there are specialized receptors in the colon for biotin absorption[154]; however, primary data for this are lacking.

Iron is essential to cellular respiration as it plays a major role in electron transport via iron-sulfur centers[155] and cytochrome a, b, and c.[156] States of iron overload[157] and iron deficiency[158] have been associated with lactic acidosis. A syndrome known as GRACILE is named for the clinical findings of growth retardation, aminoaciduria, cholestasis, iron overload, lactic acidosis, and early death.

Sugar Alcohols (Fructose, Sorbitol, and Xylitol)

Fructose enters the glycolytic pathway as lactate, glucose, or glycogen.[159] Sorbitol is poorly absorbed in the intestine and is primarily converted to fructose with only a small portions metabolized to glucose.[159] Xylitol is also poorly absorbed when orally administered but increases over time, due to adaptations in oral flora.[160] Xylitol is metabolized to glucose, glycogen, lactate, and xylulose. Lactic acidosis has been reported when fructose,[161] sorbitol,[162] or xylitol[163] was used in parenteral nutrition. Lethal xylitol toxicity characterized by increased serum osmolality, increased urine output, and hemoconcentration has been demonstrated in animals.[164]

Strychnine

Formerly used as a medication to treat a variety of ailments, strychnine is still used today as a pesticide and is rarely mixed with illegal drugs.[165] Strychnine is excitatory to the central nervous system and antagonizes the inhibitory neurotransmitter, glycine, at the postsynaptic receptor sites of motor neurons in the ventral horn. This results in anti-inhibition and hyperexcitability, leading to extreme extensor muscle spasms. The resulting convulsions are thought to be the cause of the lactic acidosis. Lactate up to 32 mmol/L was recorded in one patient.[166]

Malaria

Malaria has been a major cause of death in illness, particularly in sub-Saharan Africa, for centuries.[167] Lactic acidosis is used as a prognostic indicator in acute malarial infection.[168] Etiology of lactate elevation is unclear but may be related to decreased liver blood flow[169] and decreased lactate clearance,[170] lactate production of parasites in red blood cells via anaerobic glycolysis,[171] or mismatch between VO_2 and oxygen demand.[172] N-acetylcysteine administered to adults with severe malaria resulted in a rapid lowering of lactate,[173] but it is unknown whether or not it would improve mortality.

Valproic Acid

Valproic acid inhibits oxidative phosphorylation[174] by decreasing activity of cytochrome aa_3[175] and cytochrome c,[176] by inhibiting succinate transport,[177] and by changing conformation of mitochondrial membrane proteins.[178] Reports of lactic acidosis have been associated with valproic acid use in individuals with underlying mitochondrial abnormalities[179] and in valproate overdose.[180] Withdrawal of the medication,[181] hemodialysis,[180] and supportive care resulted in good outcome.

Cocaine and Methamphetamine

In the mid-1980s, two elite athletes, Len Bias and Don Rogers, died from cocaine use. Death from cocaine is typically due to seizures, lactic acidosis, hyperthermia, myocardial infarctions, and arrhythmias.[182,183] Cocaine stimulates adrenergic activity, leading to increased glycolysis and lactic acid production.[184] Reports of methamphetamine-related lactic acidosis have emerged.[185] Acute methamphetamine intoxication can present with coma, shock, convulsions, hyperthermia, renal failure, and acidosis.[186]

Methamphetamine decreases complex I activity in the mitochondria.[187] It also induces a decrease in proliferation, increase in apoptosis, and disruption of mitochondrial networks resulting in mitochondrial fragmentation.[188]

Cyanogenic Compounds—Cyanide, Aliphatic Nitriles, and Nitroprusside

Cyanide or cyanide-releasing chemicals are found in insulation; pesticides; metal-stripping and metal-plating solutions; the pits of apricots, cherries, and peaches; and cassava roots, almonds, and bamboo shoots.[189] Aliphatic nitriles are used in the manufacture of synthetic fibers, resins, plastics, pharmaceuticals, and vitamins. The two most studied nitriles, methacrylonitrile and acrylonitrile, release cyanide during metabolism of these substances via epoxidation in the liver.[190] Sodium nitroprusside is a medication used for its vasodilatory effect. It is composed of one iron molecule bound to five cyanide molecules and one molecule of nitric oxide.[191] Risk of cyanide toxicity from nitroprusside infusion increases with high doses over a prolonged period of time. This risk is also higher when given to individuals with malnutrition or pre-existing renal impairment.[192] Cyanide binds to cytochrome aa_3, inhibiting cytochrome-c oxidase activity.[193] This inhibition of oxidative metabolism results in decreased tissue extraction of oxygen and a shift of cellular metabolism to anaerobic glycolysis. A decrease in the arteriovenous oxygen difference should increase suspicion for cyanide intoxication. Treatment of suspected cyanide toxicity involves supportive care and treatment with a methemoglobin-forming agent and subsequently a sulfur donor. Amyl nitrite or sodium nitrite form methemoglobin,[194] which has a high affinity for cyanide, dissociating it from cytochrome oxidase and thereby restoring oxidative phosphorylation. Sodium thiosulfate is then given as a sulfur-donating substrate for conversion of cyanide a less toxic form, thiocyanate, which is then renally excreted.[195] Dialysis, in particular continuous venovenous hemodiafiltration, may also be helpful as an additional measure in severe poisonings.[191] In the case of nitroprusside-induced cyanide toxicity, addition of hydroxocobalamin may decrease the toxicity.[196]

General Anesthetics: Diethyl Ether and Halothane

Diethyl ether is commonly used as a laboratory solvent and is used in the production of cellulose plastics. It was used as a general anesthetic until nonflammable, less-toxic inhaled anesthetics, such as halothane, became available. Diethyl ether and halothane are reported as causative agents in lactic acidosis,[197] but the mechanisms have not been well described. Diethylether, diethylether derivatives, and halothane have been shown to disrupt oxidative phosphorylation.[198]

5-Fluorouracil

Reports of lactic acidosis, hyperammonemia, and encephalopathy with 5-fluorouracil (5-FU) infusions are rare.[199] Administration of 5-FU in individuals with inborn deficiencies of dihydropyrimidine dehydrogenase and dihydropyrimidinase is lethal.[200] In electron micrographs, degradation and alteration in mitochondrial structure is noted[201] and likely related to 5-FU's inhibition of DNA and RNA synthesis.[202]

TYPE B3—INBORN ERRORS OF METABOLISM

There are many genetic abnormalities known to cause syndromes of lactic acidosis. Conditions resulting in deficiency in oxidative phosphorylation, such as Kearns-Sayre syndrome; Pearson syndrome; MERRF; and mitochondrial encephalomyopathy, lactic acidosis, and stroke syndrome (MELAS), are mitochondrial encephalomyopathies commonly associated with lactic acidosis.[203] Management of these individuals is typically supportive.[204] A trial attempting to use DCA to lower lactic acid in patients with MELAS resulted in peripheral nerve toxicity and was discontinued.[205] Fructose-1,6-diphosphatase deficiency results in life-threatening hypoglycemia and lactic acidemia only when fasting occurs[206] as gluconeogenesis is impaired. This is more pronounced in glycogen storage disease type I, also known as von Gierke disease. A deficiency of glucose-6-phosphatase, glucose-6-phosphate translocase, or the endoplasmic reticulum phosphate translocase results in compromised glycogenolysis and gluconeogenesis. PDH deficiency can be due to several mutations with a gradation in phenotype.[207] The impairment may range from fatal infantile lactic acidosis to ataxia as the primary impairment. Pyruvate carboxylase deficiency also has different phenotypic expressions depending on the degree of impairment. It is also characterized by hypoglycemia, lactic acidosis, and ketosis.[208] The type C phenotype lacks the psychomotor retardation seen in type A. Unlike in type B, where infants typically die by age 3 months,[208] these individuals survive into adulthood with episodes of lactic acidemia.[209] Methylmalonic aciduria is caused by a deficiency of methylmalonyl-CoA mutase or by defects in the transport, uptake, or synthesis of 5'-deoxyadenosylcobalamin.[210] Clinical presentation varies but may include lactic acidosis, hypoglycemia, ketosis, and hyperammonemia. Dialysis has been used to clear the acidemia during metabolic crises, but there has been little success in curtailing the end-organ damage, which results from the accumulation of the toxic organic acids.[211]

D-LACTIC ACIDOSIS

D-lactate is the optical isomer of L-lactate. Elevated levels of D-lactate are usually due to bacterial production in the intestinal tract, although they can also be due to D-lactate ingestion, from endogenous production via the methylglyoxylase pathway[212] or from infusion of DL-lactate solutions in peritoneal dialysis. The clinical presentation is unique for unusual neurologic manifestations, ranging from slurred speech to abusive behavior[213] that lasts from a few hours to several days. High-glucose meals have been shown to exacerbate symptoms.[214] Severe metabolic acidosis is also present, but L-lactate levels are normal. D-lactate must be ordered to make the diagnosis. Most patients presenting with D-lactic acidosis have short bowel syndrome.[215] It is theorized that the neurologic symptoms manifest as a result of D-lactate toxicity to the brain, which lacks D-2-hydroxyacid dehydrogenase, the enzyme that converts D-lactic acid to pyruvate. Treatment of this condition includes a low-carbohydrate diet, saline enema when constipated, and poorly absorbed oral antibiotics in an effort to decrease D-lactate producing intestinal bacteria. During episodes of acidosis, insulin administration may decrease fatty acid levels, which may result in increased D-lactate oxidation and clearance.[216] In severe cases, hemodialysis may be used.[217]

REFERENCES

1. Kompanje EJ, Jansen TC, van der Hoven B, et al. The first demonstration of lactic acid in human blood in shock by Johann Joseph Scherer (1814–1869) in January 1843. Intensive Care Med 2007;33(11):1967–71.
2. Fletcher WM. Lactic acid in amphibian muscle. J Physiol 1907;35(4):247–309.
3. Huckabee WE. Relationship of pyruvate and lactate during anaerobic metabolism. IV. Local tissue components of total body O2-debt. Am J Physiol 1959; 196(2):253–60.
4. Huckabee WE. Relationships of pyruvate and lactate during anaerobic metabolism. III. Effect of breathing low-oxygen gases. J Clin Invest 1958;37(2):264–71.

5. Huckabee WE. Relationships of pyruvate and lactate during anaerobic metabolism. II. Exercise and formation of O-debt. J Clin Invest 1958;37(2):255–63.

6. Huckabee WE. Relationships of pyruvate and lactate during anaerobic metabolism. I. Effects of infusion of pyruvate or glucose and of hyperventilation. J Clin Invest 1958;37(2):244–54.

7. Huckabee WE. Abnormal resting blood lactate. I. The significance of hyperlactatemia in hospitalized patients. Am J Med 1961;30:840–8.

8. Woods HF, Cohen R. Clinical and biochemical aspects of lactic acidosis. Oxford: Blackwell Scientific; 1976.

9. Gladden LB. Lactate metabolism: a new paradigm for the third millennium. J Physiol 2004;558(Pt 1):5–30.

10. Philp A, Macdonald AL, Watt PW. Lactate—a signal coordinating cell and systemic function. J Exp Biol 2005;208(Pt 24):4561–75.

11. Levy B. Lactate and shock state: the metabolic view. Curr Opin Crit Care 2006; 12(4):315–21.

12. De Backer D, Creteur J, Zhang H, et al. Lactate production by the lungs in acute lung injury. Am J Respir Crit Care Med 1997;156(4 Pt 1):1099–104.

13. Borregaard N, Herlin T. Energy metabolism of human neutrophils during phagocytosis. J Clin Invest 1982;70(3):550–7.

14. Mizock BA. Hyperlactatemia in acute liver failure: decreased clearance versus increased production. Crit Care Med 2001;29(11):2225–6.

15. De Backer D, Creteur J, Silva E, et al. The hepatosplanchnic area is not a common source of lactate in patients with severe sepsis. Crit Care Med 2001;29(2):256–61.

16. Levraut J, Ciebiera JP, Chave S, et al. Mild hyperlactatemia in stable septic patients is due to impaired lactate clearance rather than overproduction. Am J Respir Crit Care Med 1998;157(4 Pt 1):1021–6.

17. Bellomo R. Bench-to-bedside review: lactate and the kidney. Crit Care 2002; 6(4):322–6.

18. Bihari D, Gimson AE, Lindridge J, et al. Lactic acidosis in fulminant hepatic failure. Some aspects of pathogenesis and prognosis. J Hepatol 1985;1(4):405–16.

19. Vary TC. Sepsis-induced alterations in pyruvate dehydrogenase complex activity in rat skeletal muscle: effects on plasma lactate. Shock 1996;6(2):89–94.

20. Levy B, Sadoune LO, Gelot AM, et al. Evolution of lactate/pyruvate and arterial ketone body ratios in the early course of catecholamine-treated septic shock. Crit Care Med 2000;28(1):114–9.

21. Revelly JP, Tappy L, Martinez A, et al. Lactate and glucose metabolism in severe sepsis and cardiogenic shock. Crit Care Med 2005;33(10):2235–40.

22. Dellinger RP, Levy MM, Carlet JM, et al. Surviving Sepsis Campaign: international guidelines for management of severe sepsis and septic shock: 2008. Crit Care Med 2008;36(1):296–327.

23. Weil MH, Afifi AA. Experimental and clinical studies on lactate and pyruvate as indicators of the severity of acute circulatory failure (shock). Circulation 1970; 41(6):989–1001.

24. Cady LD Jr, Weil MH, Afifi AA, et al. Quantitation of severity of critical illness with special reference to blood lactate. Crit Care Med 1973;1(2):75–80.

25. Stacpoole PW, Wright EC, Baumgartner TG, et al. Natural history and course of acquired lactic acidosis in adults. DCA-Lactic Acidosis Study Group. Am J Med 1994;97(1):47–54.

26. Trzeciak S, Dellinger RP, Chansky ME, et al. Serum lactate as a predictor of mortality in patients with infection. Intensive Care Med 2007;33(6):970–7.

27. Shapiro NI, Howell MD, Talmor D, et al. Serum lactate as a predictor of mortality in emergency department patients with infection. Ann Emerg Med 2005;45(5): 524–8.

28. Shapiro NI, Howell MD, Donnino M, et al. Occult hypoperfusion and mortality in patients with suspected infection. Intensive Care Med 2007;33(11):1892–9.

29. Mikkelsen ME, Miltiades AN, Gaieski DF, et al. Serum lactate is associated with mortality in severe sepsis independent of organ failure and shock. Crit Care Med 2009;37(5):1670–7.

30. Jansen TC, van Bommel J, Woodward R, et al. Association between blood lactate levels, sequential organ failure assessment subscores, and 28-day mortality during early and late intensive care unit stay: a retrospective observational study. Crit Care Med 2009;37(8):2369–74.

31. Chuang CK, Wang TJ, Yeung CY, et al. Interference and blood sample preparation for a pyruvate enzymatic assay. Clin Biochem 2006;39(1):74–7.

32. Suistomaa M, Ruokonen E, Kari A, et al. Time-pattern of lactate and lactate to pyruvate ratio in the first 24 hours of intensive care emergency admissions. Shock 2000;14(1):8–12.

33. Bakker J, Coffernils M, Leon M, et al. Blood lactate levels are superior to oxygen-derived variables in predicting outcome in human septic shock. Chest 1991;99(4):956–62.

34. Bakker J, Gris P, Coffernils M, et al. Serial blood lactate levels can predict the development of multiple organ failure following septic shock. Am J Surg 1996; 171(2):221–6.

35. Abramson D, Scalea TM, Hitchcock R, et al. Lactate clearance and survival following injury. J Trauma 1993;35(4):584–8 [discussion: 588–9].

36. McNelis J, Marini CP, Jurkiewicz A, et al. Prolonged lactate clearance is associated with increased mortality in the surgical intensive care unit. Am J Surg 2001; 182(5):481–5.

37. Husain FA, Martin MJ, Mullenix PS, et al. Serum lactate and base deficit as predictors of mortality and morbidity. Am J Surg 2003;185(5):485–91.

38. Nguyen HB, Rivers EP, Knoblich BP, et al. Early lactate clearance is associated with improved outcome in severe sepsis and septic shock. Crit Care Med 2004; 32(8):1637–42.

39. Stacpoole PW, Nagaraja NV, Hutson AD. Efficacy of dichloroacetate as a lactate-lowering drug. J Clin Pharmacol 2003;43(7):683–91.

40. Stacpoole PW, Kerr DS, Barnes C, et al. Controlled clinical trial of dichloroacetate for treatment of congenital lactic acidosis in children. Pediatrics 2006; 117(5):1519–31.

41. Bersin RM, Stacpoole PW. Dichloroacetate as metabolic therapy for myocardial ischemia and failure. Am Heart J 1997;134(5 Pt 1):841–55.

42. Stacpoole PW, Lorenz AC, Thomas RG, et al. Dichloroacetate in the treatment of lactic acidosis. Ann Intern Med 1988;108(1):58–63.

43. Stacpoole PW, Wright EC, Baumgartner TG, et al. A controlled clinical trial of dichloroacetate for treatment of lactic acidosis in adults. The Dichloroacetate-Lactic Acidosis Study Group. N Engl J Med 1992;327(22):1564–9.

44. Gallagher EJ, Rodriguez K, Touger M. Agreement between peripheral venous and arterial lactate levels. Ann Emerg Med 1997;29(4):479–83.

45. Lavery RF, Livingston DH, Tortella BJ, et al. The utility of venous lactate to triage injured patients in the trauma center. J Am Coll Surg 2000;190(6):656–64.

46. Marko P, Gabrielli A, Caruso LJ. Too much lactate or too little liver? J Clin Anesth 2004;16(5):389–95.

47. Noritomi DT, Soriano FG, Kellum JA, et al. Metabolic acidosis in patients with severe sepsis and septic shock: a longitudinal quantitative study. Crit Care Med 2009;37(10):2733–9.
48. Didwania A, Miller J, Kassel D, et al. Effect of intravenous lactated Ringer's solution infusion on the circulating lactate concentration: Part 3. Results of a prospective, randomized, double-blind, placebo-controlled trial. Crit Care Med 1997;25(11):1851–4.
49. Warburg O. On the origin of cancer cells. Science 1956;123(3191):309–14.
50. Baysal BE, Ferrell RE, Willett-Brozick JE, et al. Mutations in SDHD, a mitochondrial complex II gene, in hereditary paraganglioma. Science 2000;287(5454): 848–51.
51. Tomlinson IP, Alam NA, Rowan AJ, et al. Germline mutations in FH predispose to dominantly inherited uterine fibroids, skin leiomyomata and papillary renal cell cancer. Nat Genet 2002;30(4):406–10.
52. Bellance N, Lestienne P, Rossignol R. Mitochondria: from bioenergetics to the metabolic regulation of carcinogenesis. Front Biosci 2009;14:4015–34.
53. Friedenberg AS, Brandoff DE, Schiffman FJ. Type B lactic acidosis as a severe metabolic complication in lymphoma and leukemia: a case series from a single institution and literature review. Medicine (Baltimore) 2007;86(4):225–32.
54. Colombo GM, Del Vecchio LR, Sacco T, et al. Fatal lactic acidosis due to widespread diffusion of melanoma. Minerva Med 2006;97(3):295.
55. Manuel B, Suresh V, Saphwat E. Refractory metabolic acidosis in small cell cancer of the lung. South Med J 2006;99(7):782–3.
56. Field M, Block JB, Levin R, et al. Significance of blood lactate elevations among patients with acute leukemia and other neoplastic proliferative disorders. Am J Med 1966;40:528–47.
57. Ustun C, Fall P, Szerlip HM, et al. Multiple myeloma associated with lactic acidosis. Leuk Lymphoma 2002;43(12):2395–7.
58. Kachel RG. Metastatic reticulum cell sarcoma and lactic acidosis. Cancer 1975; 36(6):2056–9.
59. Varanasi UR, Carr B, Simpson DP. Lactic acidosis associated with metastatic breast carcinoma. Cancer Treat Rep 1980;64(12):1283–5.
60. Colman LK, Baker TM. Lactic acidosis with extensive oat cell carcinoma of the lung–not necessarily a poor prognostic sign: case report. Mil Med 1983;148(5):440.
61. Cheng JC, Esparza SD, Knez VM, et al. Severe lactic acidosis in a 14-year-old female with metastatic undifferentiated carcinoma of unknown primary. J Pediatr Hematol Oncol 2004;26(11):780–2.
62. Wall BM, Mansour N, Cooke CR. Acute fulminant lactic acidosis complicating metastatic cholangiocarcinoma. Am J Med Sci 2000;319(2):126–9.
63. Bischof T, Gunthard H, Straumann E, et al. [Splenic infarct, lactate acidosis, and pulmonary edema as manifestations of a pheochromocytoma]. Schweiz Med Wochenschr 1997;127(7):261–5 [in German].
64. Sillos EM, Shenep JL, Burghen GA, et al. Lactic acidosis: a metabolic complication of hematologic malignancies: case report and review of the literature. Cancer 2001;92(9):2237–46.
65. Coleman RA, Sommerville HM, Friedman HS, et al. Insulin therapy for ketolactic acidosis complicating malignancy. J Pediatr 1982;100(4):584–7.
66. Fraley DS, Adler S, Bruns FJ, et al. Stimulation of lactate production by administration of bicarbonate in a patient with a solid neoplasm and lactic acidosis. N Engl J Med 1980;303(19):1100–2.

67. Hurtado FJ, Gutierrez AM, Silva N, et al. Role of tissue hypoxia as the mechanism of lactic acidosis during *E. coli* endotoxemia. J Appl Physiol 1992;72(5): 1895–901.
68. Gore DC, Jahoor F, Hibbert JM, et al. Lactic acidosis during sepsis is related to increased pyruvate production, not deficits in tissue oxygen availability. Ann Surg 1996;224(1):97–102.
69. Vary TC. Increased pyruvate dehydrogenase kinase activity in response to sepsis. Am J Physiol 1991;260(5 Pt 1):E669–74.
70. Brown SD, Clark C, Gutierrez G. Pulmonary lactate release in patients with sepsis and the adult respiratory distress syndrome. J Crit Care 1996;11(1):2–8.
71. Severin PN, Uhing MR, Beno DW, et al. Endotoxin-induced hyperlactatemia results from decreased lactate clearance in hemodynamically stable rats. Crit Care Med 2002;30(11):2509–14.
72. Funk GC, Doberer D, Kneidinger N, et al. Acid-base disturbances in critically ill patients with cirrhosis. Liver Int 2007;27(7):901–9.
73. Tsai MH, Chen YC, Lien JM, et al. Hemodynamics and metabolic studies on septic shock in patients with acute liver failure. J Crit Care 2008;23(4): 468–72.
74. Bernal W, Donaldson N, Wyncoll D, et al. Blood lactate as an early predictor of outcome in paracetamol-induced acute liver failure: a cohort study. Lancet 2002;359(9306):558–63.
75. Burcham PC, Harman AW. Acetaminophen toxicity results in site-specific mitochondrial damage in isolated mouse hepatocytes. J Biol Chem 1991;266(8): 5049–54.
76. Donnelly PJ, Walker RM, Racz WJ. Inhibition of mitochondrial respiration in vivo is an early event in acetaminophen-induced hepatotoxicity. Arch Toxicol 1994; 68(2):110–8.
77. Esterline RL, Ray SD, Ji S. Reversible and irreversible inhibition of hepatic mitochondrial respiration by acetaminophen and its toxic metabolite, N-acetyl-p-benzoquinoneimine (NAPQI). Biochem Pharmacol 1989;38(14):2387–90.
78. Kraut JA, Kurtz I. Toxic alcohol ingestions: clinical features, diagnosis, and management. Clin J Am Soc Nephrol 2008;3(1):208–25.
79. Brooks DE, Wallace KL. Acute propylene glycol ingestion. J Toxicol Clin Toxicol 2002;40(4):513–6.
80. Wilson KC, Reardon C, Theodore AC, et al. Propylene glycol toxicity: a severe iatrogenic illness in ICU patients receiving IV benzodiazepines: a case series and prospective, observational pilot study. Chest 2005;128(3):1674–81.
81. Demey HE, Daelemans RA, Verpooten GA, et al. Propylene glycol-induced side effects during intravenous nitroglycerin therapy. Intensive Care Med 1988;14(3): 221–6.
82. Bedichek E, Kirschbaum B. A case of propylene glycol toxic reaction associated with etomidate infusion. Arch Intern Med 1991;151(11):2297–8.
83. Miller MA, Forni A, Yogaratnam D. Propylene glycol-induced lactic acidosis in a patient receiving continuous infusion pentobarbital. Ann Pharmacother 2008;42(10):1502–6.
84. Yahwak JA, Riker RR, Fraser GL, et al. Determination of a lorazepam dose threshold for using the osmol gap to monitor for propylene glycol toxicity. Pharmacotherapy 2008;28(8):984–91.
85. Parker MG, Fraser GL, Watson DM, et al. Removal of propylene glycol and correction of increased osmolar gap by hemodialysis in a patient on high dose lorazepam infusion therapy. Intensive Care Med 2002;28(1):81–4.

86. Zar T, Yusufzai I, Sullivan A, et al. Acute kidney injury, hyperosmolality and meta- bolic acidosis associated with lorazepam. Nat Clin Pract Nephrol 2007;3(9): 515–20.

87. Shibuyama S, Gevorkyan A, Yoo U, et al. Understanding and avoiding antiretro- viral adverse events. Curr Pharm Des 2006;12(9):1075–90.

88. ter Hofstede HJ, Willems HL, Koopmans PP. Serum L-lactate and pyruvate in HIV-infected patients with and without presumed NRTI-related adverse events compared to healthy volunteers. J Clin Virol 2004;29(1):44–50.

89. Birkus G, Hitchcock MJ, Cihlar T. Assessment of mitochondrial toxicity in human cells treated with tenofovir: comparison with other nucleoside reverse transcrip- tase inhibitors. Antimicrob Agents Chemother 2002;46(3):716–23.

90. Moyle G. Clinical manifestations and management of antiretroviral nucleoside analog-related mitochondrial toxicity. Clin Ther 2000;22(8):911–36 [discussion: 898].

91. Hocqueloux L, Alberti C, Feugeas JP, et al. Prevalence, risk factors and outcome of hyperlactataemia in HIV-infected patients. HIV Med 2003;4(1): 18–23.

92. Lactic Acidosis International Study Group. Risk factors for lactic acidosis and severe hyperlactataemia in HIV-1-infected adults exposed to antiretroviral therapy. AIDS 2007;21(18):2455–64.

93. Schambelan M, Benson CA, Carr A, et al. Management of metabolic complica- tions associated with antiretroviral therapy for HIV-1 infection: recommendations of an International AIDS Society-USA panel. J Acquir Immune Defic Syndr 2002; 31(3):257–75.

94. Cote HC, Brumme ZL, Craib KJ, et al. Changes in mitochondrial DNA as a marker of nucleoside toxicity in HIV-infected patients. N Engl J Med 2002; 346(11):811–20.

95. Misbin RI. Phenformin-associated lactic acidosis: pathogenesis and treatment. Ann Intern Med 1977;87(5):591–5.

96. Owen MR, Doran E, Halestrap AP. Evidence that metformin exerts its anti-dia- betic effects through inhibition of complex 1 of the mitochondrial respiratory chain. Biochem J 2000;348(Pt 3):607–14.

97. Dell'aglio DM, Perino LJ, Kazzi Z, et al. Acute metformin overdose: examining serum pH, lactate level, and metformin concentrations in survivors versus non- survivors: a systematic review of the literature. Ann Emerg Med 2009;54(6): 818–23.

98. Misbin RI, Green L, Stadel BV, et al. Lactic acidosis in patients with diabetes treated with metformin. N Engl J Med 1998;338(4):265–6.

99. Stades AM, Heikens JT, Erkelens DW, et al. Metformin and lactic acidosis: cause or coincidence? A review of case reports. J Intern Med 2004;255(2):179–87.

100. Seidowsky A, Nseir S, Houdret N, et al. Metformin-associated lactic acidosis: a prognostic and therapeutic study. Crit Care Med 2009;37(7):2191–6.

101. Fodale V, La Monaca E. Propofol infusion syndrome: an overview of a perplexing disease. Drug Saf 2008;31(4):293–303.

102. Kang TM. Propofol infusion syndrome in critically ill patients. Ann Pharmacother 2002;36(9):1453–6.

103. Merz TM, Regli B, Rothen HU, et al. Propofol infusion syndrome—a fatal case at a low infusion rate. Anesth Analg 2006;103(4):1050.

104. Mehta N, DeMunter C, Habibi P, et al. Short-term propofol infusions in children. Lancet 1999;354(9181):866–7.

105. Wolf A, Weir P, Segar P, et al. Impaired fatty acid oxidation in propofol infusion syndrome. Lancet 2001;357(9256):606–7.

106. Motsch J, Roggenbach J. [Propofol infusion syndrome]. Anaesthesist 2004; 53(10):1009–22 [in German].
107. Pharmacia & Upjohn. Zyvox (linezolid) package insert. (Revised July 2008). Available at: http://media.pfizer.com/files/products/uspi_zyvox.pdf; 2000. Accessed August 24, 2009.
108. Narita M, Tsuji BT, Yu VL. Linezolid-associated peripheral and optic neuropathy, lactic acidosis, and serotonin syndrome. Pharmacotherapy 2007;27(8): 1189–97.
109. Apodaca AA, Rakita RM. Linezolid-induced lactic acidosis. N Engl J Med 2003; 348(1):86–7.
110. Kopterides P, Papadomichelakis E, Armaganidis A. Linezolid use associated with lactic acidosis. Scand J Infect Dis 2005;37(2):153–4.
111. Wiener M, Guo Y, Patel G, et al. Lactic acidosis after treatment with linezolid. Infection 2007;35(4):278–81.
112. De Vriese AS, Coster RV, Smet J, et al. Linezolid-induced inhibition of mitochondrial protein synthesis. Clin Infect Dis 2006;42(8):1111–7.
113. Palenzuela L, Hahn NM, Nelson RP Jr, et al. Does linezolid cause lactic acidosis by inhibiting mitochondrial protein synthesis? Clin Infect Dis 2005;40(12):e113–6.
114. Pea F, Scudeller L, Lugano M, et al. Hyperlactacidemia potentially due to linezolid overexposure in a liver transplant recipient. Clin Infect Dis 2006;42(3): 434–5.
115. Bernard L, Stern R, Lew D, et al. Serotonin syndrome after concomitant treatment with linezolid and citalopram. Clin Infect Dis 2003;36(9):1197.
116. Madias NE, Goorno WE, Herson S. Severe lactic acidosis as a presenting feature of pheochromocytoma. Am J Kidney Dis 1987;10(3):250–3.
117. Bundgaard H, Kjeldsen K, Suarez Krabbe K, et al. Endotoxemia stimulates skeletal muscle Na+-K+-ATPase and raises blood lactate under aerobic conditions in humans. Am J Physiol Heart Circ Physiol 2003;284(3): H1028–34.
118. James JH, Luchette FA, McCarter FD, et al. Lactate is an unreliable indicator of tissue hypoxia in injury or sepsis. Lancet 1999;354(9177):505–8.
119. Levy B, Mansart A, Bollaert PE, et al. Effects of epinephrine and norepinephrine on hemodynamics, oxidative metabolism, and organ energetics in endotoxemic rats. Intensive Care Med 2003;29(2):292–300.
120. Eichenholz A, Mulhausen RO, Redleaf PS. Nature of acid-base disturbance in salicylate intoxication. Metabolism 1963;12(2):164–75.
121. Singer RB. The acid-base disturbance in salicylate intoxication. Medicine (Baltimore) 1954;33(1):1–13.
122. Fromenty B, Pessayre D. Inhibition of mitochondrial beta-oxidation as a mechanism of hepatotoxicity. Pharmacol Ther 1995;67(1):101–54.
123. Vessey DA, Hu J, Kelley M. Interaction of salicylate and ibuprofen with the carboxylic acid: CoA ligases from bovine liver mitochondria. J Biochem Toxicol 1996;11(2):73–8.
124. Kaplan EH, Kennedy J, Davis J. Effects of salicylate and other benzoates on oxidative enzymes of the tricarboxylic acid cycle in rat tissue homogenates. Arch Biochem Biophys 1954;51(1):47–61.
125. Haas R, Parker WD Jr, Stumpf D, et al. Salicylate-induced loose coupling: protonmotive force measurements. Biochem Pharmacol 1985;34(6):900–2.
126. Tarui S, Kono N, Kuwajima M, et al. Hereditary and acquired abnormalities in erythrocyte phosphofructokinase activity: the close association with altered 2,3-diphosphoglycerate levels. Hemoglobin 1980;4(5–6):581–92.

127. Sallis RE. Management of salicylate toxicity. Am Fam Physician 1989;39(3): 265–70.
128. Klotz U. Clinical pharmacokinetics of sulphasalazine, its metabolites and other prodrugs of 5-aminosalicylic acid. Clin Pharmacokinet 1985;10(4):285–302.
129. Dunn RJ. Massive sulfasalazine and paracetamol ingestion causing acidosis, hyperglycemia, coagulopathy, and methemoglobinemia. J Toxicol Clin Toxicol 1998;36(3):239–42.
130. Alvarez FG, Guntupalli KK. Isoniazid overdose: four case reports and review of the literature. Intensive Care Med 1995;21(8):641–4.
131. Goli AK, Goli SA, Byrd RP Jr, et al. Simvastatin-induced lactic acidosis: a rare adverse reaction? Clin Pharmacol Ther 2002;72(4):461–4.
132. Neale R, Reynolds TM, Saweirs W. Statin precipitated lactic acidosis? J Clin Pathol 2004;57(9):989–90.
133. Earthman TP, Odom L, Mullins CA. Lactic acidosis associated with high-dose niacin therapy. South Med J 1991;84(4):496–7.
134. Gustafson PR. Profound lactic acidosis in a young woman treated with nalidixic acid. Tex Med 1985;81(2):53–4.
135. Maher JR, Speyer JF, Levine M. Studies on the mode of action of isoniazid. I. The role of trace metals in the inhibition of bovine liver catalase by isoniazid. Am Rev Tuberc 1958;77(3):501–5.
136. Ghirlanda G, Oradei A, Manto A, et al. Evidence of plasma CoQ10-lowering effect by HMG-CoA reductase inhibitors: a double-blind, placebo-controlled study. J Clin Pharmacol 1993;33(3):226–9.
137. Mann NS, Russman HB, Mann SK, et al. Lactulose and severe lactic acidosis. Ann Intern Med 1985;103(4):637.
138. Mukunda BN. Lactic acidosis caused by thiamine deficiency in a pregnant alcoholic patient. Am J Med Sci 1999;317(4):261–2.
139. Cho YP, Kim K, Han MS, et al. Severe lactic acidosis and thiamine deficiency during total parenteral nutrition–case report. Hepatogastroenterology 2004; 51(55):253–5.
140. Klein M, Weksler N, Gurman GM. Fatal metabolic acidosis caused by thiamine deficiency. J Emerg Med 2004;26(3):301–3.
141. Fattal-Valevski A, Kesler A, Sela BA, et al. Outbreak of life-threatening thiamine deficiency in infants in Israel caused by a defective soy-based formula. Pediatrics 2005;115(2):e233–8.
142. Van den Berg PJ, Bijlstra PJ, Brekelmans GJ. Thiamine deficiency as a single cause of life-threatening lactic acidosis in a patient with acute axonal polyneuropathy. Intern Emerg Med 2009;4(6):539–41.
143. Song Q, Singleton CK. Mitochondria from cultured cells derived from normal and thiamine-responsive megaloblastic anemia individuals efficiently import thiamine diphosphate. BMC Biochem 2002;3:8.
144. Singleton CK, Martin PR. Molecular mechanisms of thiamine utilization. Curr Mol Med 2001;1(2):197–207.
145. Hakim AM. The induction and reversibility of cerebral acidosis in thiamine deficiency. Ann Neurol 1984;16(6):673–9.
146. Berthon HA, Kuchel PW, Nixon PF. High control coefficient of transketolase in the nonoxidative pentose phosphate pathway of human erythrocytes: NMR, antibody, and computer simulation studies. Biochemistry 1992;31(51):12792–8.
147. Navarro D, Zwingmann C, Chatauret N, et al. Glucose loading precipitates focal lactic acidosis in the vulnerable medial thalamus of thiamine-deficient rats. Metab Brain Dis 2008;23(1):115–22.

148. Visser CM, Kellogg RM. Biotin. Its place in evolution. J Mol Evol 1978;11(2): 171–87.

149. Wessman GE, Werkman CH. Biotin in the assimilation of heavy carbon in Oxalacetate. Arch Biochem 1950;26(2):214–8.

150. Sydenstricker VP, Singal SA, Briggs AP, et al. Preliminary observations on "Egg White Injury" in man and its cure with a biotin concentrate. Science 1942; 95(2459):176–7.

151. Gyorgy P, Rose CS. Cure of egg-white injury in rats by the "Toxic" fraction (avidin) of egg white given parenterally. Science 1941;94(2437):261–2.

152. Carlson GL, Williams N, Barber D, et al. Biotin deficiency complicating long-term total parenteral nutrition in an adult patient. Clin Nutr 1995;14(3):186–90.

153. Mikati MA, Zalloua P, Karam P, et al. Novel mutation causing partial biotinidase deficiency in a Syrian boy with infantile spasms and retardation. J Child Neurol 2006;21(11):978–81.

154. Said HM, Ortiz A, McCloud E, et al. Biotin uptake by human colonic epithelial NCM460 cells: a carrier-mediated process shared with pantothenic acid. Am J Physiol 1998;275(5 Pt 1):C1365–71.

155. Moreadith RW, Batshaw ML, Ohnishi T, et al. Deficiency of the iron-sulfur clusters of mitochondrial reduced nicotinamide-adenine dinucleotide-ubiquinone oxidoreductase (complex I) in an infant with congenital lactic acidosis. J Clin Invest 1984;74(3):685–97.

156. Mathews CK, van Holde KE. Biochemistry. Redwood City (CA): The Benjamin/ Cummings Publishing Company; 1990.

157. Fellman V. The GRACILE syndrome, a neonatal lethal metabolic disorder with iron overload. Blood Cells Mol Dis 2002;29(3):444–50.

158. Finch CA, Gollnick PD, Hlastala MP, et al. Lactic acidosis as a result of iron deficiency. J Clin Invest 1979;64(1):129–37.

159. Wang YM, van Eys J. Nutritional significance of fructose and sugar alcohols. Annu Rev Nutr 1981;1:437–75.

160. Wekell MM, Hartman WJ, Dong FM. Incidence of increased numbers of Clostridium perfringens in the intestinal tract of rats fed xylitol. J Nutr 1980; 110(10):2103–8.

161. Craig GM, Crane CW. Lactic acidosis complicating liver failure after intravenous fructose. Br Med J 1971;4(5781):211–2.

162. Batstone GF, Alberti KG, Dewar AK. Reversible lactic acidosis associated with repeated intravenous infusions of sorbitol and ethanol. Postgrad Med J 1977; 53(623):567–9.

163. Korttila K, Mattila MA. Increased serum concentrations of lactic, pyruvic and uric acid and bilibubin after postoperative xylitol infusion. Acta Anaesthesiol Scand 1979;23(3):273–7.

164. Wang YM, King SM, Patterson JH, et al. Mechanism of xylitol toxicity in the rabbit. Metabolism 1973;22(7):885–94.

165. Facts about strychnine. Emergency preparedness and response. Available at: http://www.bt.cdc.gov/agent/strychnine/basics/facts.asp; 2006. Accessed August 24, 2009.

166. Boyd RE, Brennan PT, Deng JF, et al. Strychnine poisoning. Recovery from profound lactic acidosis, hyperthermia, and rhabdomyolysis. Am J Med 1983; 74(3):507–12.

167. Snow RW, Guerra CA, Noor AM, et al. The global distribution of clinical episodes of Plasmodium falciparum malaria. Nature 2005;434(7030):214–7.

168. Krishna S, Waller DW, ter Kuile F, et al. Lactic acidosis and hypoglycaemia in children with severe malaria: pathophysiological and prognostic significance. Trans R Soc Trop Med Hyg 1994;88(1):67–73.
169. Molyneux ME, Looareesuwan S, Menzies IS, et al. Reduced hepatic blood flow and intestinal malabsorption in severe falciparum malaria. Am J Trop Med Hyg 1989;40(5):470–6.
170. Pukrittayakamee S, Krishna S, Ter Kuile F, et al. Alanine metabolism in acute falciparum malaria. Trop Med Int Health 2002;7(11):911–8.
171. Mi-Ichi F, Takeo S, Takashima E, et al. Unique properties of respiratory chain in Plasmodium falciparum mitochondria. Adv Exp Med Biol 2003;531: 117–33.
172. Planche T, Agbenyega T, Bedu-Addo G, et al. A prospective comparison of malaria with other severe diseases in African children: prognosis and optimization of management. Clin Infect Dis 2003;37(7):890–7.
173. Watt G, Jongsakul K, Ruangvirayuth R. A pilot study of N-acetylcysteine as adjunctive therapy for severe malaria. QJM 2002;95(5):285–90.
174. Haas R, Stumpf DA, Parks JK, et al. Inhibitory effects of sodium valproate on oxidative phosphorylation. Neurology 1981;31(11):1473–6.
175. Ponchaut S, van Hoof F, Veitch K. Cytochrome aa3 depletion is the cause of the deficient mitochondrial respiration induced by chronic valproate administration. Biochem Pharmacol 1992;43(3):644–7.
176. Ponchaut S, Van Hoof F, Veitch K. Valproate and cytochrome c oxidase deficiency. Eur J Pediatr 1995;154(1):79.
177. Rumbach L, Cremel G, Marescaux C, et al. Succinate transport inhibition by valproate in rat renal mitochondria. Eur J Pharmacol 1989;164(3):577–81.
178. Rumbach L, Mutet C, Cremel G, et al. Effects of sodium valproate on mitochondrial membranes: electron paramagnetic resonance and transmembrane protein movement studies. Mol Pharmacol 1986;30(3):270–3.
179. Lin CM, Thajeb P. Valproic acid aggravates epilepsy due to MELAS in a patient with an A3243G mutation of mitochondrial DNA. Metab Brain Dis 2007;22(1):105–9.
180. Blayac D, Roch A, Michelet P, et al. [Deep lactic acidosis after valproate self-poisoning]. Ann Fr Anesth Reanim 2004;23(10):1007–10 [in French].
181. Lam CW, Lau CH, Williams JC, et al. Mitochondrial myopathy, encephalopathy, lactic acidosis and stroke-like episodes (MELAS) triggered by valproate therapy. Eur J Pediatr 1997;156(7):562–4.
182. Jonsson S, O'Meara M, Young JB. Acute cocaine poisoning. Importance of treating seizures and acidosis. Am J Med 1983;75(6):1061–4.
183. Isner JM, Estes NA 3rd, Thompson PD, et al. Acute cardiac events temporally related to cocaine abuse. N Engl J Med 1986;315(23):1438–43.
184. Giammarco RA. The athlete, cocaine, and lactic acidosis: a hypothesis. Am J Med Sci 1987;294(6):412–4.
185. Burchell SA, Ho HC, Yu M, et al. Effects of methamphetamine on trauma patients: a cause of severe metabolic acidosis? Crit Care Med 2000;28(6): 2112–5.
186. Lan KC, Lin YF, Yu FC, et al. Clinical manifestations and prognostic features of acute methamphetamine intoxication. J Formos Med Assoc 1998;97(8):528–33.
187. Thrash B, Karuppagounder SS, Uthayathas S, et al. Neurotoxic effects of methamphetamine. Neurochem Res 2009;35(1):171–9.
188. Tian C, Murrin LC, Zheng JC. Mitochondrial fragmentation is involved in methamphetamine-induced cell death in rat hippocampal neural progenitor cells. PLoS One 2009;4(5):e5546.

189. Public health statement for cyanide. [Cited 2007 September 4]. Available at: http://www.atsdr.cdc.gov/toxprofiles/phs8.html. 2007. Accessed August 24, 2009.

190. El Hadri L, Chanas B, Ghanayem BI. Comparative metabolism of methacrylonitrile and acrylonitrile to cyanide using cytochrome P4502E1 and microsomal epoxide hydrolase-null mice. Toxicol Appl Pharmacol 2005;205(2):116–25.

191. Nessim SJ, Richardson RM. Dialysis for thiocyanate intoxication: a case report and review of the literature. ASAIO J 2006;52(4):479–81.

192. Johanning RJ, Zaske DE, Tschida SJ, et al. A retrospective study of sodium nitroprusside use and assessment of the potential risk of cyanide poisoning. Pharmacotherapy 1995;15(6):773–7.

193. Krab K, Slater EC. Ferrocyanide as electron donor to cytochrome aa3. Cytochrome c requirement for oxygen uptake. Biochim Biophys Acta 1979;547(1):58–69.

194. Chen KK, Rose CL. Nitrite and thiosulfate therapy in cyanide poisoning. J Am Med Assoc 1952;149(2):113–9.

195. Baskin SI, Horowitz AM, Nealley EW. The antidotal action of sodium nitrite and sodium thiosulfate against cyanide poisoning. J Clin Pharmacol 1992;32(4):368–75.

196. Cottrell JE, Casthely P, Brodie JD, et al. Prevention of nitroprusside-induced cyanide toxicity with hydroxocobalamin. N Engl J Med 1978;298(15):809–11.

197. Dobkin AB. Anaesthesia with azeotropic mixture of nalothane and diethyl ether; the effect on acid-base balance, electrolyte balance, cardiac rhythm and circulatory dynamics. Br J Anaesth 1959;31(2):53–65.

198. Kumar B, Kumar A, Pandey BN, et al. Role of mitochondrial oxidative stress in the apoptosis induced by diospyrin diethylether in human breast carcinoma (MCF-7) cells. Mol Cell Biochem 2009;320(1–2):185–95.

199. Valik D. Encephalopathy, lactic acidosis, hyperammonaemia and 5-fluorouracil toxicity. Br J Cancer 1998;77(10):1710–2.

200. Ito T. Children's toxicology from bench to bed—liver injury (1): drug-induced metabolic disturbance–toxicity of 5-FU for pyrimidine metabolic disorders and pivalic acid for carnitine metabolism. J Toxicol Sci 2009;34(Suppl 2):SP217–22.

201. Zelickson AS, Mottaz J, Weiss LW. Effects of topical fluorouracil on normal skin. Arch Dermatol 1975;111(10):1301–6.

202. Noordhuis P, Holwerda U, Van der Wilt CL, et al. 5-Fluorouracil incorporation into RNA and DNA in relation to thymidylate synthase inhibition of human colorectal cancers. Ann Oncol 2004;15(7):1025–32.

203. DiMauro S, Schon EA. Mitochondrial respiratory-chain diseases. N Engl J Med 2003;348(26):2656–68.

204. DiMauro S, Mancuso M. Mitochondrial diseases: therapeutic approaches. Biosci Rep 2007;27(1–3):125–37.

205. Kaufmann P, Engelstad K, Wei Y, et al. Dichloroacetate causes toxic neuropathy in MELAS: a randomized, controlled clinical trial. Neurology 2006;66(3):324–30.

206. van den Berghe G. Disorders of gluconeogenesis. J Inherit Metab Dis 1996;19(4):470–7.

207. Robinson BH. Lactic acidemia and mitochondrial disease. Mol Genet Metab 2006;89(1–2):3–13.

208. Robinson BH, Oei J, Saudubray JM, et al. The French and North American phenotypes of pyruvate carboxylase deficiency, correlation with biotin containing protein by 3H-biotin incorporation, 35S-streptavidin labeling, and Northern blotting with a cloned cDNA probe. Am J Hum Genet 1987;40(1):50–9.

209. Hamilton J, Rae MD, Logan RW, et al. A case of benign pyruvate carboxylase deficiency with normal development. J Inherit Metab Dis 1997;20(3):401–3.
210. Morath MA, Okun JG, Muller IB, et al. Neurodegeneration and chronic renal failure in methylmalonic aciduria—a pathophysiological approach. J Inherit Metab Dis 2008;31(1):35–43.
211. Kolker S, Sauer SW, Surtees RA, et al. The aetiology of neurological complications of organic acidaemias—a role for the blood-brain barrier. J Inherit Metab Dis 2006;29(6):701–4 [discussion: 705–6].
212. Thornalley PJ. Pharmacology of methylglyoxal: formation, modification of proteins and nucleic acids, and enzymatic detoxification—a role in pathogenesis and antiproliferative chemotherapy. Gen Pharmacol 1996;27(4):565–73.
213. Uribarri J, Oh MS, Carroll HJ. D-lactic acidosis. A review of clinical presentation, biochemical features, and pathophysiologic mechanisms. Medicine (Baltimore) 1998;77(2):73–82.
214. Hudson M, Pocknee R, Mowat NA. D-lactic acidosis in short bowel syndrome—an examination of possible mechanisms. Q J Med 1990;74(274):157–63.
215. Oh MS, Phelps KR, Traube M, et al. D-lactic acidosis in a man with the short-bowel syndrome. N Engl J Med 1979;301(5):249–52.
216. Halperin ML, Kamel KS. D-lactic acidosis: turning sugar into acids in the gastrointestinal tract. Kidney Int 1996;49(1):1–8.
217. Zhang DL, Jiang ZW, Jiang J, et al. D-lactic acidosis secondary to short bowel syndrome. Postgrad Med J 2003;79(928):110–2.
218. Brooks GA. The lactate shuttle during exercise and recovery. Med Sci Sports Exerc 1986;18:360–8.

Mean Arterial Pressure: Therapeutic Goals and Pharmacologic Support

David S. Shapiro, MD[a,b,c,*], Laurie A. Loiacono, MD, FCCP, FCCM[a,b]

KEYWORDS

- Mean arterial pressure • Sepsis • Septic shock
- Blood pressure • Vasopressors

Early goal-directed therapy in sepsis, including the optimization of hemodynamic parameters, has been demonstrated to improve end points of resuscitation, limit organ dysfunction, improve mortality, and contribute to decreases in resource consumption.[1] The Surviving Sepsis Campaign[2] targets central venous pressure (CVP), mean arterial pressure (MAP), and central venous oxygen saturation (Scvo$_2$) as guides for resuscitation.[3] These measurements, achieved with fluid resuscitation and vasoactive medications, are guidelines for goals of resuscitation, and help to guide the clinicians' decision-making regarding the success of such measures. Further, it has been demonstrated that the achievement of supranormal physiologic parameters, compared with the normal values as the targets of resuscitation, leads to an increase in mortality.[4,5] A MAP greater than or equal to 65 mm Hg is imperative to maintain perfusion pressure and adequate flow at the arteriolar level. At pressures below this number, autoregulation can be dysfunctional in many tissue beds.[2] Patients with septic shock require vasoactive therapy to achieve adequate tissue perfusion.[6,7] The use of norepinephrine is recommended to maintain MAP of 65 mm Hg, and has been shown to preserve tissue perfusion.[7] Although adequate volume resuscitation should be achieved before instituting vasoactive medications, their use may be required simultaneously with volume resuscitation early in the resuscitation to escape patient demise. The Surviving Sepsis Campaign guidelines are listed in **Box 1**.[2]

Therapy for septic shock should include the maintenance of organ perfusion and cardiac output; infectious source control; and, when possible, an interruption of the cascade of events propagating the septic state. Organ perfusion must be maintained during the administration of antibiotics, procedures to achieve surgical drainage, and other interventions. Therapeutics must be targeted at circulatory support from the

[a] Department of Surgery, University of Connecticut School of Medicine, Farmington, CT, USA
[b] Saint Francis Hospital and Medical Center, Department of Surgery, 114 Woodland Street, Hartford, CT 06106, USA
[c] Saint Francis Medical Group, 1000 Asylum Avenue, Suite 4320, Hartford, CT 06105, USA
* Corresponding author. Saint Francis Medical Group, 1000 Asylum Avenue, Suite 4320, Hartford, CT 06105.
E-mail address: davidscottshapiro@gmail.com

Crit Care Clin 26 (2010) 285–293
doi:10.1016/j.ccc.2009.12.005
0749-0704/10/$ – see front matter © 2010 Elsevier Inc. All rights reserved.

Box 1
The Surviving Sepsis Campaign guidelines

1. MAP maintained $\geq$65 mm Hg.

2. Use of norepinephrine or dopamine as the first choice vasopressor agent to correct hypotension in septic shock (administered through a central catheter as soon as one is available).

3. Epinephrine, phenylephrine, or vasopressin should not be administered as the initial vasopressor in septic shock. Vasopressin (0.03 U/min) may be subsequently added to norepinephrine with anticipation of an effect equivalent to norepinephrine alone.

4. Epinephrine is the first chosen alternative agent in septic shock, which is refractory to norepinephrine or dopamine.

---

outset of intervention. Although the phenomenon of organ dysfunction in sepsis is complex, the maintenance of organ perfusion in the septic state depends partly on MAP. Maintenance of MAP as a therapeutic target for vasoactive medications is a mainstay in the care of the septic patient.[1,8]

This article identifies the nature of arterial pressure and the maintenance of blood flow and cardiac output during sepsis and septic shock, and suggests means of supportive measures when possible.

DEFINING MAP

Circulatory pressure is derived from the ejection of blood from the left ventricle. Ventricular acceleration of blood into a normal arterial system results in elastic distention of the vessel walls. Potential energy is generated by this elasticity and subsequent recoil, in a normal arterial system, resulting in continuous pressured flow of blood, even during diastole.[9] Blood pressure is measured traditionally as a systolic number, the highest pressure occurring as a result of left ventricular contraction, over a diastolic number, which is the result of continuous forward flow during the period of cardiac filling and rest. The MAP is not an arithmetic mean, and instead is derived to represent the proportion of time in systole and diastole.[10]

The vascular circuit maintains blood pressure with the cardiac function acting as pump, and the blood vessels serving as conduit. The circuit is composed of arteries, capillaries, and veins. The pulmonary circuit is similarly composed, but is not discussed here. The flow through these conduits at rest is near 5 to 8 L/min. The flow is dependent on the pressure gradient between both ends of the circuit, and the resistance to flow within each conduit.

The MAP can be measured by invasive or noninvasive monitoring,[9] but is defined as the area under the blood pressure curve divided by the time of the cardiac cycle:

$$MAP = \int P \, dt/\Delta t$$

An approximation can be made of the MAP from the systolic blood pressure and diastolic blood pressure:

$$MAP = (2\,DBP + SBP)/3$$

where DBP is the diastolic blood pressure and SBP is the systolic blood pressure. As described previously, however, this formula approximates a MAP, and depends on normal physiology of the ration of time in each portion of the cardiac cycle. The formula assumes a resting heart rate of 60 beats per minute. At this rate, diastole occupies two thirds of duration of the cardiac cycle. In normal physiology, the heart rate is unfixed and varies greatly during the septic state. Patients with heart rates greater than 100 beats per minute may have diastole lasting for less than half the cardiac cycle. MAP is then falsely elevated by this formula, and organ perfusion may be ineffective despite a measured MAP within a target range. Additionally, MAP is maintained at the aortic and arterial level, but as the intravascular volume progresses toward arterioles and capillaries, a significant pressure gradient exists.[9]

Blood flow through the circuit can only occur if a pressure gradient exists. CVP is 0 to 4 mm Hg, whereas the aortic MAP is around 70 to 90 mm Hg. This difference produces a pressure gradient from central arteries, dispersing the pressure through every patent vascular network, down to the value of the CVP. The rate of flow is determined by the degree of gradient between tissue beds, not by only the inflow and outflow absolute values.

MONITORING THE MAP

The first measurement of arterial pressure was made by Reverend Stephen Hales in 1731. Reverend Hales' rudimentary but effective measurement was performed in an equine artery cannulated with a goose quill, which was in turn connected to an 8-ft glass column of water. This methodology was impractical, but demonstrated pressure was present within the circulatory system.[11] In 1847, Carl Ludwig's kymograph recorded human blood pressure invasively. The device featured a u-shaped manometer fixed to a brass pipe. A float would sketch a rudimentary blood pressure curve on a rotating drum, which became the first blood pressure recording device. In 1855, Karl Vierordt demonstrated with an inflatable cuff that pressure in a human artery could be obliterated. Just a few years later, Etienne Jules Mary and Samuel Siegfried Karl Ritter von Basch independently contributed to the sphygmomanometer. The pressure required to obliterate pressure in an artery was measured and recorded. The devices were inaccurate, but the largest advance came with Scipione Riva-Rocci, who demonstrated the device using mercury as a measuring fluid. He proposed using the sphygmomanometer with distal palpation in 1896. Korotkoff, in 1905, proposed the use of auscultation in addition to sphygmomanometry. These techniques were simple, safe, and effective. Although the medical community was initially reluctant to adopt routine blood pressure monitoring, by 1930 it had become the standard of care.[12]

By the 1960s, the standard measurement of blood pressure was by mercury sphygmomanometer. Subsequently, continuous intra-arterial monitoring was reintroduced with electromechanical transducers replacing Hales' glass column.

MAP may be measured or estimated. Most electronic recording devices measure the MAP by integration of the area under the pressure curve and division by the cardiac cycle duration. This provides far more accurate a measure, because the estimation method, mentioned previously, does not provide for variation in the duration of the cardiac cycle.

Noninvasive Monitoring

In most circumstances, blood pressure is measured by manual or automatic noninvasive sphygmomanometry. Also in most situations, auscultation, palpation, and oscillometry measurements coincide, but systolic pressures measured indirectly may be up to 20 mm Hg lower than invasive monitors demonstrate, and diastolic pressures may be higher than invasive pressures. The noninvasive monitors also leave to chance the operator variability inherent to human interventions.[13,14]

Noninvasive monitoring devices use an air bladder to exert pressure in a cuff wrapped circumferentially, usually on the upper arm, measuring pressure transmitted through the brachial artery. The air bladder is positioned directly over the artery. The cuff is then inflated to a pressure above the disappearance of the distally palpated pulse. When positioned properly, inflation of the air bladder compresses the artery against the adjacent bone, decreasing and eventually stopping the flow of blood. This should result in both the absence of distal palpable pulsations and the absence of Korotkoff sounds, which are low-frequency sounds occurring during the occlusion of flow. The cuff is then deflated during auscultation, allowing for gradual return of flow. Turbulent flow of blood is restored as the cuff deflates, and sounds return, noted by the examiner or the device. In patients with normal physiology, vibrations associated with turbulent flow result in tapping Korotkoff sounds, correlating with systolic pressure. As the pressure of the cuff continues to decrease, more flow returns and Korotkoff sounds continue in a deformed blood vessel, and the character of the sounds develops from "tapping" to "popping," and as the pressure approaches diastolic pressure, the sounds become muffled and eventually disappear. The disappearance of sound correlates with diastolic pressure. This method, despite astounding advances in technology, survives today as the most common method for deriving blood pressure.[15]

Currently, most hospitals use automatic oscillometric machines to acquire blood pressure measurements. In turn, these machines calculate the MAP by the estimation formula mentioned previously, rather than by derivation. Machines can be calibrated to repeat the measurement at intervals, and are widely used in operating rooms, hospitals, and intensive care units around the world.

Although the noninvasive method is quite safe, there are pitfalls, including reasons for falsely elevated or falsely diminished measurements. A cuff that is inappropriately small may render a falsely high blood pressure reading. Also, obesity and measurements taken with the arm lower than the phlebostatic axis may contribute to falsely high readings. Similarly, falsely low readings can be obtained from too large a cuff or from the arm being measured too high above the phlebostatic axis. Human error may also contribute, with misinterpreted sounds, noisy environments, and artifact contributing to falsely high or low measurements.

Invasive Monitoring

Patients with septic shock, sepsis, or those who have the potential for sepsis should be monitored continuously and with invasive monitoring. The choice of catheter is a concern when monitoring blood pressure. According to the Poiseuille-Hagen formula, flow is directly proportional to radius, and inversely proportional to length and to fluid viscosity. This means that as the lumen diameter decreases, and as the length or viscosity increase, the flow diminishes. In the physiologic milieu of a septic patient, peripheral vasoconstriction provides an incremental increase in systemic blood pressure, but eventually the lumen diameter decreases to the point of flow insufficient for organ perfusion, and end-organ injury occurs. Similarly, the catheter chosen to measure pressure invasively contributes to the value monitored. Resistance in a system is the mathematical inverse of flow. Flow is expressed as:

$$Q = \frac{\pi r2}{8\eta L}$$

where η is the fluid viscosity, L is the length of the tube, and r is the radius.

It is imperative at this juncture to mark a distinction between pressure and flow. The use of vasoconstrictors to increase blood pressure in septic shock is widely acceptable, but the vasoconstrictive effects of the agent chosen may also be the culprit in limiting blood flow at the end-organ level. Quite often, demonstration of an adequately maintained target MAP does not translate into organ blood flow.

Invasive monitoring is the most reliable method of continuous monitoring, and offers the advantage of relatively pain-free and low-risk access for blood sampling. Fluid-filled electronic monitoring is the most commonly used device for measuring blood pressure directly.

The fluid-filled system is composed of a catheter, a fluid-filled conduit, a transducer, an amplifier, and a recorder-monitor. The catheter, placed within a blood-filled vessel, can transmit the pressure through a static column of similar fluid, usually a crystalloid, to reach a transducer. The transducer converts the detected pressure into an electrical signal, which is delivered to the amplifier and to the monitor for display.

MAP AND THE PHYSIOLOGY OF SEPSIS

Intrinsic mechanisms to increase systemic blood pressure are the result of vasoconstriction by the catecholamine effect. The increase in measured blood pressure incompletely reflects perfusion pressure in different tissue beds. The resistance to blood flow in each tissue is in constant flux, changing in response to these intrinsic and other extrinsic phenomena. Poiseuille's law describes resistance to laminar flow in a rigid tube:

$$R = 8\eta \, L/\pi \, r^4$$

where η is the viscosity, L is the length of the tube, and r is the radius. Applied to the vascular system, the resistance in this simplified representation depends both on the blood composition and on the characteristics of the tube, or the blood vessel itself. Resistance is subject to viscosity changes, caused by hematocrit and protein concentration changes, and vessel radius, which is under autoregulatory and endogenous nervous system control. Poiseuille's law provides only an approximation of resistance, however, because blood vessels are not rigid, flow is not laminar, and distribution of flow is not uniform.

Blood vessel radius, especially of the arterial tree, is the primary variable in the regulation of blood pressure. The resistances of the coronary, cerebral, and renal vascular beds are primarily controlled by autoregulatory means, and are less contributory to systemic vascular resistance. Most of the control is the arterial diameter in mesenteric, cutaneous, and skeletal muscle vascular beds. This blood vessel radius is under particularly influential control of circulating hormones, especially epinephrine, norepinephrine, angiotensin II, and vasopressin.[9]

PHARMACOLOGIC SUPPORT OF MAP IN SEPSIS

Support of septic patient begins with an adequately secured airway, appropriate ventilation parameters to optimize oxygenation and ventilation, and aggressive support of end-organ perfusion. Source control must be considered from the onset of interventions, and broad-spectrum antimicrobial coverage instituted. Although adequate volume resuscitation is imperative to the maintenance of organ perfusion in shock, refractory patients may require the use of vasopressors early or even from the initiation of care, concomitant with aggressive fluid resuscitation. Resuscitation end points may not be necessarily discrete; instead, appropriate goals of resuscitation target interventions toward restoration of tissue perfusion, and subsequent resuscitation is tapered to maintain, and not overshoot, those goals. Signs of adequate resuscitation, according to the Surviving Sepsis Campaign, include an appropriate volume resuscitation to a CVP between 8 and 12 mm Hg, appropriate perfusion pressures demonstrated as MAP greater than 65 mm Hg, evidence of organ perfusion including urine output above 0.5 mL/kg/h, and evidence of adequate oxygen use with a superior vena cava oxygen saturation above 70% or mixed venous oxygen saturation greater than 65%.[1,16]

These end points of resuscitation in sepsis have been widely discussed and reported. The goals of therapy are to eliminate the source of sepsis, control its influence on the cascade of events leading to sepsis, and support the organism through these events. The optimum level of blood pressure is still unknown. The target of 65 mm Hg translates to higher perfusion pressures, and is thought to be the most optimum of goals.[7,16,17] Vascular tone is mediated by three interwoven systems, each of which is affected by sepsis: (1) the sympathetic nervous system, (2) endogenous vasopressin, and (3) plasma angiotensin. The goal of pharmacotherapy for septic shock is to increase perfusion pressure to a point where blood flow is optimized.

Sympathetic tone can be restored with exogenous adrenergic agonists and the vasopressin repleted. Vasodilatory shock is a complex interaction between vasodilation, relative and absolute hypovolemia, myocardial dysfunction, and altered perfusion, each of which may be attributed to the systemic inflammatory response to injury.[18,19] Many vasoactive agents have come in and out of fashion since the mid-twentieth century. Few randomized controlled trials exist to demonstrate their efficacy and contribution to improved outcome.[20] Further, the Cochrane Database of Systematic Reviews describes that sufficient evidence is not yet suited to inform clinical practice absolutely, and that one particular vasopressor is no better than other agents in treatment of fluid-refractory shock.[20]

Agents useful in septic shock are described next. Many agents are available, each with its unique profile of effects.

Norepinephrine

Norepinephrine is a potent α-adrenergic agonist and less potent β-adrenergic agonist. It is useful to increase MAP in patients with hypotension caused by sepsis.[21] Norepinephrine is equivalent in effect on increasing MAP,[6,22,23] oxygen consumption, and oxygen delivery compared with other catecholamine pressors. At least one study has suggested that norepinephrine has greater potency compared with dopamine and more substantially improves the hemodynamic parameters of shock.

Martin and coworkers[24] in a small randomized study of patients with hyperdynamic sepsis observed that 93% of patients receiving norepinephrine (1.5 $\pm$ 1.2 µg/kg/min) had normalization of MAP compared with only 31% who were receiving dopamine (10–25 µg/kg/min). In addition, norepinephrine has been shown to be effective rescue therapy when other catecholamine pressures have failed to maintain MAP. In one recent study, Martin and colleagues[25] have suggested that norepinephrine use in patients with septic shock is also associated with a reduced mortality rate (relative risk = 0.68; 95% confidence interval, 0.54–0.87) compared with those patients treated with other catecholamine pressors. The etiology of the mortality difference is unclear but may relate to the side effect profile of norepinephrine compared with other agents.

Despite its greater potency and vasoconstricting potential, end-organ damage may be less prevalent in septic patients treated with norepinephrine compared with those treated with other catecholamine pressors. The addition of norepinephrine to other catecholamine pressors was observed by Redl-Wenzl and others to increase urine output and creatinine clearance.[24] The mechanism is unclear but may be secondary to vasoconstriction of the efferent arteriole of the glomerulus, which leads to increased filtration through the kidney. Unpredictable effects occur in the splanchnic circulation with some patients developing ischemia secondary to vasoconstriction. Preservation of cardiac output with the use of norepinephrine (and ionotropes), however, may preserve splanchnic flow. In addition, gastric pHi has been observed to increase (not decrease) in septic patients treated with norepinephrine alone. As a result of improved end-organ blood flow, Martin and colleagues[24] observed reduced lactate levels after treatment (4.8 $\pm$ 1.6–2.9 $\pm$ 0.8 mmol/L), suggesting improved tissue oxygenation and lactate clearance, the latter of which has been associated with improved survival.[3]

Although the achievement of supraphysiologic MAP has been associated with increased mortality, evidence exists that increasing norepinephrine doses benefits tissue oxygenation.[4,5,25] Jhanji and colleagues[25] recently demonstrated that patients with septic shock had an increase in global oxygen delivery, cutaneous microvascular flow, and tissue oxygenation increasing MAP with norepinephrine. Although the effect was demonstrated in a small number of patients, and the incremental increase in oxygenation was of questionable clinical significance, if oxygen delivery and use are the answers to the morbidity of sepsis, these small increases may be useful. Further work is required.

Epinephrine

Epinephrine is also a potent α-adrenergic and β-adrenergic agent that contributes to increasing MAP by both an increase in vascular tone and an increase in cardiac index. Epinephrine increases the delivery of oxygen to organ beds, but the use of epinephrine can increase oxygen consumption. The administration of epinephrine can treat hypotension resistant to other agents, but it should be considered a second-line agent because of its effects on splanchnic circulation and increases in lactate concentration. Because epinephrine is a potent β-adrenergic agent, tachyarrhythmias are often a complication.

Vasopressin

Vasopressin is a peptide hormone synthesized in the hypothalamus and transported to and stored in the pituitary. Vasopressin is released in response to decreased blood volume and osmolality. Vascular smooth muscle cells are directly affected by vasopressin through V1 receptors, and also acts to enhance the vascular response to catecholamines.[26]

Under nonseptic conditions, vasopressin has little effect on blood pressure. During hypovolemia, it may prevent aberrancies in the vascular response to shock.[22,27] The Vasopressin Vs Norepinephrine in Septic Shock Study reported there was no difference in 28-day mortality in groups with septic shock treated with each agent. Vasopressin fared better in a subgroup analysis of less severely affected patients. Further, vasopressin added to norepinephrine in a moderate dose (0.03 U/min) is as safe and effective as norepinephrine alone in fluid-resuscitated patients with septic shock. In this setting, patients may benefit from lower doses of norepinephrine with vasopressin, than with higher doses of norepinephrine alone.

Phenylephrine

Phenylephrine is a selective α_1-adrenergic agonist, which mediates elevation in MAP by vasoconstriction. Phenylephrine has relatively selective vasoconstrictive effect, without direct inotropic activity. Although this makes it an attractive agent in the management of vasodilatory shock, caution must be observed in its use because of the potential to reduced cardiac output in this population.[6] Without β-adrenergic agonism, there may be a role for phenylephrine in patients with tachyarrythmias related to other vasopressors, but its role in septic shock has not been extensively studied.

Increased doses of phenylephrine demonstrated an increase in MAP without a significant increase in cardiac index. Phenylephrine may be of selective use in small doses, and for unsustained use. If oxygen use is unaffected, then perhaps phenylephrine requires revisitation as an option in the septic patient. Linear increases in MAP without significant increases in cardiac index have been demonstrated in a study of septic patients, but these increases were met with unpredictable oxygen delivery and use.[23] Dose-response studies are required to safely administer phenylephrine routinely.

Dopamine

Dopamine is the precursor of norepinephrine and epinephrine and has well-known distinctly dose-dependent effects. At doses of less than 5 μg/kg/min, dopamine receptors are activated with renal and mesenteric vasodilation. An increase to 5 to 10 μg/kg/min results in β_1-adrenergic receptor stimulation and an increase in inotropic and chronotropic effect. At doses greater than 10 μg/kg/min, α_1-adrenergic effects predominate, with vasoconstriction and increased MAP. Dopamine increases MAP in septic patients who remain hypotensive after volume resuscitation, but oxygen consumption may be affected adversely.[24]

The use of dopamine in septic shock may be optimal in patients with cardiac dysfunction. Tachycardia and a propensity for arrhythmias more than other agents make dopamine a good choice in the appropriate circumstance.

REFERENCES

1. Rivers E, Nguyen B, Havstad S, et al. Early goal-directed therapy in the treatment of severe sepsis and septic shock. N Engl J Med 2001;345:1368–77.
2. Dellinger RP, Levy MM, Carlet JM, et al. Surviving Sepsis Campaign: international guidelines for management of severe sepsis and septic shock. Intensive Care Med 2008;34:17–60.
3. Varpula M, Tallgren M, Saukkonen K, et al. Hemodynamic variables related to outcome in septic shock. Intensive Care Med 2005;31:1066–71.
4. Hayes MA, Timins AC, Yau EH, et al. Elevation of systemic oxygen delivery in the treatment of critically ill patients. N Engl J Med 1994;330:1717–22.
5. Gattinoni L, Brazzi L, Pelosi P, et al. A trial of goal-oriented hemodynamic therapy in critically ill patients: svO2 Collaborative Group. N Engl J Med 1995;333: 1025–32.
6. Hollenberg SM, Ahrens TS, Annane D, et al. Practice parameters for hemodynamic support of sepsis in adult patients: 2004 update. Crit Care Med 2004; 32:1928–48.
7. LeDoux D, Astiz ME, Carpati CM, et al. Effects of perfusion pressure on tissue perfusion in septic shock. Crit Care med 2000;28:2729–32.
8. DiGiantomasso D, May CN, Bellomo R. Vital organ blood flow during sepsis. Chest 2003;124:1053–9.
9. Schlame M, Blanck TJJ. Cardiovascular system. In: Gabrielli A, Layon AJ, Mihae Y, editors. Civetta Taylor and Kirby's critical care. 4th edition. Philadelphia (PA): Lippincott Williams & Wilkins; 2009. p. 693–5.
10. Darovic GO. Cardiovascular anatomy and physiology. In: Darovi GO, editor. Hemodynamic monitoring: invasive and noninvasive clinical application. 2nd edition. Philadelphia (PA): WB Saunders; 2002. p. 103–5.

11. Magner LN. A history of the life sciences. Philadelphia (PA): Marcel Dekker, Inc; 2002. p. 223–5.
12. Marino PL. The ICU book. Philadelphia (PA): Lippincott Williams & Wilkins; 2007. p. 151–4.
13. Bur A, Hirschl M, Vleck M, et al. Factors influencing the accuracy of oscillometric blood pressure measurements in critically ill patients. Crit Care Med 2003;31: 793–9.
14. Davis RF. Clinical comparison of automated auscultatory and oscillometric and catheter-transducer measurements of arterial pressure. J Clin Monit 1985;1: 114–9.
15. Shlyakhto E, Conrady A. Korotkoff sounds: what do we know about its discovery? J Hypertens 2005;23:3–4.
16. Leone M, Martin C. Vasopressor use in septic shock: an update. Curr Opin Anesthesiol 2008;21:141–7.
17. Bourgoin A, Leone M, Delmas A, et al. Increasing mean arterial pressure in patients with septic shock: effects on oxygen variables and renal function. Crit Care Med 2005;33:780–6.
18. Holmes CL, Walley KR. Vasoactive drugs for vasodilatory shock in ICU. Curr Opin Crit Care 2009;15:398–402.
19. Beale RJ, Hollenberg SM, Vincent JL, et al. Vasopressor and inotropic support in septic shock: an evidence based review. Crit Care Med 2004;32:S455–65.
20. Müllner M, Urbanek B, Havel C, et al. Vasopressors for shock. Cochrane Database Syst Rev 2004;(3):CD003709.
21. Levy B, Bollaert PE, Charpentier C, et al. Comparison of norepinephrine and dobutamine to epinephrine for hemodynamics, lactate metabolism, and gastric tonometric variables in septic shock: a prospective, randomized study. Intensive Care Med 1997;23:282–7.
22. Wakatsuki T, Nakaya Y, Inoue I. Vasopressin modulates K+ channel activities of cultured smooth muscle cells from porcine coronary artery. Am J Physiol 1992; 263:H491–6.
23. Flancbaum L, Dick M, Dasta JF, et al. A dose-response study of phenyleprhine in critically ill, septic surgical patients. Eur J Clin Pharmacol 1997;51:461–5.
24. Martin C, Papazian L, Perrin G, et al. Norepinephrine or dopamine for the treatment of hyperdynamic septic shock. Chest 1993;103:1826–31.
25. Jhanji S, Stirling S, Patel N, et al. The effect of increasing doses of norepinephrine on tissue oxygenation and microvascular flow in patients with septic shock. Crit Care Med 2009;37:1961–6.
26. Holmes CL, Patel BM, Russell JA, et al. Physiology of vasopressin relevant to management of septic shock. Chest 2001;120:989–1002.
27. Barrett BJ, Parfrey PS. Clinical practice: preventing nephropathy induced by contrast medium. N Engl J Med 2006;34:379–86.

Static Measures of Preload Assessment

Richard A. Nahouraii, MD, Susan E. Rowell, MD*

KEYWORDS

- Preload • Central venous pressure
- Pulmonary artery occlusion pressure
- Volumetric measurement
- Right ventricular end-diastolic volume
- Global end-diastolic volume

The identification of relative intravascular volume insufficiency in the hemodynamically unstable patient and the restoration of optimal intravascular volume remain among the core challenges in the ICU. By the Frank-Starling mechanism, the normal heart automatically adjusts stroke volume (SV) for changes in ventricular end-diastolic volume load via the relationship between initial sarcomere length (preload) and force of contraction. Hence, myocardial preload clinically may be considered the end-diastolic volume of the right or left ventricle and, in turn, is a reflection of the relative intravascular volume of the patient. Unlike skeletal muscle however, the heart normally functions not at the maximal, or plateau, portion of its force versus length (ie, preload) cardiac function curve but rather on a roughly linear or ascending portion of the curve.[1] Volume resuscitation will increase SV in the hypovolemic patient only while on the ascending portion of the cardiac function curve; fluid administered once the plateau is reached will contribute to tissue and pulmonary edema, right ventricular dysfunction, and increased intra-abdominal pressure. In practice, the clinician is faced with the challenge of not only identifying intravascular volume deficiency but also restoring the volume of the intravascular space while avoiding overresuscitation.

Generally, techniques for the assessment of cardiac preload attempt to measure—either directly or, more commonly, indirectly—the end-diastolic volume of the right or left ventricle or both in combination. These may be static measurements, such as the central venous pressure (CVP) (right ventricle), the pulmonary artery occlusion pressure (Ppao) (left ventricle), assessments of right ventricular end-diastolic volume (RVEDV) or global end-diastolic volume (GEDV) via thermodilution, or echocardiographic measurement of left ventricle end-diastolic area (LVEDA).[2] Alternatively, dynamic measurement indices have been developed in which respiratory variations in systolic pressure, pulse pressure, or SV are used to assess preload status and fluid

Division of Trauma, Critical Care and Acute Care Surgery, Department of Surgery, Oregon Health and Science University, 3181 SW Sam Jackson Park Road, Portland, OR 97239, USA
* Corresponding author.
E-mail address: rowells@ohsu.edu

Crit Care Clin 26 (2010) 295–305
doi:10.1016/j.ccc.2009.12.008
0749-0704/10/$ – see front matter © 2010 Elsevier Inc. All rights reserved.

responsiveness.[3,4] This article focuses on static methods for determining preload, specifically pressure and volumetric indices measured at the bedside. Dynamic measurement techniques are addressed in a separate article in this issue.

PRESSURE MEASUREMENTS: CVP AND Ppao

CVP is the simplest and most common invasive method of assessing ventricular preload.[5] Given the nature of CVP, only right heart pressures (right atrial pressure as a surrogate for right ventricular end-diastolic pressure [RVEDP]) and, hence, right ventricular preload (RVEDV) are assessed. Whether right-sided measurements are superior or inferior to left-sided measurements for optimizing preload is still debated and is beyond the scope of this article. However, it is clear that given the steady-state requirement of cardiac output (CO) equaling venous return, and the fact that the right heart is the interaction point of the venous return system with the cardiac system, the right heart's function is crucial to the optimization of the left. Furthermore, the high compliance of veins (compared with arteries) and the capacitance nature of the venous system are such that the left-sided arterial pressures are not the primary force returning blood to the right heart; the regulation of right atrial pressure (CVP) by the right heart determines venous return and hence right ventricular preload and subsequent cardiac output. This effective regulation of CO through the right heart's determination of venous return, independent of the left heart's function, gives rise to Magder's[6] maxim "no left-sided success without right-sided success."

CVP is universally measured throughout ICUs for preload assessments in critically ill patients and is even incorporated into formal resuscitative algorithms and guidelines such as the Surviving Sepsis Campaign.[7] Although convenient and accessible given the wide use of central venous catheters, the measurement of CVP for assessing preload is complicated by several factors.

External Reference Landmark

First, the CVP depends on the external reference landmark used for the zero point in its measurement. This zero point is the position in the circulatory system where the CVP varies little, if at all, with postural changes. This point theoretically lies within the right atrium. Accordingly, the transducer's external reference point (in practice, the stopcock of the transducer, the point at which the transducer can be "zeroed" by opening the stopcock to atmospheric pressure, the reference point for all hemodynamic catheter measurements) should be placed co-level ("leveled") with this point.[8] The classic position used is that of the phlebostatic axis, taken as the line where a coronal plane midway between the back and sternum (in practice, the midaxillary line) intersects a cross-sectional plane through the fourth intercostal space.[9] An alternative zero point, advocated by Magder's group, is a point 5 cm vertically below the sternal angle (at the junction of the sternum and the second rib costal cartilage).[10,11] This point is within the right atrium and essentially remains within the right atrium regardless of the incline of the patient's head and torso from the supine position.[11] In reality, changes in the angle of the patient's position do have a small effect on CVP measurements because of changes in the position of the heart in the chest (and hence the CVP zero point) relative to the anatomic landmark used to set the transducer's external reference point.[12,13] Given these variations, Magder recommends the midaxillary-fourth intercostal space be used only when the patient is supine.[8] Whatever technique used, the importance of an agreed upon zero point and consistent, identical leveling of the transducer by all staff cannot be overstated. In a recent study, Figg and Nemergut[14] tested 50 health care providers (registered nurses, anesthesiology residents, and anesthesiology attendings) as they placed a CVP transducer at a specified level on the same mock patient in three patient positions (supine, 30 degrees head up, and 15 degrees head down). At a repeat session 6 months later, the same 50 health care providers repeated the exercise on the same mock patient in the same three patient positions but now were given a laser level to identify anatomic landmarks and place the transducer at the proper level. The results of the study were revealing. The initial session resulted in variations in zero-level positioning that corresponded to standard deviations in CVP measurements of 3.2, 4.8, and 3.2 mm Hg in the supine, 30 degrees head up, and 15 degrees head down positions, respectively. Even more revealing, the repeat test using laser levels showed no change in the variance of the positioning, with corresponding pressure measurement standard deviations of 2.9, 4.3, and 2.6 mm Hg, respectively. The investigators concluded that hospital-wide standardization of appropriate zero-point levels and staff education are required to minimize systematic errors in CVP measurement from interprovider variability.

The Effects of the Respiratory Cycle

The effects of the respiratory cycle must be considered when determining CVP (and Ppao). During spontaneous inspiration, the CVP falls as the pleural pressure declines relative to the external atmosphere and, during positive pressure ventilation, CVP rises as pleural pressure increases with inspiration. Hence, a respiratory variation is seen in CVP and Ppao measurements.[9] However, the relevant pressure for determining intra-vascular volumes (such as preload) is the transmural pressure. Thus, it is the difference between the intravascular and the extravascular (ie, pleural) pressure that correlates with volume. Given the complexity and impracticality of determining pleural pressure (various approaches have involved measuring intraesophageal pressures or measuring variations in Ppao in patients with pulmonary artery catheters[15]), hemodynamic pressures such as CVP and Ppao are measured at end-expiration when the pleural pressure is closest to zero relative to atmosphere (the reference point for all hemodynamic catheter measurements) and intravascular pressure most closely approximates transmural pressure. Even this technique is imperfect, however, because positive end-expiratory pressure (PEEP) (both intrinsic and extrinsic), active expiration, pericardial fluid or mediastinal edema, and increased intra-abdominal pressure (IAP) will alter pleural pressure in ways that are difficult to quantify.[16] Theoretically, assuming chest wall (C_W) and lung compliance (C_L) are known, the proportion of airway pressure (P_{aw}) transmitted to pleural pressure (P_{pl}) is given by $P_{pl} = P_{aw}(C_L/C_L + C_W)$. In practice, when considering PEEP (ie, P_{aw} at end expiration), some comfort may be taken from the fact that approximately half of the airway pressure in normal lungs is transmitted to the pleural space; in diseased lungs (stiffer, less compliant lungs) less than half is transmitted. Thus, in diseased lungs, especially when ventilated with low lung volumes and low levels of PEEP, the increase in end-expiratory CVP (and in the approximation of transmural pressure) is likely to be small: less than 4 to 5 cm water at a total PEEP of 10 cm H_2O.[8,11] Higher PEEP levels will have a greater effect but, even then, the magnitude will depend on the percentage of pressure transmission: with low lung compliance the heart may or may not see much transmitted pleural pressure and even that amount may vary in the respiratory cycle as lung recruitment around the heart occurs. Even more concerning is the effect of active expiration. Active use of the muscles of the thorax and abdomen by a ventilated patient during expiration, particularly if the patient actively expires throughout the whole expiratory cycle (as opposed to active force only at the beginning of the cycle with passive flow for the remainder) will result in a pleural pressure that is elevated above atmospheric pressure throughout expiration. Hence, at no point in the respiratory cycle (and definitely not at end-expiration) will the pleural pressure be close to zero. In such instances, which are common in ventilated patients, an accurate measurement of CVP cannot be made.[8,9,16] A similar effect is seen with IAP, in which investigators have demonstrated the transmission of IAP to the chest and quantified its effects on end-expiratory measurements of CVP and even intracranial pressure.[17] Indeed, taking this effect into account and applying it to the previously discussed problem of forced expiratory efforts confounding CVP determination, Qureshi and colleagues[18] demonstrated that in spontaneously breathing patients with active expiratory effort, subtracting the respiratory change in IAP from the end-expiratory CVP corrects for the expiratory effort and gives an accurate estimation of transmural pressure. In short, just as both lung and chest wall compliance affect the pleural pressure, so does the abdominal compliance, and efforts to measure end-expiratory CVP as a guide to resuscitation must take into account elevated IAP.[17] Finally, it should be noted that measuring hemodynamic pressures such as CVP and Ppao at end-expiration requires the interpretation of pressure tracings. Although arguably the most accurate measure of transmural pressures is through pressure tracings, such readings have been shown to have high interobserver variability and require expertise for proper assessment.[19] Because of these challenges, many practitioners use the mean pressures obtained over the respiratory cycle, calculated by software in the transducer's computer system and displayed on the monitor. This approach avoids the problems of interobserver variability and the difficulties of tracing interpretation.[20] However, there is the risk of allowing artifacts from the respiratory and cardiac cycles to skew the measurements.

Effects of the Cardiac Cycle

The cardiac cycle also affects the proper measurement of CVP and Ppao. Just as the optimal measurement of CVP and Ppao should be performed at end-expiration, the relationship of ventricular diastole and systole should be considered when interpreting CVP (and Ppao) pressure tracings. The normal CVP waveform contains three waves: a, corresponding to atrial contraction during ventricular diastole; c, corresponding to the bulging of the tricuspid valve into the right atrium during right ventricular systole (isovolumic contraction); and v, corresponding to venous filling of the right atrium during late ventricular systole while the tricuspid valve is closed. When the CVP is measured to estimate preload, the pressure just at the onset of the c-wave (the base of the c-wave) represents the final atrial pressure (and the ventricular end-diastolic pressure) before closure of the tricuspid valve and the beginning of ventricular systole. Thus, when measured at end-expiration, the base of the c-wave yields the CVP measurement that best represents the transmural end-diastolic pressure, or preload. As the c-wave is not always visible, the base of the a-wave may be used instead as an estimator; alternatively, the R-wave of the EKG on the monitor may be used to find the end of diastole or beginning of systole on the CVP tracing.[21] Again, although more representative of transmural pressures, measurements from pressure tracings are subject to interobserver variability and are more difficult to obtain than the mean pressure.

Physiologic and Anatomic Properties of the Heart

Physiologic and anatomic properties of the heart affect the CVP. Changes in right-ventricular compliance (such as from heart failure or acute myocardial infarction) and venous tone (eg, hyperadrenergic states), or conditions such as pulmonary hypertension, may have profound effects on CVP independent of the patient's intravascular volume status. Additionally, valvular disorders, such as tricuspid insufficiency, "ventricularize" the CVP waveform, resulting in an elevated mean CVP; careful pressure waveform reading before the ventricularized v-wave (ie, before the regurgitant systolic wave, best marked by the time of the EKG R-wave) is necessary to obtain an accurate CVP. Similarly, tricuspid stenosis elevates the mean CVP, resulting in a gradient between the RAP and the RVEDP.[21] To illustrate just how fine the distinction between a pathologic CVP and a CVP indicative of normovolemia can be, Magder and colleagues[22] demonstrated that a y-descent greater than 4 mm Hg correlated with a low likelihood of response to a fluid bolus, indicating a volume-loaded ventricle, while the loss of the y-descent (along with the loss of the x-descent) is a sign of tamponade.[8]

Like CVP, which measures RAP as a surrogate for RVEDP and RVEDV, Ppao measures left atrial pressure as a surrogate for left ventricular end-diastolic pressure and volume (LVEDP and LVEDV). The pulmonary artery catheters (PA catheters) used for such measurements entail additional risks in their use above those of standard central venous catheters. However, they enable the measurement not only of Ppao but also CVP and CO; more modern catheters even allow determination of RVEDV and right ventricle ejection fraction (RVEF).[23] Nevertheless, measurements of Ppao through PA catheters are subject to the same complicating factors already discussed for CVP measurements: much as the CVP is a reflection of RAP, the Ppao is a "delayed, damped reflection of left atrial pressure."[24] Hence, Ppao will be affected by the respiratory and cardiac cycles and by anatomic or physiologic factors (eg, mitral regurgitation and mitral stenosis; compliance changes from hypertrophy or ischemia; elevated pleural pressure from PEEP or forced expirations) in the same manner as the CVP (eg, the complexities of PEEP and the difficulty in determining its transmission to pleural and pericardial pressures). Attempts to more accurately measure Ppao in the face of hyperinflation secondary to PEEP led to measuring Ppao at end-expiration while the airway was briefly (<3 seconds) disconnected. Assuming no airway obstruction, the lung rapidly returns to its resting functional residual capacity, and the subsequently measured "nadir Ppao" provides an accurate measurement of the on-PEEP LVEDP when total PEEP is less than 15 cm H_2O.[25] In addition to the obvious inconvenience of transient airway disconnection, the subsequent alveolar collapse after disconnection argues against this technique (Teboul and colleagues[26] subsequently developed a corrective index of transmission I_T that allowed an estimation of transmural Ppao without airway disconnection). Also, accurate measurement of Ppao usually requires that the tip of the PA catheter lie within West zone 3 of the lung where CVP exceeds alveolar pressure, otherwise Ppao will reflect alveolar pressure rather than LAP.[27] Even a properly positioned PA catheter, however, only reflects LAP and not capillary pressure; that is, Ppao does not equal pulmonary capillary pressure. True pulmonary capillary pressure can be determined from the inflection point of the Ppao curve after balloon inflation as the measured occlusion pressure drops through the pulmonary arterial and pulmonary venous resistances in series. Its clinical significance serves as another warning of the complexities of Ppao: in conditions such as acute respiratory distress syndrome, increased pulmonary venous resistance can result in elevated pulmonary capillary pressures with low Ppao pressures, resulting in pulmonary edema in the face of a low Ppao.[28]

Putting aside the difficulties inherent in the accurate measurement of CVP and Ppao, the larger problem of their usefulness as measures of preload and as predictors of fluid responsiveness is a separate question. In a prospective observational study of 83 patients admitted to a medical-surgical ICU, most of whom were nonseptic patients after cardiac surgery and all of whom had a PA catheter inserted, Magder and Bafaqeeh[29] investigated fluid responsiveness over a range of CVP values in an attempt to identify a threshold CVP above which volume expansion was unlikely to increase cardiac output. Using fluid challenges that increased CVP by at least 2 mm

Hg (measured exclusively by pressure tracings from carefully zeroed and leveled transducers), a response was defined as an increase in CO of 300 mL/min/m^2 or more. Of the 66 patients in whom the CVP increased by at least 2 mm Hg with fluid challenges, there were 40 responders and 26 nonresponders. No patient responded when the CVP was greater than 13 mm Hg. Only 3 of the 12 patients with an initial CVP greater than 10 mm Hg responded to fluids on their first trial. Nonresponders, however, were identified at all initial CVP levels. They concluded that a CVP of greater than 10 mm Hg (measured with a transducer leveled 5 cm below the sternal angle) indicates a low likelihood of improving CO in response to fluid challenge, with the caveat that nonresponders will still be found at CVPs less than 10 mm Hg. Hence, CVP is best viewed as a negative predictor of fluid responsiveness. Similarly, Jellinek and colleagues[30] showed that, in response to increasing PEEP challenges, a CVP less than 10 mm Hg predicted a decrease in cardiac output. However, the response in patients with a CVP greater than 10 mm Hg was unpredictable: increases, decreases, and no changes in CO were observed. Thus, CVP as a predictor of CO change in response to PEEP challenge functioned as a "one-way" test.[28]

Further evidence against the utility of CVP measurements comes from a recent meta-analysis of 24 studies incorporating 830 medical and surgical patients that examined both CVP and changes in CVP as predictors of intravascular blood volume and fluid responsiveness.[31] None of the studies calculated transmural pressures, factored in PEEP, or used end-expiratory pressure tracings in their determinations of CVP; mean pressures were used as is common practice in most clinical settings. In none of the studies was CVP able to predict either blood volume or fluid responsiveness. The pooled correlation coefficient between the CVP and intravascular blood volume (5 studies) was 0.16 (95% CI, 0.03–0.28); between CVP and stroke index (10 studies) was 0.18 (95% CI, 0.08–0.28); between change in CVP and stroke index (7 studies) was 0.11 (95% CI, 0.01–0.21); and the pooled area under the ROC curve (AUC) of CVP and fluid responsiveness (10 studies) was 0.56 (95% CI, 0.51–0.61). The AUC of CVP for predicting fluid responsiveness effectively suggests that CVP is barely better than a coin toss.

Multiple studies have examined Ppao as a predictor of fluid responsiveness and preload over the prior 3 decades. In 2002, Michard and Teboul[32] reviewed 12 studies examining both static and dynamic measures of preload as predictors of fluid responsiveness in ICU patients, 9 of which included pulmonary artery occlusion pressures (all measured at end-expiration without adjustment for PEEP). Although the studies used different criteria and protocols for volume expansion, in 7 studies the preinfusion, baseline Ppao was not significantly lower in responders versus nonresponders. Of the 3 studies finding a difference in Ppao before and after volume infusion, 1 study[33] found a higher preinfusion Ppao in responders compared with nonresponders and a poor correlation ($r = 0.42$) between Ppao and cardiac index (CI). In the other 2 studies,[22,34] preinfusion baseline Ppao was found to be lower in responders than nonresponders, with Tousignant and colleagues[34] finding no correlation between Ppao and SV ($r = 0.15$) after fluid challenge, while Wagner and Leatherman[23] identified a moderate ($r = 0.58$) negative correlation between change in SV and Ppao. None of the studies were able to identify a clear Ppao threshold value that predicted fluid responsiveness. More recently (2007), Osman and colleagues[35] retrospectively analyzed prospective data on 150 fluid challenges in 96 patients with severe sepsis. Defining a response as a 15% or greater increase in CI, responders and nonresponders showed increases in Ppao and CVP after fluid challenge, with a baseline (preinfusion) Ppao difference that was slightly but statistically significantly lower in the responder group. The optimum threshold value of a preinfusion Ppao of less than 11 mm Hg predicted fluid responsiveness with a sensitivity of 77% (95% CI, 65%–87%), a specificity of 51% (95% CI, 40%–62%), a positive predictive value of 54%, and a negative predictive value of 74%. The AUC was only 0.63 (95% CI, 0.55–0.70).

Further difficulties with Ppao and CVP as predictors of fluid responsiveness were demonstrated by Kumar and colleagues[36] in a prospective study of 45 healthy normal volunteers. Using PA catheterization, radionuclide cineangiography, and volumetric echocardiography, they assessed ventricular filling volumes, cardiac performance, and fluid responsiveness during 3 L of normal saline infusion over 3 hours. They demonstrated no predictable relationship between Ppao or CVP and volumetric preload indexes (RVEDVI and LVEDVI) or cardiac performance measures (CI and SV index [SVI]). In addition, increases in neither Ppao nor CVP predicted the response of either SVI or end-diastolic volume-to-volume expansion.

The interplay of anatomic and physiologic characteristics of the heart, coupled with the effects of the respiratory cycle and the cardiac cycle on the measurement of Ppao (and CVP) complicates the use of static pressure measurements to predict fluid responsiveness. Pinsky[37] highlights some of the underlying problems with Ppao: (1) the nonlinear relationship between Ppao and preload (LVEDV) and its variation among subjects implies that no set Ppao, or change in Ppao, can reliably predict a specific preload or change in preload; (2) the effect of juxtapericardial and pleural pressures such as forced expiration, tamponade, and PEEP; and (3) changes in compliance of the left ventricle from ischemia and arrhythmias or, in the right ventricle, from pulmonary embolus or acute onset pulmonary hypertension, all of which can have a rapid onset. Hence, the complex physiology of the cardiothoracic system conspires against predicting its function from isolated, static pressure measurements.

VOLUMETRIC MEASUREMENTS: CONTINUOUS RVEDV AND GEDV

The practical measurement of preload via volumetric techniques began in the 1980s. Bing and colleagues[38] first proposed the idea of quantifying right ventricular volume by indicator dilution in 1951. The mounting of fast-response thermistors on PA catheters allowed the measurement of beat-to-beat pulmonary artery temperature changes from a cold injectate or, in the current generation of devices, a heated filament that emits a pulse of thermal boluses. Regardless of the technique, the resultant thermodilution allows the measurement of SV, CO, and RVEF. RVEDV is then calculated from RVEF and SV.[39] That RVEDV is calculated from SV and, hence, CO gives rise to the possibility of "mathematical coupling," in which a significant portion of any correlation between RVEDV and CO may arise from a computational, as opposed to a truly physiologic, relationship.

Multiple investigators have assessed RVEDV and its index RVEDVI as measures of preload and predictors of fluid responsiveness. Diebel and colleagues[33] in a study of 29 patients with trauma or sepsis found that RVEDI correlated with CI significantly better than Ppao and was a far better predictor of fluid responsiveness and failure to respond than Ppao. In a second study of 32 critically ill trauma patients with a more stringent definition of fluid responsiveness (an increase in CI of at least 20% as opposed to 10% in their earlier study), Diebel and colleagues[40] again found RVEDVI to be superior to Ppao in predicting fluid responsiveness, with RVEDVI cutoff values of less than 90, 90 to 140, and greater than 140 mL/m^2 predicting fluid responsiveness in 64%, 27%, and 0%, respectively, of test subjects.

Durham and colleagues[41] similarly compared REVDVI and Ppao and found a better correlation between RVEDVI and CI than Ppao and CI, even after correcting for mathematical coupling. They also constructed ventricular function curves for each patient and established that RVEDVI was a better clinical indicator of preload than Ppao. Cheatham and colleagues[42] studied the effects of PEEP on RVEDVI, Ppao, and CI in mechanically ventilated patients. They concluded that there was a higher correlation between RVEDVI and CI than between Ppao and CI at all PEEP levels. Wiesenack and colleagues[43] recently evaluated RVEDVI, Ppao, and LVEDA index (LVEDAI; measured with transesophageal echocardiography [TEE]) in patients undergoing elective cardiac surgery and found RVEDVI to more reliably reflect preload than Ppao or LVEDAI; however, RVEDVI did not predict fluid responsiveness. LVEDAI did correlate with fluid responsiveness (change in SV index), but only weakly ($r^2 = 0.38$, $P<.01$). In another recent multicenter study involving liver transplantation, Della Rocca and colleagues[44] showed that RVEDVI better reflected preload than CVP and Ppao, and they were able to demonstrate an increase in SVI of 0.25 mL/m^2 for an increase in RVEDVI of 1 mL/m^2. No strong correlation between SVI and CVP or Ppao was noted. Della Rocca and colleagues[45] again investigated RVEDVI in liver transplant patients, this time including LVEDAI via TEE in addition to CVP and Ppao. Both RVEDVI and LVEDAI demonstrated a superior correlation with SVI then either CVP or Ppao, although only RVEDVI reached statistical significance, with an increase in SVI of 0.21 mL/m^2 for each increase of 1 mL/m^2 in RVEDVI.

GEDV and GEDV index (GEDVI), and the closely related intrathoracic blood volume and index (ITBV and ITBVI), are another set of volumetric estimates of cardiac preload. Using a thermistor-tipped arterial catheter (usually placed in the femoral artery) and a central venous catheter (subclavian or internal jugular) devices such as the PiCCO system (Pulsion Medical Systems, Germany) allow the measurement of GEDVI and ITBVI via single-indicator transpulmonary thermodilution from a cold injectate of saline through the central venous catheter (earlier versions of the technique used a plasma-bound indicator dye in addition to the temperature injectate and were thus known as double-indicator dilution techniques). The GEDV measures the largest volume of blood in the four chambers of the heart. The ITBV is the GEDV plus the volume of blood within the pulmonary vessels.[46] In addition to such measures of preload, the PiCCO also provides a continuous pulse contour-derived CO and an estimation of extravascular lung water.

Numerous investigators have studied GEDVI and ITBVI as measures of preload and predictors of fluid responsiveness. In an article by Della Rocca and colleagues,[47] 18 studies comparing GEDVI or ITBVI with CI or SVI in diverse patient populations (eg, neurosurgery, cardiac surgery, abdominal and laparoscopic surgery, and intensive care patients) were examined. In all of these studies, ITBVI was a better measure of cardiac preload than CVP or Ppao. The question of mathematical coupling arises again, given that GEDV and CO are derived from the same thermo-dilution curve. Evidence to the contrary however was provided by Michard and colleagues[48] in a study of 36 patients with septic shock. GEDVI and CVP were compared with SVI and CI in separate series of fluid challenges and dobutamine infusions. GEDVI, CVP, SVI, and CI significantly increased after volume loading, and the changes in GEDVI were correlated with changes in SVI whereas changes in CVP were not. Moreover, after dobutamine infusion SV increased as expected but no increase was seen in GEDVI, thus arguing against mathematical coupling as the cause of the correlation between GEDVI and SVI. The good correlation between changes in GEDVI and changes in SVI was also confirmed by Hofer and colleagues[49] in a study of 20 elective cardiac surgery patients in whom RVEDI (via modified PA catheter) and LVEDAI (via TEE) were also monitored. Changes in GEDVI correlated with changes in SVI better ($r^2 = 0.576$) than changes in RVEDI correlated with changes in SVI ($r^2 = 0.267$).

Overall, the use of transpulmonary thermodilution-derived indices such as GEDVI and ITBVI appear to correlate better with preload and changes in CO or SVI than traditional pressure measurements. Even so, the correlations are generally moderate. Whether this imperfect correlation is due to rapid changes in cardiovascular physiology during illness or is due to flaws in the assumptions underlying thermodilution-derived volumetric measurements requires further study.[3] Furthermore, the use of the PiCCO may be precluded by patient factors known to interfere with transpulmonary thermodilution, such as valvular disease or a thoracic aneurysm (which increases transit time) or by contraindications to the placement of a femoral arterial catheter, in which case the axillary artery is an alternative site.[47]

SUMMARY

The use of static preload measurements should be approached with a careful appreciation of the weaknesses inherent in their measurement and their ability to reflect both preload and volume responsiveness. Given that volume responsiveness is the usual clinical question at hand, it is not simply the preload but also the underlying ventricular function that will determine where the patient's position on their Frank-Starling ventricular function curve and, hence, the patient's response to a fluid challenge. Later articles in this issue will address more advanced, dynamic methods of preload assessment and volume responsiveness.[50] However, at the bedside, the most readily available methods still remain pressure-derived preload assessments, particularly the CVP. The proper interpretation and use of such measures, coupled with an understanding of their limitations and knowledge of alternative methods, is necessary to guide properly volume resuscitation in the critically ill.

REFERENCES

1. Despopoulos A, Silbernagl S. Coloratlas of physiology. 5th edition. Stuttgart (Germany): Georg Thieme Verlag; 2003. p. 67–204.
2. Scheuren K, Wente MN, Hainer C, et al. Left ventricular end-diastolic area is a measure of cardiac preload in patients with early septic shock. Eur J Anaesthesiol 2009;26(9):759–65.
3. Benington S, Ferris P, Nirmalan M. Emerging trends in minimally invasive haemodynamic monitoring and optimization of fluid therapy. Eur J Anaesthesiol 2009; 26(11):893–905.
4. Magder S. Clinical usefulness of respiratory variations in arterial pressure. Am J Respir Crit Care Med 2004;169:151–5.
5. Boldt J, Lenz M, Kumle B, et al. Volume replacement strategies on intensive care units: results from a postal survey. Intensive Care Med 1998;24:147–51.
6. Magder S. More respect for the CVP. Intensive Care Med 1998;24:651–3.
7. Dellinger RP, Levy MM, Carlet JM, et al. Surviving Sepsis Campaign: international guidelines for management of severe sepsis and septic shock: 2008 [published correction appears in Crit Care Med 2008; 36:1394–96]. Crit Care Med 2008;36: 296–327.
8. Magder S. Central venous pressure monitoring. Curr Opin Crit Care 2006;12: 219–27.
9. Marino PL. The ICU book. 3rd edition. Philadelphia: Lippincott Williams & Wilkins; 2007. p. 181, 183.
10. Bates B, Hoekelman RA, Thompson JE. A guide to physical examination and history taking. 5th edition. Philadelphia: J.B. Lippincott; 1991. p. 286–7.

11. Magder S. Central venous pressure: a useful but not so simple measurement. Crit Care Med 2006;34(8):2224–7.

12. McGee SR. Physical examination of venous pressure: a critical review. Am Heart J 1998;136(1):10–8.

13. Haywood GA, Joy MD, Camm AJ. Influence of posture and reference point on central venous pressure measurement. BMJ 1991;303:626–7.

14. Figg KK, Nemergut EC. Error in central venous pressure measurement. Anesth Analg 2009;108:1209–11.

15. Bellemare P, Goldberg P, Magder SA. Variations in pulmonary artery occlusion pressure to estimate changes in pleural pressure. Intensive Care Med 2007;33:2004–8.

16. Magder S. How to use central venous pressure measurements. Curr Opin Crit Care 2005;11:264–70.

17. Malbrain ML, Wilmer A. The polycompartment syndrome: towards an understanding of the interactions between different compartments. Intensive Care Med 2007;33:1869–72.

18. Qureshi AS, Shapiro RS, Leatherman JW. Use of bladder pressure to correct for the effect of expiratory muscle activity on central venous pressure. Intensive Care Med 2007;33(11):1907–12.

19. Komadina KH, Schenk DA, LaVeau P, et al. Interobserver variability in the interpretation of pulmonary artery catheter pressure tracings. Chest 1991;100:1647–54.

20. Holcroft JW, Anderson JT. Cardiovascular monitoring. In: Souba WW, Fink MP, Jurkovich GJ, et al, editors. ACS surgery: principles and practice. 6th edition. New York: WebMD; 2007. p. 1502–15.

21. Mark JB. Getting the most from a CVP catheter. In: 52nd Annual Refresher Course Lectures, Clinical updates and basic science reviews of the American Society of Anesthesiologists 2001;231:1–7.

22. Magder S, Erice F, Lagonidis D. Determinants of the 'y' descent and its usefulness as a predictor of ventricular filling. J Intensive Care Med 2000;15:262–9.

23. Wagner JG, Leatherman JW. Right ventricular end-diastolic volume as a predictor of the hemodynamic response to a fluid challenge. Chest 1998;113:1048–54.

24. Mark JB. CVP and PAC Monitoring. In: 58th Annual Refresher Course Lectures, clinical updates and basic science reviews of the American Society of Anesthesiologists 2007;102:1–6.

25. Pinsky MR, Vincent JL, DeSmet JM. Estimating left ventricular filling pressure during positive end expiratory pressure in humans. Am Rev Respir Dis 1991;143:25–31.

26. Teboul JL, Pinsky MR, Mercat A, et al. Estimating cardiac filling pressure in mechanically ventilated patients with hyperinflation. Crit Care Med 2000;28:3631–6.

27. Teboul JL, Besbes M, Andrivet P, et al. A bedside index assessing the reliability of PA occlusion pressure measurments during mechanical ventilation with PEEP. J Crit Care 1992;7:22–9.

28. Pinsky MR. Hemodynamic monitoring in the intensive care unit. Clin Chest Med 2003;24:549–60.

29. Magder S, Bafaqeeh F. The clinical role of central venous pressure measurements. J Intensive Care Med 2007;22(1):44–51.

30. Jellinek H, Krafft P, Fitzgerald RD, et al. Right atrial pressure predicts hemodynamic response to apneic positive airway pressure. Crit Care Med 2000;28(3):672–8.

31. Marik E, Baram M, Vahid B. Does central venous pressure predict fluid responsiveness? Chest 2008;134:172–8.
32. Michard F, Teboul J. Predicting fluid responsiveness in ICU patients. Chest 2002; 121:2000–8.
33. Diebel LN, Wilson RF, Tagett MG, et al. End-diastolic volume: a better indicator of preload in the critically ill. Arch Surg 1992;127:817–22.
34. Tousignant CP, Walsh F, Mazer CD. The use of transesophageal echocardiography for preload assessment in critically ill patients. Anesth Analg 2000;90:351–5.
35. Osman D, Ridel C, Patrick R, et al. Cardiac filling pressures are not appropriate to predict hemodynamic response to volume challenge. Crit Care Med 2007;35:64–8.
36. Kumar A, Anel R, Bunnell E, et al. Pulmonary artery occlusion pressure and central venous pressure fail to predict ventricular filling volume, cardiac performance, or the response to volume infusion in normal subjects. Crit Care Med 2004;32(3):691–9.
37. Pinsky MR. Clinical significance of pulmonary artery occlusion pressure. Intensive Care Med 2003;29:175–8.
38. Bing R, Heimbecker R, Falholt W. An estimation of residual volume blood in the right ventricle of normal and diseased human hearts in vivo. Am Heart J 1951; 42:483–502.
39. Boldt J. Right ventricular end-diastolic volume. In: Pinsky MR, Payden D, editors. Functional hemodynamic monitoring. New York: Springer-Verlag; 2005. p. 269–81.
40. Diebel LN, Wilson RF, Heins J, et al. End-diastolic volume versus pulmonary artery wedge pressure in evaluating cardiac preload in trauma patients. J Trauma 1994;37(6):950–5.
41. Durham R, Neunaber K, Vogler G, et al. Right ventricular end-diastolic volume as a measure of preload. J Trauma 1995;39(2):218–23.
42. Cheatham ML, Nelson LD, Chang MC, et al. Right ventricular end-diastolic volume index as a predictor of preload status in patients on positive end-expiratory pressure. Crit Care Med 1998;26:1801–6.
43. Wiesenack C, Fiegl C, Keyser A, et al. Continuously assessed right ventricular end-diastolic volume as a marker of cardiac preload and fluid responsiveness in mechanically ventilated cardiac surgical patients. Crit Care 2005;9(3): R226–33.
44. Della Rocca G, Costa MG, Feltracco P, et al. Continuous right ventricular end diastolic volume and right ventricular ejection fraction during liver transplantation: a multicentre study. Liver Transpl 2008;14:327–32.
45. Della Rocca G, Costa MG, Coccia C, et al. Continuous right ventricular end-diastolic volume in comparison with left ventricular end-diastolic area. Eur J Anaesthesiol 2009;26(4):272–8.
46. Marik PE. Techniques for assessment of intravascular volume in critically ill patients. J Intensive Care Med 2009;24(5):329–37.
47. Della Rocca G, Costa MG, Pietropaoli P. How to measure and interpret volumetric measures of preload. Curr Opin Crit Care 2007;13:297–302.
48. Michard F, Alaya S, Zarka V, et al. Global end-diastolic volume as an indicator of cardiac preload in patients with septic shock. Chest 2003;124:1900–8.
49. Hofer CK, Furrer L, Matter-Ensner S, et al. Volumetric preload measurement by thermodilution: a comparison with transoesophageal echocardiography. Br J Anaesth 2005;94:748–55.
50. De Hert SG. Perioperative assessment of volume status: measurement of preload is not measurement of preload responsiveness. Eur J Anaesthesiol 2009;26: 269–71.

Dynamic Indices of Preload

T. Miko Enomoto, MD[a],*, Louise Harder, MD[b]

KEYWORDS

- Dynamic preload indicator
- Fluid responsiveness • Volume overload

Hypotension and shock are important issues confronting the intensivist. The question that confronts most intensive care providers on a daily basis is: will fluid increase perfusion to end organs, or will it worsen pulmonary or systemic edema? This can be especially true when treating septic patients, where volume expansion is often one of the cornerstones of early resuscitation. Volume overload can have dire consequences such as decreased gas exchange and increased myocardial dysfunction. Several studies suggest that even experienced intensivists using traditional parameters are correct only about 50% of the time when determining preload responsiveness.[1–6]

As the importance of early goal directed therapy in the successful treatment of septic shock becomes increasingly apparent, it is all the more imperative that goals be based in science and supported by evidence. Clearly, static measurements have failed as a meaningful endpoint for fluid resuscitation.

Clinically, many practitioners rely on the central venous pressure (CVP), pulmonary artery occlusion pressure (PAOP), or other static measurements to determine the volume status of a patient. Studies in recent years have confirmed that these filling pressures have little correlation with fluid responsiveness.[5–9]

In many patients, a rapid fluid bolus is a reasonable diagnostic and potentially therapeutic option, but in others (eg, acute respiratory distress syndrome [ARDS]), it has the potential to cause harm, and may delay institution of appropriate therapy. Ideally, it would be possible to determine if a patient will be preload responsive before the volume is given. The poor predictive value of static measures and clinical examination has led to investigation of the dynamic measures of fluid responsiveness. In contrast to static measures, dynamic indices rely on the changing physiology of heart lung interactions to determine whether a patient will benefit from increased preload.

---

[a] Department of Anesthesiology and Perioperative Medicine, Oregon Health Sciences University, Mail Code UHS-2, 3181 SW Sam Jackson Park Road, Portland, OR 97239-3098, USA
[b] Department of Critical Care Medicine, Oregon Health and Sciences University, Mail Code UHN 67, 3181 SW Sam Jackson Park Road, Portland, OR 97239-3098, USA
* Corresponding author.
E-mail address: enomotot@ohsu.edu

Crit Care Clin 26 (2010) 307–321
doi:10.1016/j.ccc.2009.12.004
0749-0704/10/$ – see front matter © 2010 Elsevier Inc. All rights reserved.

PHYSIOLOGIC RATIONALE OF DYNAMIC INDICES

Preload of the heart is defined as the wall stress at the end of diastole.[10] Direct measurement of wall stress in vivo is difficult; end diastolic volumes or pressures have been used as proxies, but both have significant limitations. Perhaps most importantly, an accurate measure of preload at a point in time does not necessarily reflect preload responsiveness.

An understanding of the Frank-Starling curve is fundamental to understanding the concept of preload responsiveness. The slope of the relationship between ventricular preload and stroke volume (SV) depends on ventricular contractility. As contractility increases, the Starling curve shifts upwards and to the left and increases its slope. Decreasing contractility has the opposite effect. Increasing preload serves to augment ventricular output predominantly on the steep portion of the curve. As seen in **Fig. 1**, augmenting preload on the flat portion of the curve produces minimal increases in SV.

As a ventricle fails, its contractility and therefore the slope of its Frank-Starling curve decreases, and a preload that would indicate volume responsiveness in the normal heart may not apply to a failing heart. Therefore even a precise measurement of left ventricular (LV) preload does not determine if that LV is fluid-responsive (ie, if it will increase cardiac output in response to increased volume). Additionally, the relationship between preload and SV is curvilinear rather than linear.

Dynamic indices apply a controlled and reversible preload variation and measure the hemodynamic response. This can be done by observing the cardiovascular response to positive pressure ventilation, or to reversible preload-increasing maneuvers, such as passive leg raising.

Cavallaro has proposed a useful classification of dynamic indices that predict volume responsiveness. Group A consists of indices based on cyclic variation in SV or SV-related hemodynamic parameters determined by mechanical ventilation-induced cyclic variation in intrathoracic pressure, and includes such metrics as pulse pressure variation (PPV), its derivatives, and aortic blood flow. Group B is made up of indices based on cyclic variations of nonstroke volume-related hemodynamic parameters determined by mechanical ventilation, and includes vena cava diameter or

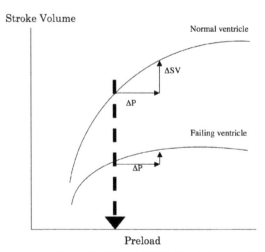

Fig. 1. Frank-Starling curves demonstrating relationship between change in preload to change in SV in a normal and failing ventricles. A given change in preload may cause variable changes in SV, depending on the slope of the curve.

ventricular pre-ejection period. Group C consists of indices based on preload redistribution maneuvers; mechanical ventilation is not required, and group C includes passive leg raising and Valsalva maneuvers.[11]

Group A and B techniques are based on the physiologic interaction of the heart and lungs within a closed thoracic cavity, and rely on the phasic changes in SV created by changing intrathoracic pressure due to positive pressure mechanical ventilation. During positive pressure inspiration, preload to the right heart is decreased because of increased intrathoracic pressure, both from compression of the vena cava (decreased venous return) and increased right atrial pressure. This decrease in right ventricular (RV) preload leads to a decrease in RV output, which subsequently leads to a decrease in pulmonary artery blood flow, LV filling, and LV output.[12] Other mechanisms postulated to increase LV SV variation with PPV include the following changes during inspiration, caused by increased transpulmonary pressure

Increased RV afterload
Increased LV preload
Decreased LV afterload.[12]

The end result of these pressure changes is that LV SV increases, while RV SV decreases during positive pressure inspiration. The delay of pulmonary blood transit time results in decreased RV SV translating to a decreased LV SV a few heartbeats later (ie, usually during expiration).[8]

These phasic differences are exaggerated in the setting of hypovolemia for several reasons:

The underfilled vena cava is more collapsible
The underfilled right atrium is more susceptible to increased intrathoracic pressure
More of the lung demonstrates the physiology of West Zones 1 and 2 (in West Zone 1 the alveolar pressure is greater then the arteriolar pressure, which is greater than venous pressure; in West Zone 2 the arteriolar pressure is greater than alveolar pressure, which is greater than venous pressure), which effectively increases RV afterload
Larger changes are seen when operating on the steeper portion of the Frank-Starling curve.[12]

This increased variation in pressures between the inspiratory phase and the expiratory phase can be used to identify hypovolemia and volume responsiveness, and is the basis for Cavallaro's group A and B indices, including stroke volume variation (SVV) and pulse pressure variation.

SVV

SVV examines the difference between the SV during the inspiratory and expiratory phases of ventilation, and requires a means to directly or indirectly assess SV. This eliminates arterial compliance as a variable, but until recently, has required invasive monitoring such as aortic flow probes. Now, the PiCCO (Pulsion Medical Systems, Munich, Germany), LiDCO (LiDCO Group PLC, London, England) and FloTrac sensor (Edwards Lifesciences, Irvine, CA, USA) monitors uses pulse contour analysis through a proprietary formula to measure cardiac output and SVV. Because arterial compliance is not a factor in this index, it should most closely represent the change in cardiac output during the respiratory cycle, and also be the most predictive of volume responsiveness. Indeed, some studies do suggest that SVV, as measured by pulse contour technique, can be helpful as a fluid responsiveness predictor.[13] This has not been consistently reproducible, however, and other studies find poor predictive value.[14,15]

Systolic Pressure Variation

Systolic pressure variation (SPV) is the difference between the maximum and the minimum systolic pressure over a single respiratory cycle and can be expressed in millimeters of mercury (SPmax − SPmin) or as a percent (SPV(%) = $100 \times (SP_{max} - SP_{min})/[(SP_{max} + SP_{min})/2]$). Increased SPV was the first of these indices to be recognized to correlate with hypovolemia and was later shown to have a sensitivity of 82%, specificity of 86%, and area under the receiver operator characteristic (ROC) curve (AUC) of 0.92, using a threshold of 8.5 mm Hg.[16,17]

SPV can be broken down into delta up (dUp) and delta down (dDown). These two components are calculated using a reference systolic pressure measured during an end–expiratory pause according to the following equations:

dUp = SPmax − SPref
dDown = SPref − SPmin

where SPmax is the maximum systolic pressure in a single respiratory cycle; SPref is the reference systolic pressure at end–expiration, and SPmin is the minimum systolic pressure measured in a single respiratory cycle.

dUp reflects the inspiratory increase in systolic pressure, resulting from an increase in extramural aortic pressure (increase in diastolic pressure) and an increase in LV SV. As the extramural aortic pressure component seems more significant in many patients,[18] increased dUp is not a reliable indicator of fluid responsiveness. Indeed, in animal models, dUp is increased in congestive heart failure[19] and with increasing volume resuscitation in the presence of cardiac ischemic dysfunction.[20]

dDown reflects the expiratory decrease in LV SV related to the inspiratory decrease in RV SV.[12]

PPV

Arterial pulse pressure is the difference between arterial systolic and diastolic pressure. This difference is influenced by SV and the arterial compliance. Comparison of the pulse pressure during inspiration with pulse pressure during expiration demonstrates the degree to which the pulse pressure is preload-limited. As comparison is being made during a single respiratory cycle, change in arterial compliance theoretically should be minimal. Analysis of the PPV thus can be used to predict volume responsiveness, and is expressed as a percentage: PPV(%) = $100 \times (PPmax - PPmin)/[(PPmax + PPmin)/2]$.

Several studies have demonstrated the utility of increased PPV as a predictor of fluid responsiveness. Michard and colleagues found that in mechanically ventilated patients with septic shock, a PPV of 13% identified patients who had a greater than or equal to 15% increase in cardiac output in response to volume expansion with 500 mL of 6% hydroxyethylstarch, with a sensitivity of 94% and specificity of 96%. Additionally, this group found that using ROC analysis, PPV was a more accurate predictor of volume responsiveness than SPV.[21] Auler and colleagues[22] had similar findings in a population of patients mechanically ventilated after cardiac surgery.

dDown and PPV since have been demonstrated to be more sensitive and specific predictors of volume responsiveness than SPV. At a threshold of 5 mm Hg, dDown has a sensitivity and specificity of 86% in patients undergoing cardiac surgery, and an AUC of 0.92%.[19] In another study, Tavernier and colleagues[23] found that in successive volume loading steps in 15 septic and mechanically ventilated patients, a dDown of 5 mm Hg had a 95% positive predictive value and 93% negative predictive value, with an area under the ROC of 0.97 (95% confidence interval [CI] 0.9 to 1.0). PPV was not evaluated in this study, but SPV was found to have an area under the ROC of 0.91 (95% CI of 0.76 to 0.98).

Kubitz and colleagues compared SPV and PPV with aortic flow probe-derived SVV in pigs undergoing pharmaceutical alteration of blood pressure with phenyl-ephrine and adenosine. At decreased pressures, SPV decreased compared with baseline, while PPV stayed the same across the range of decreased and increased pressures. Both SPV and PPV showed good correlation with SVV at baseline and decreased pressures, and slightly less correlation at increased pres-sures, although both maintained significance. Bland-Altman analysis found a mean bias of SPV and SVV of 5.35% (standard error [SE] 0.42, limits of agreement 8.31% and 2.40%). Similar analysis of PPV and SVV revealed a mean bias of 1.41% (SE 0.58, limits of agreement 5.46% and −2.63%). From this, the authors concluded that PPV is a more reliable value than SPV when blood pressure is being augmented by vasoconstrictors. This study did not include a volume expan-sion component to the experiment.[24]

Plethmysography

Examining amplitude variation between inspiration and expiration phases has been extended to the plethysmographic waveform. Although this technique has several similarities to arterial pulse pressure variation, there are several important differences. The plethysmographic waveform obtained from a standard pulse oximeter probe is based on transmission and reflection of infrared wavelengths of light by tissue. The pulsatility is a function of changing tissue volume between systole and diastole, producing the familiar wave tracing.[25]

The pulse oximeter as a gauge of volume status first was suggested by Partridge[26] in 1987. Variation in the plethysmographic waveform has been referred to by many names: change in pulse oximetry plethysmography (dPOP), ventilation-induced plethysmo-graphic variation (VPV), and DP$_{PLET}$. For the sake of this article, the authors will refer to VPV (VPV(%) = 100 × ([Max amplitude − Min amplitude]/[(Max amplitude − Min amplitude)/2])). Cannesson and colleagues[27] reported the strong correlation (r^2 = .82, P<.001) of VPV with PPV in 22 mechanically ventilated patients. It should be noted that the precision of this correlation appears to decrease as variation increases. The Cannesson study did not demonstrate volume responsiveness, but only that VPV of greater than or equal to 15% was predictive of having PPV greater than or equal to 13%, the threshold value for volume responsiveness sited in many studies. Wyffels and colleagues[28] reported that in 32 postoperative cardiac surgery patients, PPV and VPV reliably predicted at least a 15% increase in cardiac index in response to adminis-tration of 500 mL 6% hydroxyethylstarch with an AUC (95% CI) of 0.937 (0.792 to 0.991) and 0.892 (0.731 to 0.972), respectively. Feissel and colleagues[29] demonstrated in 23 septic patients that a VPV of 14% allowed discrimination of volume responders and nonresponders with a sensitivity of 84% and specificity of 80%.

Several concerns have been raised regarding the use of VPV in clinical care. Land-sverk and colleagues showed large inter- and intra-individual variation in VPV in 14 mechanically ventilated intensive care unit (ICU) patients. In addition, Bland-Altman analysis demonstrated poor agreement between VPV and PPV.[30] There is also acknowledgment by several authors that proprietary signal processing by different manufacturers may alter the raw data such that it interferes with the use of the waveform for purposes other than oxygen saturation monitoring. For example, the auto–gain function on most pulse oximeters will conceal amplitude changes.[25]

Some monitors allow this function to be turned off, while others do not. As there is no accepted standard of signal processing between manufacturers, this may prevent the reproduction of results between institutions using different monitors, as well as reliable clinical use of this technique.

Although the obvious and tantalizing advantage to the use of the pulse oximeter to determine fluid responsiveness is the complete noninvasiveness of the technique, at this time, evidence does not support reliance on this method.

Respiratory variability of the superior and inferior vena cava

The inferior and superior venae cavae are distensible blood vessels whose diameters and flow vary with respiration.[31] These variations are reflected by changes in aortic flow within a few beats of the heart.[32] The IVC enters the right atrium almost immediately after crossing the diaphragm. Therefore its extramural pressure is equivalent to abdominal pressure, and its intramural pressure is close to right atrial pressure. The transmural pressure versus volume relationship of the venae cavae is nonlinear, with a steep slope at low distention and a plateau at full volume.[33,34] In PPV, the increase in pleural pressure is transmitted fully to the right atrium, and partially transmitted to the abdomen via depression of the diaphragm, causing an overall increase in transmural pressure of the IVC. Because the IVC is distensible, this increase in pressure causes an increase in diameter of the IVC. In hypovolemic patients (ie, those on the steep part of the pressure volume curve), these diameter changes should be larger than if the IVC is full (ie, on the flat part of the pressure volume curve).[31–33,35,36]

Unlike the IVC, the course of the SVC is mainly intrathoracic. Positive pressure ventilation then should cause a decrease in transmural pressure, and subsequent decrease in the diameter of the SVC, especially in hypovolemic patients.[33]

Using different indices as reference standards, three groups tested the hypothesis that changes in the diameter of the IVC and the SVC with PPV are predictive of fluid responsiveness, and independently concluded that respiratory variations in IVC and SVC diameter during mechanical ventilation could be used to determine preload responsiveness in sedated, mechanically ventilated patients.

Barbier and colleagues determined that the distensibility index of the IVC (dIVC), defined as (Dmax − Dmin)/Dmin and expressed as a percentage, was predictive of fluid responsiveness with a sensitivity of 90% and a specificity of 90%. Twenty-three septic patients were evaluated with subcostal images of the IVC and cardiac index measured by esophageal Doppler. They concluded that a dIVC above 18% was predictive of an increase in cardiac index of at least 15% with fluid loading.

Feissel and colleagues used a slightly different index to reach similar conclusions. Using subcostal imaging of the IVC, they measured the maximum and minimum IVC diameters over a single respiratory cycle in fully sedated, mechanically ventilated patients without arrhythmias. They calculated DD_{IVC} as maximal IVC diameter − minimum IVC diameter divided by the mean of the two values and expressed as a percentage. Cardiac output was measured by volume time integral (VTI) of aortic blood flow via transthoracic echocardiography. Defining responders as those whose cardiac output increased by at least 15%, they found that DD_{IVC} of 12% predicted fluid responsiveness with a positive predictive value of 93% and negative predictive value of 92%.[32]

Viellard-Baron studied the effect of PPV on the SVC and the ability to predict volume responsiveness. They studied 66 mechanically ventilated patients in septic shock with acute lung injury. An SVC collapsibility index (maximum diameter on expiration − minimum diameter on inspiration/maximum diameter on expiration) threshold of 36% allowed discrimination between nonresponders and responders with sensitivity of 90% and specificity of 100%.[36]

The dIVC and DD$_{IVC}$ are appealing, because both techniques are noninvasive and relatively easy to learn. The SVC collapsibility index requires esophageal Doppler placement, which is not routine in many ICUs. In all of these studies, the patients were sedated and fully ventilated in volume control mode with an average tidal volume close to 8 mL/kg. It is unclear how smaller or larger tidal volumes would affect the results. Patients with arrhythmias were excluded. Only 7 out of 123 patients in the three studies were excluded, because the examiners were unable to obtain adequate imaging. Certainly in some ICU patient populations (postlaparotomy, morbidly obese), one would anticipate more difficulty obtaining images.[31] It is also unclear how elevated intra-abdominal pressures would affect the validity of dIVC and DD$_{IVC}$.

Using respiratory variation in IVC and SVC diameter has potential for predicting preload responsiveness in septic patients. Phasic variation of SVC diameter may be more accurate, as it is not influenced by intra-abdominal pressure. However, it necessitates a transesophageal, rather than transthoracic, approach. Further validation of these concepts in large, multicenter trials is warranted.

Cautions Regarding Cavallaro Group A and B Indices

There are several important caveats to keep in mind when using these dynamic indices to predict fluid responsiveness:

Positive pressure, controlled ventilation is required to obtain meaningful values for any of the Cavallaro group A or B indices. Spontaneous respiratory efforts, even when supported by the ventilator, alter the mechanics such that these numbers lose their reliability.

Sinus rhythm is required. Arrhythmia or frequent extra systoles result in altered SV and invalidate these tools to predict volume responsiveness.

Many of these techniques require invasive arterial blood pressure monitoring with a catheter, and as such, they are prone to the same errors in measurement associated with invasive blood pressure monitoring: air bubbles in the catheter tubing, excessive tubing length, kinks in the tubing, excessively compliant tubing, and other errors.

A single value never should replace clinical judgment. A high PPV value in a normotensive patient with evidence of normal tissue perfusion does not mean that person requires volume expansion.

Further investigation of these techniques in the setting of vasoactive medications is needed. Animal data suggest that group A dynamic indicators are useful even in the setting of high doses of vasoconstricting agents. In a swine model, PPV appears to maintain more fidelity to SVV measured by aortic flow probe than SPV when blood pressure is modified pharmacologically using phenylephrine and adenosine.[24] Nouira and colleagues[37] observed a decrease in SPV and PPV with norepinephrine infusion after hemorrhage in anesthetized dogs. Further investigation is needed in people.

How extremes of ventilation (ie, low tidal volume, high respiratory rate, high positive end-expiratory pressure [PEEP]) affect group A and B indices is not yet clear. Most of the early data came from patients ventilated with at least 10 mL/kg tidal volumes. Huang and colleagues[38] found that PPV remains a valuable indicator of volume responsiveness in patients with ARDS and ventilated with a lung protective strategy, although the area under the ROC curve, at 0.768, was smaller than in the studies using 8 to 12 mL/kg tidal volumes. Mean tidal volume in the Huang study was 6.4 mL/kg with a standard deviation of 0.7. Interestingly, in another trial by De Backer and colleagues[39] involving 17 hypovolemic patients ventilated with low (14 to 16 breaths per minute) and high (30 to 40 breaths per minute) respiratory rates, the authors concluded that respiratory variation in SV and its derivates is affected by respiratory rate, and caution against using these indices as predictors of volume responsiveness at high respiratory rates. Mean tidal volumes in this study were 8.5 mL/kg (8.2 to 9.2) ideal body weight.

Further investigation of these indicators in the setting of the open abdomen or open thorax is needed before their use should be relied upon in these populations.

Passive Leg Raising

Passive leg raising (PLR) is a form of reversible volume challenge that can be used to evaluate which patients will benefit from intravenous fluid and increased preload. Elevating a patient's legs allows a passive transfer of blood from the lower part of the body toward the central circulation. The amount of blood transferred from the legs is variable and has been estimated to be between 150 to 750 mL depending on technique and study.[1,40–42] If the heart is preload-responsive, the shift of fluid from the lower part of the body to the thorax should result in increased cardiac output. This requires that both the right and left ventricles be preload-dependent. If the right ventricle cannot increase cardiac output with increased preload, the left ventricle will not see the increased preload, and cardiac output will not improve.[43]

Several studies have determined that PLR is effective in determining which patients are preload-responsive.[1–4,43,44] Importantly, PLR can be used in spontaneously breathing patients and in patients not in sinus rhythm.[1] The increase in preload from the maneuver is reversed completely when the legs are returned to horizontal,[1,43,44] meaning it is safe even in cases in which increasing blood volume may be harmful, such as ARDS. International consensus guidelines now recommend PLR to evaluate fluid responsiveness in patients with shock.[45]

Boulain and colleagues[44] was the first to demonstrate the utility of PLR clinically. He demonstrated that in sedated, mechanically ventilated patients in sinus rhythm, PLR induced changes in radial arterial pulse pressure correlated with subsequent volume-induced changes in SV. This study, however, gave no threshold value to distinguish between those who responded to an intravenous fluid bolus and those who did not.

In 2002, Monnet and colleagues[1] evaluated PLR to assess fluid responsiveness in spontaneously breathing patients and those with arrhythmias. Using esophageal Doppler measurements of aortic blood flow as a surrogate of cardiac output, Monnet found that an increase in aortic blood flow of at least 10% with PLR predicted volume responsiveness with a sensitivity of 97% and specificity of 94%. Changes in aortic blood flow were rapid (within 30 seconds of PLR) and transient. The authors found that the PLR-induced changes in aortic blood flow and arterial pulse pressure variation were predictive of volume responsiveness, but the former was more accurate than the latter. Of note, this is the first study in which the starting position of the patients before PLR was semirecumbent, rather than supine.

Jabot and colleagues confirmed that maximal fluid shifts, and therefore better predictive value, are obtained when patients are shifted from the semirecumbent (chair) position to supine with legs elevated 45°. Elevating the legs of a horizontal supine patient may still be helpful, but sensitivity is decreased.[42]

In follow-up to Monnet's study, Maizel and colleagues[4] examined the predictive value of PLR in spontaneously breathing patients using transthoracic echocardiographic measures of SV and cardiac output. Patients with arrhythmias were excluded. He found that in increase of cardiac output or SV of greater than 12% with PLR predicted volume responsiveness. There was no change in heart rate with PLR, indicating lack of catecholamine response to any stimulus the PLR maneuver may have created in these awake patients. This confirms earlier findings of Gaffney and colleagues[41] in healthy volunteers.

In the largest study to date, Thiel and colleagues measured SV changes with PLR in 89 medical ICU patients determined to need volume expansion by their attending clinician. Using a transthoracic Doppler device (USCOM Limited, Sydney, Australia), they determined that a greater than or equal to 15% increase in SV with PLR predicted volume responsiveness with sensitivity and specificity of 81% and 93%, respectively. Less than 50% of the patients given fluid boluses were volume-responsive, once again confirming the poor ability to determine preload responsiveness clinically.[3]

Because the hemodynamic response to PLR is rapid and transient,[5,41,46] real-time assessment of cardiac output is needed, which generally means some form of invasive monitoring. It is not clear how much blood is autotransfused, how much this varies between patients and patient populations, and if the variation is significant. Importantly, the characterization of responders versus nonresponders has not been defined clearly. Vasoconstrictors, increased intra-abdominal pressures, and elastic compression stockings all may have an impact on validity of PLR; further studies are needed to clarify these issues. It would be prudent to avoid PLR in patients with increased intracranial pressure.

Respiratory Systolic Variation Test

The respiratory systolic pressure variation (RSVT) is a technique whereby three or four consecutive pressure-controlled breaths of increasing peak inspiratory pressures are administered over a brief period of time to intubated, sedated patients. The minimum systolic blood pressure (SBP) value following each of these breaths is recorded, and the results plotted against their respective airway pressures. A steeper slope (ie, larger decrease in SBP with increasing tidal volume) implies that the patient will be fluid-responsive, whereas less of a slope implies the patient's ventricles are on the flat part of the Frank-Starling curve, and the patient will not increase cardiac output with fluid loading.[19,47]

Two studies have demonstrated the potential utility of the RSVT to predict fluid responsiveness. Preisman and colleagues[20] compared several different dynamic preload indicators, including RSVT, before and after fluid loading. Eighteen patients undergoing elective coronary artery bypass graft (CABG) were evaluated preoperatively after induction of anesthesia, and again postoperatively before transfer to the ICU. Operators used transesophageal echocardiography to measure LV end–diastolic area index (LVEDAI) and fractional area change (FAC), and a PiCCO femoral arterial catheter to measure intrathoracic blood volume index (ITBVI), LV stroke volume index (LVSVI), systolic pressure variation (SPV), dDown, PPV, and SVV along with the RSVT (**Fig. 2**). Area under ROC curve was used to evaluate the ability of the tested hemodynamic parameters to predict fluid responsiveness. Patients were considered volume-responsive if the LVSVI increased by at least 15%. Forty-six percent of study patients were responders. SVV, PPV, SPV, dDown, and RSVT were all very good predictors of fluid responsiveness. RSVT had similar predictive value as PPV, with area under ROC curve of 0.96 and 0.95 respectively. The predictive value of CVP was little better than chance.

Perel and colleagues[47] studied 14 patients after abdominal aortic surgery. They also found that steeper RSVT slopes were associated with a greater than or equal to 15% increase in cardiac index after fluid administration with a sensitivity of 87.5% and a specificity of 83%.

The accuracy with which many of the dynamic preload indicators predict fluid responsiveness can be affected by variations in tidal volume.[47,48] The main advantage

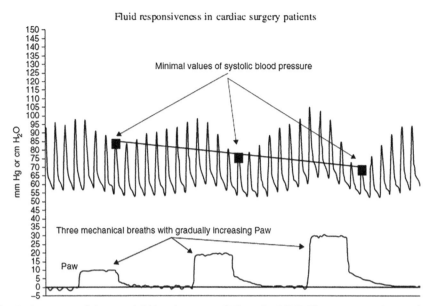

Fig. 2. Response of the arterial blood pressure (BP) to the RSVT. Three consecutive mechanical pressure-controlled breaths are delivered with inspiratory pressures of 10, 20, and 30 cm H_2O. Minimal values of SBP in response to each breath are recorded, and then the slope of the relationship between the decrease in BP and inspiratory pressure is calculated. (*From* Preisman S, Kogan S, Berkenstadt H, et al. Predicting fluid responsiveness in patients undergoing surgery: functional haemodynamic parameters including the Respiratory Systolic Variation Test and static preload indicators. Br J Anaesth 2005;95:746–55; with permission.)

of RSVT is that it is independent of set tidal volume. A complex respiratory maneuver is required, combined with complicated off-line measurements and calculations, making it unsuitable for routine clinical practice. Newer ventilators that are able to perform the RSVT while integrating with hemodynamic monitors may make this feasible in the near future.[19]

End–Expiratory Occlusion Pressure

Recently, Monnet and colleagues proposed a promising new dynamic indicator of fluid responsiveness. Positive pressure ventilation increases intrathoracic pressure and impedes venous return, which in turn reduces cardiac preload. Monnet hypothesized that an end–expiratory occlusion (EEO) may abolish the inspiratory increase in intrathoracic pressure, prevent the cyclic drop in cardiac preload, and allow an increase in venous return, thus acting like a fluid challenge.[49] They tested whether this could serve as a functional test for fluid responsiveness in patients with circulatory failure.

Thirty-four mechanically ventilated patients with shock in whom volume expansion was planned by their clinician were studied. Blood pressure and cardiac index (pulse contour-derived via PiCCO) were measured at baseline, during PLR, during the last 5 seconds of EEO, and after 500 mL normal saline. Hemodynamic measurements obtained during the 15-second EEO were compared with those obtained during PLR. All patients were ventilated in volume-assist controlled mode with tidal volumes of 6.8 ± 1.1 mL/kg. Thirty two percent had arrhythmias. The remainder had some spontaneous breathing effort, but mild enough that it did not interrupt the 15-second EEO. Ten patients were excluded, because they triggered the ventilator during occlusion. Responders to volume expansion were defined as those with an increase in cardiac index of at least 15%. Twenty-three patients were responders. An increase in arterial pulse pressure or cardiac index of at least 5% during EEO was both sensitive and specific for volume responsiveness, as was an increase in cardiac index of at least10% with PLR.

Because the duration of the EEO in this experiment encompassed several cardiac cycles, determination of fluid responsiveness would perhaps be independent from cardiac arrhythmias. Patients with spontaneous breathing were included, as long as they did not trigger the ventilator during the test.

This appears to be a new and novel test for volume responsiveness with several advantages. It is simple to perform, and can be used in patients with arrhythmias and those with some spontaneous respiratory effort. As yet, it only has been demonstrated in one small study, and needs further validation, but it does offer promise as a useful clinical tool.

Valsalva Maneuver

The physiologic response to the Valsalva maneuver is complex, but its main hemodynamic effect is to impair venous return to the right ventricle by rapidly increasing intrathoracic pressure. If both ventricles are preload-dependent (ie, on the steep part of the Frank-Starling curve), LV SV, and hence cardiac output, should decrease. In this way, the Valsalva maneuver theoretically could be used, like PLR, as a reversible gauge of preload dependency.

Garcia and colleagues tested this hypothesis on 30 spontaneously breathing, nonintubated patients in a mixed ICU. Patients with arrhythmias were excluded, as were those who could not achieve at least 20 cm H_2O of airway pressure. Cardiac outputs and SVs were measured via FloTrac (Edwards LifeSciences) sensor attached to an arterial line.[50] PPV and SPV were measured during a 10-second Valsalva maneuver, and after a 500 mL colloid bolus. Responders were classified as those with an increase in SV index of at least 15% after the fluid bolus. A threshold PPV during Valsalva of 52% predicted fluid responsiveness with a sensitivity and specificity of 91% and 95% respectively. For a cutoff SPV of 30%, sensitivity was 73% and specificity

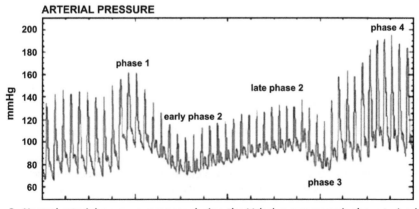

Fig. 3. Normal arterial pressure response during the Valsalva maneuver is characterized by a sinusoidal pattern due to a fall in arterial pressure during phase 2 and overshot during phase 4. (*From* Garcia S, Cano A, Monrove J. Arterial pressure changes during the Valsalva maneuver to predict fluid responsiveness in spontaneously breathing patients. Intensive Care Med 2009;35:77–84; with permission.)

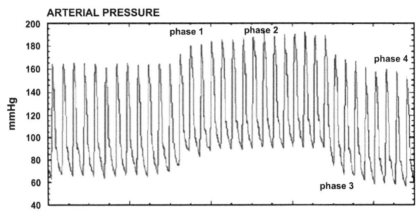

Fig. 4. Abnormal arterial response is characterized by absence of decreased pulse pressure during phase 2, producing the typical square wave pattern. (*From* Garcia M, Cano A, Monrove J. Arterial pressure changes during the Valsalva maneuver to predict fluid responsiveness in spontaneously breathing patients. Intensive Care Med 2009;35:77–84; with permission.)

79%. The authors conclude that the arterial pressure response to a 10-second Valsava maneuver could be a useful clinical tool to measure preload responsiveness in spontaneously ventilating patients.

There are limitations to this study. Study patients were deemed to need fluid based on hypotension, tachycardia, or oliguria. No data were presented on urine output, but the average SBP before Valsalva or fluid was nearly 130, mean arterial pressure 90, and heart rate 83 beats per minute. These data would not trigger fluid administration in most ICUs. Although there were statistically significant differences between responders and nonresponders with respect to SPV with Valsalva, there remained considerable overlap between the two groups. Proper interpretation of the measurements required measuring PPV during early phase 2 of the Valsalva response (**Figs. 3 and 4**). Although the Valsalva maneuver is relatively simple and noninvasive, and may easily be performed at the bedside,[51] it requires active cooperation of the patient. Ultimately, the ability to accurately assess preload responsiveness in nonintubated patients would be of great use, and the concept deserves further exploration.

SUMMARY

Dynamic indices repeatedly have been shown to be superior to static measures for determining preload responsiveness in critically ill patients. The number of options for assessing fluid responsiveness available to the clinician is increasing; however, few have been evaluated in large, multicenter trials. Currently there are no data on whether managing patients using dynamic indices affects outcomes. It is important to remember that preload responsiveness does not equate to needing more preload. Healthy individuals are preload-responsive, and will increase their cardiac output in response to a fluid challenge, but they do not require increased blood volume. Therefore even with accurate measures of preload responsiveness, clinical judgment remains essential.

REFERENCES

1. Monnet X, Rienzo M, Osman D, et al. Passive leg raising predicts fluid response in the critically ill. Crit Care Med 2006;34(5):1402–7.

2. Lafanechere A, Pene F, Goulenok C, et al. Changes in aortic blood flow induced by passive leg raising predict fluid responsiveness in critically ill patients. Crit Care 2006;10(5):R132.

3. Thiel S, Kollef M, Isakow W. Noninvasive stroke volume measurement and passive leg raising predict volume responsiveness in medical ICU patients: an observational cohort study. Crit Care 2009;13:R111.

4. Maizel J, Airapetian N, Lorne E, et al. Diagnosis of central hypovolemia by using passive leg raising. Intensive Care Med 2007;33:1133–8.

5. Michard F, Teboul JL. Predicting fluid responsiveness in ICU patients, a critical analysis of the evidence. Chest 2002;121:2000–8.

6. Marik PE, Baram M, Vahid B. Does the central venous pressure predict fluid responsiveness? A systematic review of the literature and the tale of seven mares. Chest 2008;134:172–8.

7. Osman D, Ridel C, Ray P, et al. Cardiac filling pressures are not appropriate to predict hemodynamic response to volume challenge. Crit Care Med 2007;35:64–8.

8. Bendjelid K, Romand JA. Fluid responsiveness in mechanically ventilated patients: a review of indices used in intensive care. Intensive Care Med 2003; 29:352–60.

9. Vincent JL, Weil MH. Fluid challenge revisited. Crit Care Med 2006;34(5):1333–7.

10. Libby P, Bonow RO, Mann DL, et al. Braunwald's heart disease: a textbook of cardiovascular medicine. 8th edition. Philadelphia (PA): Saunders, Elsevier; 2008.

11. Cavallaro F, Sandroni C, Antonelli M. Functional hemodynamic monitoring and dynamic indices of fluid responsiveness. Minerva Anestesiol 2008;74:123–35.

12. Michard F. Changes in arterial pressure during mechanical ventilation. Anesthesiology 2005;103:419–28.

13. Reuter DA, Felbinger TW, Schmidt C, et al. Stroke volume variation for assessment of cardiac responsiveness to volume loading in mechanically ventilated patients after cardiac surgery. Intensive Care Med 2002;28:392–8.

14. Wiesenak C, Prasser C, Rodig G, et al. Stroke volume variation as an indicator of fluid responsiveness using pulse contour analysis in mechanically ventilated patients. Anesth Analg 2003;96:1254–7.

15. Pinsky MR. Probing the limits of arterial pulse contour analysis to predict preload responsiveness. Anesth Analg 2003;96:1245–7.

16. Rick JJ, Burke SS. Respiratory paradox. South Med J 1978;71:1376–8.

17. Preisman S, Kogan S, Berkenstadt H, et al. Predicting fluid responsiveness in patients undergoing cardiac surgery: functional hemodynamic parameters including the Respiratory Systolic Variation Test and static preload indicators. Br J Anaesth 2005;95:746–55.

18. Tavernier B, Robin E, Granet F. Inspiratory increases in systolic blood pressure ("Delta-up") and pulse pressure are not equivalent. Anesthesiology 2008;109: 934–5.

19. Pizov R, Ya'ari Y, Perel A. The arterial pressure waveform during acute ventricular failure and synchronized external chest compression. Anesth Analg 1989;68: 150–6.

20. Preisman S, DiSegni E, Vered Z, et al. Left ventricular preload and function during graded hemorrhage and retransfusion in pigs: analysis of arterial pressure waveform and correlation with echocardiography. Br J Anaesth 2002;88:716–8.

21. Michard F, Boussat S, Chemla D, et al. Relation between respiratory changes in arterial pulse pressure and fluid responsiveness in septic patients with acute circulatory failure. Am J Respir Crit Care Med 2000;162:134–8.

22. Auler JO, Galas F, Jajjar L, et al. Online monitoring of pulse pressure variation to guide fluid therapy after cardiac surgery. Anesth Analg 2008;106:1201–6.
23. Tavernier B, Makhotine O, Leguffe G, et al. Systolic pressure variation as a guide to fluid therapy in patients with sepsis-induced hypotension. Anesthesiology 1998;89:1313–21.
24. Kubitz JC, Forkl S, Annecke T, et al. Systolic pressure variation and pulse pressure variation during modifications of arterial pressure. Intensive Care Med 2008;34:1520–4.
25. Shelley KH. Photoplethysmography: beyond the calculation of arterial oxygen saturation and heart rate. Anesth Analg 2007;105:S31–6.
26. Partridge BL. Use of pulse oximetry as a noninvasive indicator of intravascular volume status. J Clin Monit 1987;3:263–8.
27. Cannesson M, Besnard C, Durand PG, et al. Relation between respiratory variations in pulse oximetry plethysmographic waveform amplitude and arterial pulse pressure in ventilated patients. Crit Care 2005;9:R562–8.
28. Wyffels PAH, Durnez PJ, Helderweirt J, et al. Ventilation-induced plethysmographic variations predict fluid responsiveness in ventilated postoperative cardiac surgery patients. Anesth Analg 2007;105:448–52.
29. Feissel M, Teboul JL, Merlani P, et al. Plethysmographic dynamic indices predict fluid responsiveness in septic ventilated patients. Intensive Care Med 2007;33:993–9.
30. Lansverk SA, Hoiseth LO, Kvandal P, et al. Poor agreement between respiratory variation in pulse oximetry photoplethysmographic waveform amplitude and pulse pressure in intensive care unit patients. Anesthesiology 2008;109:849–55.
31. Vignon P. Evaluation of fluid responsiveness in ventilated septic patients: back to venous return. Intensive Care Med 2004;30:1699–701.
32. Feissel M, Michard F, Faller JP, et al. The respiratory variation in inferior vena cava diameter as a guide to fluid therapy. Intensive Care Med 2004;30:1834–7.
33. Feihl F, Broccard AF. Interactions between respiration and systemic hemodynamics. Part I: basic concepts. Intensive Care Med 2009;35(1):45–54.
34. Barbier C, Loubieres Y, Jardin F, et al. Author's reply to the comment by Dr. Bendjelid. Intensive Care Med 2004;30:1848.
35. Barbier C, Loubieres Y, Schmit C, et al. Respiratory changes in inferior vena cava diameter are helpful in predicting fluid responsiveness in ventilated septic patients. Intensive Care Med 2004;30:1740–6.
36. Vieillard-Baron A, Chergui K, Rabiller A, et al. Superior vena caval collapsibility as a gauge of volume status in ventilated septic patients. Intensive Care Med 2004; 30:1734–9.
37. Nouira S, Elatrous S, Dimassi S, et al. Effects of norepinephrine on static and dynamic preload indicators in experimental hemorrhagic shock. Crit Care Med 2005;33:2339–43.
38. Huang CC, Fu JY, Huu HC, et al. Predition of fluid responsiveness in acute respiratory distress syndrome patients ventilated with low tidal volume and high positive end-expiratory pressure. Crit Care Med 2008;36:2810–6.
39. De Backer D, Taccone FS, Holsten R, et al. Influence of respiratory rate on stroke volume variation in mechanically ventilated patients. Anesthesiology 2009;100: 1092–7.
40. Rutlen DL, Wackers F, Zaret B. Radionuclide assessment of peripheral intravascular capacity: a technique to measure intravascular volume changes in the capacitance circulation in man. Circulation 1991;64(1):146–52.
41. Gaffney F, Bastian B, Thai E, et al. Passive leg raising does not produce a significant or sustained autotransfusion effect. J Trauma 1982;22(3):190–3.

42. Jabot J, Teboul JL, Richard C, et al. Passive leg raising for predicting fluid responsiveness: importance of the postural change. Intensive Care Med 2009; 35:85–90.
43. Monnet X, Teboul JL. Passive leg raising. Intensive Care Med 2008;34:659–63.
44. Boulain T, Achard J, Teboul J, et al. Changes in BP induced by passive leg raising predict response to fluid loading in critically ill patients. Chest 2002;121:1245–52.
45. Antonelli M, Azoulay E, Bonten M, et al. Year in Review in Intensive Care Medicine, 2007. III. Ethics and legislation, health services, research, pharmacology and toxicology, nutrition and paediatrics. Intensive Care Med 2008;34(4): 598–609.
46. Kumar A, Anel R, Bunnell, et al. Pulmonary artery occlusion pressure and central venous pressure fail to predict ventricular filling volume, cardiac performance, or the response to volume infusion in normal subjects. Crit Care Med 2004;32: 691–9.
47. Perel A, Minkovich L, Preisman S, et al. Assessing fluid responsiveness by a standardized ventilatory maneuver: the respiratory systolic variation test. Anesth Analg 2005;100:942–5.
48. Reuter D, Bayerlein J, Goepfert M, et al. Influence of tidal volume on left ventricular stroke volume variation measured by pulse contour analysis in mechanically ventilated patients. Intensive Care Med 2003;29:476–80.
49. Monnet X, Osman D, Ridel C, et al. Predicting volume responsiveness by using the end-expiratory occlusion in mechanically ventilated intensive care unit patients. Crit Care Med 2009;37(3):951–6.
50. Garcia M, Cano A, Monrove J. Arterial pressure changes during the Valsalva maneuver to predict fluid responsiveness in spontaneously breathing patients. Intensive Care Med 2009;35:77–84.
51. Rehberg S, Ertmer C, Westphal M. Valsalva, Valsava, may you give me a clue, who needs fluids in my ICU? Intensive Care Med 2009;35:7–8.

Optimizing Hemodynamic Support in Septic Shock Using Central and Mixed Venous Oxygen Saturation

Supriya Maddirala, MD, Akram Khan, MD*

KEYWORDS

- Central venous blood gas • Mixed venous blood gas
- Sepsis • Septic shock

Severe sepsis (acute organ dysfunction secondary to infection) and septic shock (severe sepsis plus hypotension not reversed with fluid resuscitation) are major health care problems, affecting millions of individuals around the world each year, killing one in four patients (and often more), and increasing in incidence.[1] Sepsis represents a continuum from an inciting infectious event and host-pathogen interaction to the hemodynamic consequences caused by the relationship among proinflammatory, anti-inflammatory, and apoptotic mediators and is associated with circulatory insufficiency from hypovolemia, myocardial depression, increased metabolic rate, and vasoregulatory perfusion abnormalities eventually leading to an imbalance between tissue oxygen supply and demand, causing global tissue hypoxia.[2] Studies have shown a tendency for increased oxygen consumption (Vo_2) with an increased tissue oxygen extraction during initial hypodynamic or normodynamic circulation.[3] Later in the hyperdynamic circulation, when cardiac output and systemic oxygen delivery (Do_2) are augmented therapeutically to 50% to 80% above normal values, an associated elevation of global Vo_2 may be seen.[3] In nonsurvivors, oxygen extraction may be impaired at supranormal values of Do_2 in the presence of peripheral tissue hypoxia.[4] The presence of elevated blood lactate concentrations suggests tissue hypoxia and indicates continued impairment of Vo_2 with supranormal Do_2.[3] Autopsy data on patients have failed to reveal the cause of death in patients with sepsis. Necrosis

Divisions of Nephrology, Pulmonary and Critical Care, Department of Internal Medicine, Oregon Health and Science University, 3181 Southwest Sam Jackson Park Road, Portland, OR 97239, USA
* Corresponding author.
E-mail address: khana@ohsu.edu

Crit Care Clin 26 (2010) 323–333
doi:10.1016/j.ccc.2009.12.006
0749-0704/10/$ – see front matter © 2010 Elsevier Inc. All rights reserved.

criticalcare.theclinics.com

and apoptosis are quite rare in organs of patients with sepsis on autopsy except in the lymphocytes and gastrointestinal epithelial cells.[5] Prolonged global tissue hypoxia is one of the major causes of multisystem organ dysfunction (MODS).[6] In septic shock patients, tissue oxygen saturation below 78% has been shown to be associated with increased mortality at day 28.[7] Early hemodynamic optimization is associated with lower mortality and optimization efforts have a lower chance of success once MODS has set in.[8,9] Hemodynamic assessment using clinical signs and symptoms, central venous pressure (CVP), and urinary output can fail to detect early septic shock and early markers of global tissue hypoxia can help detect and treat sepsis and potentially prevent MODS.[10,11]

VENOUS OXYGEN SATURATION PHYSIOLOGY

Oxygen saturation of the venous blood can be measured either at the level of the pulmonary artery: mixed venous oxygen saturation (Svo_2), the level of the inferior vena cava, superior vena cava, or right atrium (RA): central venous oxygen saturation ($Scvo_2$). Although hemodynamic assessment using clinical signs and symptoms, CVP, and urinary output can fail to detect early septic shock, tissue hypoxia suggested by $Scvo_2$ or Svo_2, and arterial blood lactate concentration can be an early marker of sepsis or marginal circulation (**Table 1**).[10,11] It is important, however, to remember that venous oxygen saturation like cardiac output is a marker of global tissue hypoxia and does not yield information on oxygen reserves or adequate tissue oxygenation of individual organs. Normal or even supernormal Svo_2 levels can coexist with severe tissue hypoxia or impaired mitochondrial use in such conditions as hepatic failure or severe sepsis leading to arteriovenous shunting. This can limit the interpretation of absolute Svo_2 values as indicators of tissue oxygenation.[12] This is also possible in conditions disturbing the unloading of oxygen from hemoglobin through a leftward shift of the oxygen dissociation curve or blockage of the respiratory chain, such as in cyanide poisoning.[12] Based on the Fick principle,[13] both $Scvo_2$ and Svo_2 depend on the balance between arterial oxygen delivery (Do_2) and tissue oxygen consumption (Vo_2) (**Box 1**).[14] $Scvo_2$ and Svo_2 provide an indication of the degree of oxygen extracted by the organs before the blood returns to the right heart and hence gives a measure of the balance between Do_2 and Vo_2, providing an indication of the ability of the cardiac output to meet the individual's oxygenation needs. As shown in **Fig. 1**, changes in oxygen saturation (Sao_2),[15] Vo_2,[16] cardiac output,[17] or hemoglobin[16] can change oxygen extraction ratio and $Scvo_2$ and Svo_2. In pathologic situations, Svo_2 is dependent on complex interactions between these four interdependent factors all of which can be potentially altered by varying degrees of pathology and treatment (eg, an increase in cardiac output can compensate for a fall in hemoglobin from hemorrhagic

Table 1 Causes of high and low Svo_2 & $Scvo_2$	
High Svo_2 & $Scvo_2$	**Low Svo_2 & $Scvo_2$**
Late sepsis/post–cardiac arrest/cytopathic hypoxia	Early sepsis
Distributive shock	Cardiogenic shock
High cardiac output	Hypovolemia
Hypothermia	
Arteriovenus fistulae	
Cellular poisons	

> **Box 1**
> **Determinants of mixed venous oxygen saturation**
>
> Oxygen consumption (Fick equation) = Vo_2 (mL/min)
>
> $Vo_2 = CO \times (Cao_2 - Cvo_2)$
>
> Where CO = cardiac output, Cao_2 and Cvo_2 = arterial and mixed venous blood O$_2$ content
>
> $Cao_2 = Sao_2 \times 1.34 \, Hb + (Po_2 \times 0.003)$
>
> $Cvo_2 = Svo_2 \times 1.34 \times Hb + (Po_2 \times 0.003)$
>
> Where Sao_2 and Svo_2 = arterial and venous oxygen saturation respectively, Hb = hemoglobin (g/dL)
>
> Po_2 = partial pressure of oxygen, because the dissolved fraction is negligible
>
> $Vo_2 \approx CO \times 1.34 \, Hb \times (Sao_2 - Svo_2)$
>
> $Svo_2 \approx Sao_2 - (Vo_2/CO \times 1.34 \times Hb)$
>
> Thus value of Svo_2 depends on four variables: Vo_2, CO, Sao_2, and Hb.
>
> Arterial oxygen delivery= Do_2 (mL/min)
>
> $Do_2 = CO \times Cao_2$
>
> Oxygen extraction (OE) = Vo_2/ Do_2, replacing values of Vo_2 and Do_2
>
> OE = $(Sao_2 - Svo_2)/ Sao_2$.
>
> If $Sao_2 \approx 100\%$, OE = $1 - Svo_2$
>
> $Svo_2 = 1 - OE = 1 - Vo_2 / Do_2$.
>
> Under normal physiologic values: $Sao_2 = 100\%$, CO = 5 L/min, $Vo_2 = 250$ mL/min and Hb = 15 g/dL
>
> $Svo_2 \approx 75\%$

shock). Global tissue hypoxia leads to increases in tissue oxygen extraction leading to decreases in $Scvo_2$ and Svo_2. When the limits of this compensatory mechanism are reached, anaerobic metabolism ensues leading to an increase in lactate production.[10] Up to 50% of patients resuscitated from shock may have evidence suggestive of continued global tissue hypoxia (ie, increased lactate and decreased $Scvo_2$) even with the normalization of vital signs and CVP.[10] The ability to detect and resolve occult tissue hypoxia early in the course of patient care may have outcome benefit.[9]

Svo$_2$ and Scvo$_2$ Measurement

Venous O$_2$ saturations differ among organ systems because they extract different amounts of oxygen so the absolute value of the measurement depends on the site of measurement. Measurement of both Svo_2 and $Scvo_2$ can be done by repeated venous sampling or by infrared oximetry, which is based on reflection spectrophotometry and the change in color of the red blood cells (RBCs) as their oxygen content gradually decreases. Infrared light is transmitted into the blood, reflected off RBCs, and read by a photo detector. The amount of light reflected at different wavelengths varies depending on the concentration of oxyhemoglobin, desoxyhemoglobin, carboxyhemoglobin, and methemoglobin and is used to generate a value for the Svo_2 and $Scvo_2$.[18] Svo_2 measurement requires the placement of a pulmonary artery catheter (PAC), whereas $Scvo_2$ is measured with a central venous catheter. While Svo_2 is measured at the level of the pulmonary artery, $Scvo_2$ can be measured at the level of the inferior vena cava, superior vena cava, or the RA. The normal range for Svo_2

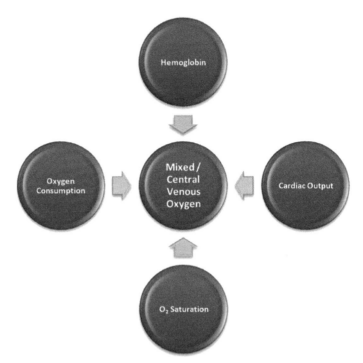

Fig. 1. Factors effecting mixed-central venous oxygen consumption.

is 65% to 75%, whereas $Scvo_2$ is generally 5% to 7% higher than Svo_2 in critically ill patients.[19,20] Although many researchers have found strong correlations between $Scvo_2$ and Svo_2,[20–23] some have suggested that these values do not always agree.[17,19,24–27] Some researchers have concluded that use of $Scvo_2$ is not a reliable surrogate at low oxygen saturations for Svo_2,[19,28,29] whereas others believe that the limits of agreement for repeated measures of $Scvo_2$ and Svo_2 may be narrow enough to allow for continuous monitoring of $Scvo_2$ as a surrogate for Svo_2 in individual patients and help guide resuscitation leading to a decrease in mortality.[9,20,30]

It is difficult to compare and contrast the multiple studies on this topic because they often differ in the number of patients studied, the number and type of comparisons, and the statistical methods used. Most authors agree, however, that $Scvo_2$ and Svo_2 have a strong correlation and are equally clinically useful.[17,27] In the largest study to date Rinehart and colleagues[20] demonstrated that $Scvo_2$ and Svo_2 changed in parallel in 90% of the 1498 instances in which Svo_2 changed more than 5% providing strong support of the clinical use of $Scvo_2$ as a surrogate for Svo_2.

RELATIONSHIP BETWEEN Svo_2 AND $Scvo_2$

Measurement of Svo_2 requires access to blood from the pulmonary artery using the distal port of a PAC or by using a PAC equipped with a fiberoptic infrared sensor. Fiberoptic catheters are also commercially available for the continuous measurement of $Scvo_2$ in the superior vena cava, and can help avoid some of the complications associated with PACs. There is a correlation between both in-vitro and in-vivo Svo_2 and $Scvo_2$ that has been shown in critically ill patients[19,20,23,29] and in animal models.[22] A 5% to 7% step-down from $Scvo_2$ measurements to Svo_2 measurements has been noted in two studies,[19,20] whereas other authors have shown that the difference may be more marked in patients with septic shock.[29] The decrease in Svo$_2$ compared with Scvo$_2$ has been postulated to be caused by myocardial extraction of oxygen as blood flows through the right ventricle, mixing with inferior vena cava blood that has lower oxygen saturation, and mixing of blood emanating from the coronary sinus and thebesian veins.[19] For patients in shock Scvo$_2$ has been shown to be consistently greater than Svo$_2$.[19,28,29] Redistribution of blood flow away from the splenic, renal, and mesenteric bed toward the cerebral and coronary circulation, including more desaturated blood from the coronary sinus, has been suggested to contribute to this observation.[28,29]

CLINICAL USES

Reductions in Scvo$_2$ have been independently associated with postoperative complications with an optimal Scvo$_2$ cutoff value for morbidity prediction of 64.4%.[31] Svo$_2$ less than 65% has been associated with complications in cardiothoracic surgery patients.[32] A fall in Svo$_2$ of more than 5% or a value below 60% predicted a period of hypotension.[32] Svo$_2$ has been shown to have diagnostic, prognostic, and therapeutic use in the treatment of critically ill patients in the medical ICU and in septic shock.[9,33–35] It has also been used in mechanically ventilated patients to determine the optimal level of positive end-expiratory pressure (PEEP) and to assist in weaning from mechanical ventilation.[36,37] In a small study of 15 patients by Suter and colleagues[36] PEEP was adjusted to optimize oxygen transport and static compliance. Svo$_2$ increased between zero PEEP and the PEEP resulting in maximum oxygen transport, but then decreased at higher end-expiratory pressures suggesting that Svo$_2$ can be used to find the optimal PEEP level for patients. In a small trial by Jubran and colleagues,[37] during a spontaneous breathing trial, patients who were successfully extubated had a decrease in cardiac index and oxygen transport, whereas those who failed the trial of spontaneous breathing had an increase in Svo$_2$ caused by an increase in oxygen extraction. The Svo$_2$ was 61.3% $\pm$ 5.8% and 65.4% $\pm$ 1.6%, in the weaning failure and success group, respectively. At the end of the trial, it decreased to 51.5% $\pm$ 7.9% in the failure group, whereas it remained unchanged in the success group suggesting that an increase in Svo$_2$ during the trial of spontaneous breathing may predict weaning failure.

CLINICAL USES OF CENTRAL VENOUS OXYGEN SATURATION MONITORING IN SEPTIC SHOCK

In sepsis and septic shock, global hypoxia is one of the major risk factors in the occurrence of MODS.[6] In a study by Rady and colleagues,[10] 50% of critically ill patients presenting in shock who were resuscitated to normal vital signs continued to have low Scvo$_2$ and increased lactate suggesting tissue hypoxia and anaerobic metabolism. This study led to the clinical use of Scvo$_2$ in early management of cardiac arrest, the postresuscitation period, trauma and hemorrhage, severe heart failure, severe sepsis, and septic shock.[10] Similarly, Scvo$_2$ monitoring during cardiac arrest has been shown to be of diagnostic and therapeutic value.[38,39] In the immediate postresuscitation period of a cardiac arrest, mixed venous hyperoxia has been shown to be associated with poor outcomes. In a study by Rivers and colleagues[4] in a group of 13 patients following cardiac arrest when Svo$_2$ was compared with Do$_2$, nonsurvivors tended to exhibit higher Svo$_2$ than survivors at the lower range of Do$_2$ suggesting an impairment of systemic oxygen use and lower oxygen extraction than survivors.

$Scvo_2$ value less 65%, measured in the first 24 hours after admission in patients with major trauma and head injury, has been shown to be associated with higher mortality and prolonged hospitalization.[40,41] In patients with cardiogenic shock caused by acutely decompensated end-stage chronic congestive heart failure presenting to the emergency department, $Scvo_2$ was significantly lower in patients with high lactic acid levels compared with those with normal lactic acid levels. There were no significant differences in age, ejection fraction, temperature, heart rate, respiratory rate, mean arterial pressure (MAP), CVP, or Killip and New York Heart Association classification among the groups, suggesting that clinical evaluation may fail to identify illness severity of congestive heart failure in a subset of patients and lactic acid and $Scvo_2$ may be helpful in identifying patients with occult cardiogenic shock.[42] Similarly, Svo_2 has been shown to be a better index of effectiveness of dobutamine in patients with congestive heart failure than cardiac index.[43]

A retrospective analysis of 111 patients by Varpula and colleagues[11] showed that the best predictive threshold level for mortality was 65 mm Hg for MAP and 70% for Svo_2 during the first 48 hours. In their study, during standard treatment the most important hemodynamic variables predicting 30-day outcome in septic shock were MAP and lactate for the first 6 hours and MAP, Svo_2, and CVP for the first 48 hours. A randomized controlled trial by Gattinoni and colleagues[44] for the Svo_2 collaborative group compared increasing the cardiac index to a supranormal or increasing mixed venous oxygen saturation to a normal level with a control group. Svo_2 was not shown to have outcome benefit as a goal-directed hemodynamic end point. This study had limitations in that 55% of patients in the cardiac-index group and 33% of those in the mixed venous oxygen-saturation group did not reach or sustained their target values during the 5 days of the study. A subgroup analysis of the patients in whom hemodynamic targets were achieved, also however, did not show a difference in mortality rates.[44] In a study by Rivers and colleagues[9] evaluating early goal-directed therapy (EGDT) using $Scvo_2$, patients presenting with severe sepsis and septic shock were randomized to 6 hours of EGDT or standard therapy before ICU admission. Patients in both groups were resuscitated to a CVP in the range of 8 to 12 mm Hg and MAP greater than 65 mm Hg, but those in the treatment group were also resuscitated to a $Scvo_2$ greater than 70% guided by continuous $Scvo_2$ monitoring. Serial end points of resuscitation, physiologic and organ dysfunction scores, mortality rate, and health care resource consumption were compared during the first 72 hours. In-hospital mortality was 30.5% in the group assigned to EGDT, as compared with 46.5% in the group assigned to standard therapy ($P = .009$). During the interval from 7 to 72 hours, the patients assigned to EGDT had a significantly higher $Scvo_2$ (70.4% $\pm$ 10.7% vs 65.3% $\pm$ 11.4%), a lower lactate concentration (3 $\pm$ 4.4 vs 3.9 $\pm$ 4.4 mmol/L), a lower base deficit (2 $\pm$ 6.6 vs 5.1 $\pm$ 6.7 mmol/L), and a higher pH (7.40 $\pm$ 0.12 vs 7.36 $\pm$ 0.12) than the patients assigned to standard therapy ($P \le .02$ for all comparisons). During the same period, mean APACHE II scores were significantly lower, indicating less severe organ dysfunction in the patients assigned to EGDT than in those assigned to standard therapy (13 $\pm$ 6.3 vs 15.9 $\pm$ 6.4, $P < .001$). This suggests that using $Scvo_2$ as a resuscitation end point in addition to MAP and CVP provides significant outcome benefit for patients with severe sepsis and septic shock over standard therapy. Key differences between the Svo_2 collaborative group and EGDT were the timing of intervention with the enrolling of patients for up to 72 hours after presentation in the Svo_2 collaborative group, whereas EGDT enrolled patients in the first 6 hours of presentation. The Svo_2 collaborative group also had a more diverse population of critically ill patients and had a higher baseline Svo_2 (low 70s) compared with the EGDT group, which had patients with septic shock and lower Scvo$_2$ (high 40s).[9,44] A meta-analysis of hemodynamic optimization trials has also suggested that early, but not late, hemodynamic optimization reduced mortality.[8] Although EGDT has been validated in multiple other prospective trials,[45,46] the use of applying the principles of EGDT outside the single United States urban hospital in which the trial was performed has been questioned.[47] In view of the fact that a few recent trials have shown that incidence of low Scvo$_2$ was uncommon at the time of admission to the ICU, it has been suggested that the EGDT study findings were the result of realignment of limited quality care back to a level considered acceptable elsewhere in the world.[48–50] The answer to this question may only be available once the results of the Australasian Resuscitation In Sepsis Evaluation and the Protocolized Care Early Severe Sepsis trials become available.[47]

BLEEDING

Scvo$_2$ monitoring can be an early indicator of bleeding, estimated blood loss, and may affect the decision to transfuse. In a study of 26 trauma patients, Scalea and colleagues[41] found that the 10 patients who had Scvo$_2$ less than 65% had more serious injuries, significantly larger estimated that losses, and required more transfusions than those patients with Scvo$_2$ greater than 65%. In this study linear regression coefficients showed that Scvo$_2$ was better than heart rate, MAP, CVP, pulse pressure, and urine output in predicting estimated blood loss.

Anemia and Blood Transfusion

Transfusion of RBCs has not, however, shown to increase Vo$_2$ in critically ill patients.[51–53] This may be related to multiple factors including storage time, increased endothelial adherence of stored RBCs, nitric oxide binding by free hemoglobin in stored blood, donor leukocytes, host inflammatory response, or reduced red cell deformability.[54] It has also been suggested that transfusion may hamper right ventricular ejection by increasing the pulmonary vascular resistance index.[53] A restrictive strategy of RBC transfusion, with hemoglobin concentrations of 7 to 9 mg/dL, was found to be at least as effective and possibly superior to a liberal transfusion strategy in critically ill patients by Herbert and coworkers.[55] This trial, however, did not specifically address patients with severe sepsis, and septic shock patients with hypovolemia and global tissue hypoxia. Transfusion to keep hematocrit greater than 30% was one of the recommendations of EGDT[9] because hemoglobin is one of the factors that can affect Scvo$_2$ and Svo$_2$. In EGDT volume resuscitation as the initial therapy was sufficient to restore a Scvo$_2$ of greater than 70% in 35.9% of patients. After fluid therapy, RBC transfusion in those patients with a hematocrit less than 30% was successful in allowing an additional 50.4% of the patients to attain a Scvo$_2$ of greater than 70%. In those patients who met volume resuscitation and hematocrit goals, inotropic therapy was required in the remainder of patients (13.7%) to reach a Scvo$_2$ of greater than 70%.[2] Microvascular alterations play a role in the development of MODS in severe sepsis. It has been shown in a small trial that sublingual microcirculation is globally unaltered by RBC transfusion in septic patients; however, it can improve in patients with altered capillary perfusion at baseline.[56]

CENTRAL VENOUS-TO-ARTERIAL CARBON DIOXIDE DIFFERENCE

Venous-to-arterial carbon dioxide (CO$_2$) difference, calculated with mixed venous blood sample (P[v-a]CO$_2$), and cardiac index is inversely correlated in case of nonseptic and septic circulatory failure.[57,58] In an animal model increased P(v-a)CO$_2$ was found to be related to the decrease in cardiac output because P(v-a)CO$_2$ was increased in ischemic hypoxia but not in hypoxic hypoxia for the same degree of O_2 supply-dependency.[59] In a recent study by Vallee and colleagues,[60] 89% of the resuscitated septic patients had a $Scvo_2$ larger than 70%. In these patients those with an initial $P(cv-a)CO_2$ lower than 6 mm Hg had a lower lactate concentration and a higher lactate clearance during the next 12 hours and a significant and larger decrease in the Sequential Organ Failure Assessment (SOFA) score on day 1 than patients who presented with an initial $P(cv-a)CO_2$ higher than 6 mm Hg. This suggests that the presence of a high $P(cv-a)CO_2$ value could also be a useful tool to identify patients who remain inadequately resuscitated despite a $Scvo_2$ larger than 70%.

SUMMARY

Global tissue hypoxia is one of the most important factors in the development of MODS. In hemodynamically unstable critically ill patients, $Scvo_2$ and Svo_2 monitoring has been shown to be a better indicator of global tissue hypoxia than vital signs and other clinical parameters alone. Svo_2 and $Scvo_2$, although not identical, are functionally equivalent. Svo_2 is probably more representative of global tissue oxygenation, whereas $Scvo_2$ is less invasive. Svo_2 values are an average of 5% to 7% lower than $Scvo_2$ values and the changes in these two parameters correlate. Svo_2 and $Scvo_2$ monitoring can have diagnostic and therapeutic uses in understanding the efficacy of interventions in treating critically ill, hemodynamically unstable patients.

REFERENCES

1. Dellinger RP, Levy MM, Carlet JM, et al. Surviving sepsis campaign: international guidelines for management of severe sepsis and septic shock: 2008. Crit Care Med 2008;36(1):296–327.
2. Otero RM, Nguyen HB, Huang DT, et al. Early goal-directed therapy in severe sepsis and septic shock revisited: concepts, controversies, and contemporary findings. Chest 2006;130(5):1579–95.
3. Edwards JD, Brown GC, Nightingale P, et al. Use of survivors' cardiorespiratory values as therapeutic goals in septic shock. Crit Care Med 1989;17(11):1098–103.
4. Rivers EP, Rady MY, Martin GB, et al. Venous hyperoxia after cardiac arrest: characterization of a defect in systemic oxygen utilization. Chest 1992;102(6):1787–93.
5. Hotchkiss RS, Karl IE. The pathophysiology and treatment of sepsis. N Engl J Med 2003;348(2):138–50.
6. Marshall JC. Inflammation, coagulopathy, and the pathogenesis of multiple organ dysfunction syndrome. Crit Care Med 2001;29(Suppl 7):S99–106.
7. Leone M, Blidi S, Antonini F, et al. Oxygen tissue saturation is lower in nonsurvivors than in survivors after early resuscitation of septic shock. Anesthesiology 2009;111(2):366–71.
8. Kern JW, Shoemaker WC. Meta-analysis of hemodynamic optimization in high-risk patients. Crit Care Med 2002;30(8):1686–92.
9. Rivers E, Nguyen B, Havstad S, et al. Early goal-directed therapy in the treatment of severe sepsis and septic shock. N Engl J Med 2001;345(19):1368–77.
10. Rady MY, Rivers EP, Nowak RM. Resuscitation of the critically ill in the ED: responses of blood pressure, heart rate, shock index, central venous oxygen saturation, and lactate. Am J Emerg Med 1996;14(2):218–25.
11. Varpula M, Tallgren M, Saukkonen K, et al. Hemodynamic variables related to outcome in septic shock. Intensive Care Med 2005;31(8):1066–71.

12. Bauer P, Reinhart K, Bauer M. Significance of venous oximetry in the critically ill. Med Intensiva 2008;32(3):134–42.
13. Fick A. Über die messung des blutquantums in den herzventrikeln. Verh Phys Med Ges Würzburg 1870;2:16–28.
14. Reinhart K, Bloos F. The value of venous oximetry. Curr Opin Crit Care 2005;11(3): 259–63.
15. Ho KM, Harding R, Chamberlain J. The impact of arterial oxygen tension on venous oxygen saturation in circulatory failure. Shock 2008;29(1):3–6.
16. Van der Linden P, Gilbart E, Engelman E, et al. Effects of anesthetic agents on systemic critical O2 delivery. J Appl Phys 1991;71(1):83–93.
17. Yazigi A, El Khoury C, Jebara S, et al. Comparison of central venous to mixed venous oxygen saturation in patients with low cardiac index and filling pressures after coronary artery surgery. J Cardiothorac Vasc Anesth 2008;22(1):77–83.
18. Rivers EP, Ander DS, Powell D. Central venous oxygen saturation monitoring in the critically ill patient. Curr Opin Crit Care 2001;7(3):204–11.
19. Chawla LS, Zia H, Gutierrez G, et al. Lack of equivalence between central and mixed venous oxygen saturation. Chest 2004;126(6):1891–6.
20. Reinhart K, Kuhn HJ, Hartog C, et al. Continuous central venous and pulmonary artery oxygen saturation monitoring in the critically ill. Intensive Care Med 2004; 30(8):1572–8.
21. Ladakis C, Myrianthefs P, Karabinis A, et al. Central venous and mixed venous oxygen saturation in critically ill patients. Respiration 2001;68(3):279–85.
22. Reinhart K, Rudolph T, Bredle DL, et al. Comparison of central-venous to mixed-venous oxygen saturation during changes in oxygen supply/demand. Chest 1989;95(6):1216–21.
23. Tahvanainen J, Meretoja O, Nikki P. Can central venous blood replace mixed venous blood samples? Crit Care Med 1982;10(11):758–61.
24. Dueck MH, Klimek M, Appenrodt S, et al. Trends but not individual values of central venous oxygen saturation agree with mixed venous oxygen saturation during varying hemodynamic conditions. Anesthesiology 2005;103(2):249–57.
25. Pieri M, Brandi LS, Bertolini R, et al. [Comparison of bench central and mixed pulmonary venous oxygen saturation in critically ill postsurgical patients]. Minerva Anestesiol 1995;61(7–8):285–91 [in Italian].
26. Ho KM, Harding R, Chamberlain J, et al. A comparison of central and mixed venous oxygen saturation in circulatory failure. J Cardiothorac Vasc Anesth 2008. [Epub ahead of print].
27. Kopterides P, Bonovas S, Mavrou I, et al. Venous oxygen saturation and lactate gradient from superior vena cava to pulmonary artery in patients with septic shock. Shock 2009;31(6):561–7.
28. Lee J, Wright F, Barber R, et al. Central venous oxygen saturation in shock: a study in man. Anesthesiology 1972;36(5):472–8.
29. Scheinman MM, Brown MA, Rapaport E. Critical assessment of use of central venous oxygen saturation as a mirror of mixed venous oxygen in severely ill cardiac patients. Circulation 1969;40(2):165–72.
30. Rivers E. Mixed vs central venous oxygen saturation may be not numerically equal, but both are still clinically useful. Chest 2006;129(3):507–8.
31. Pearse R, Dawson D, Fawcett J, et al. Changes in central venous saturation after major surgery, and association with outcome. Crit Care 2005;9(6):R694–9.
32. Krauss XH, Verdouw PD, Hughenholtz PG, et al. On-line monitoring of mixed venous oxygen saturation after cardiothoracic surgery. Thorax 1975;30(6): 636–43.

33. Birman H, Haq A, Hew E, et al. Continuous monitoring of mixed venous oxygen saturation in hemodynamically unstable patients. Chest 1984;86(5):753–6.

34. Krafft P, Steltzer H, Hiesmayr M, et al. Mixed venous oxygen saturation in critically ill septic shock patients: the role of defined events. Chest 1993;103(3):900–6.

35. Heiselman D, Jones J, Cannon L. Continuous monitoring of mixed venous oxygen saturation in septic shock. J Clin Monit 1986;2(4):237–45.

36. Suter PM, Fairley B, Isenberg MD. Optimum end-expiratory airway pressure in patients with acute pulmonary failure. N Engl J Med 1975;292(6):284–9.

37. Jubran A, Mathru M, Dries D, et al. Continuous recordings of mixed venous oxygen saturation during weaning from mechanical ventilation and the ramifications thereof. Am J Respir Crit Care Med 1998;158(6):1763–9.

38. Snyder AB, Salloum LJ, Barone JE, et al. Predicting short-term outcome of cardiopulmonary resuscitation using central venous oxygen tension measurements. Crit Care Med 1991;19(1):111–3.

39. Nakazawa K, Hikawa Y, Saitoh Y, et al. Usefulness of central venous oxygen saturation monitoring during cardiopulmonary resuscitation: a comparative case study with end-tidal carbon dioxide monitoring. Intensive Care Med 1994;20(6):450–1.

40. Di Filippo A, Gonnelli C, Perretta L, et al. Low central venous saturation predicts poor outcome in patients with brain injury after major trauma: a prospective observational study. Scand J Trauma Resusc Emerg Med 2009;17(1):23.

41. Scalea TM, Hartnett RW, Duncan AO, et al. Central venous oxygen saturation: a useful clinical tool in trauma patients. J Trauma 1990;30(12):1539–43.

42. Ander DS, Jaggi M, Rivers E, et al. Undetected cardiogenic shock in patients with congestive heart failure presenting to the emergency department. Am J Cardiol 1998;82(7):888–91.

43. Teboul JL, Graini L, Boujdaria R, et al. Cardiac index vs oxygen-derived parameters for rational use of dobutamine in patients with congestive heart failure. Chest 1993;103(1):81–5.

44. Gattinoni L, Brazzi L, Pelosi P, et al. A trial of goal-oriented hemodynamic therapy in critically ill patients. SvO2 Collaborative Group. N Engl J Med 1995;333(16):1025–32.

45. Jones AE, Focht A, Horton JM, et al. Prospective external validation of the clinical effectiveness of an emergency department-based early goal-directed therapy protocol for severe sepsis and septic shock. Chest 2007;132(2):425–32.

46. Micek ST, Roubinian N, Heuring T, et al. Before-after study of a standardized hospital order set for the management of septic shock. Crit Care Med 2006; 34(11):2707–13.

47. Bellomo R, Reade MC, Warrillow SJ. The pursuit of a high central venous oxygen saturation in sepsis: growing concerns. Crit Care 2008;12(2):130.

48. van Beest PA, Hofstra JJ, Schultz MJ, et al. The incidence of low venous oxygen saturation on admission to the intensive care unit: a multi-center observational study in The Netherlands. Crit Care 2008;12(2):R33.

49. Ho BC, Bellomo R, McGain F, et al. The incidence and outcome of septic shock patients in the absence of early-goal directed therapy. Crit Care 2006;10(3):R80.

50. ARISE, ANZICS APD Management Committee. The outcome of patients with sepsis and septic shock presenting to emergency departments in Australia and New Zealand. Crit Care Resusc 2007;9(1):8–18.

51. Gramm J, Smith S, Gamelli RL, et al. Effect of transfusion on oxygen transport in critically ill patients. Shock 1996;5(3):190–3.

52. Shah DM, Gottlieb ME, Rahm RL, et al. Failure of red blood cell transfusion to increase oxygen transport or mixed venous PO2 in injured patients. J Trauma 1982;22(9):741–6.

53. Fernandes CJ Jr, Akamine N, De Marco FV, et al. Red blood cell transfusion does not increase oxygen consumption in critically ill septic patients. Crit Care 2001; 5(6):362–7.
54. Napolitano LM, Corwin HL. Efficacy of red blood cell transfusion in the critically ill. Crit Care Clin 2004;20(2):255–68.
55. Hebert PC, Wells G, Blajchman MA, et al. A multicenter, randomized, controlled clinical trial of transfusion requirements in critical care. Transfusion Requirements in Critical Care Investigators, Canadian Critical Care Trials Group. N Engl J Med 1999;340(6):409–17.
56. Sakr Y, Chierego M, Piagnerelli M, et al. Microvascular response to red blood cell transfusion in patients with severe sepsis. Crit Care Med 2007;35(7):1639–44.
57. Mecher CE, Rackow EC, Astiz ME, et al. Venous hypercarbia associated with severe sepsis and systemic hypoperfusion. Crit Care Med 1990;18(6):585–9.
58. Bakker J, Vincent JL, Gris P, et al. Veno-arterial carbon dioxide gradient in human septic shock. Chest 1992;101(2):509–15.
59. Neviere R, Chagnon JL, Teboul JL, et al. Small intestine intramucosal PCO(2) and microvascular blood flow during hypoxic and ischemic hypoxia. Crit Care Med 2002;30(2):379–84.
60. Vallee F, Vallet B, Mathe O, et al. Central venous-to-arterial carbon dioxide difference: an additional target for goal-directed therapy in septic shock? Intensive Care Med 2008;34(12):2218–25.

The Optimal Hematocrit

Louise Harder, MD[a],*, Lynn Boshkov, MD[b]

KEYWORDS

• Blood transfusion • Hematocrit • Hemoglobin • Anemia

Blood transfusion has been a mainstay of medical therapy for vast numbers of patients worldwide for several decades. Nearly 15 million units of packed red blood cells (RBCs) and whole blood are transfused annually in the United States alone.[1] Until recently, the major risks from blood transfusion were thought to be transmission of viral infections, and overall blood transfusion was believed by most providers to be safe. Corwin and colleagues[2] demonstrated in 1995 that blood transfusion in the intensive care unit (ICU) was common, and often without clear indication.

In 1999 Hebert and colleagues[3] published the landmark TRICC (Transfusion Requirements In Critical Care) trial, a multicenter, randomized controlled clinical trial that demonstrated that a restrictive transfusion strategy was not only safe, but in certain patients possibly beneficial. Much work has been done since that time to further the understanding of the pathophysiological effects of red cell transfusion, but there is still a lack of clear guidelines for transfusion of packed red blood cells (PRBCs) in settings other than the actively hemorrhaging patient.[4]

Current guidelines recommend a transfusion threshold hemoglobin level between 7 and 8 g/dL in noncritically ill patients.[4] A notable exception are recommendations for transfusion during early sepsis,[5] based largely on the study by Rivers and colleagues[6] demonstrating improved outcomes in septic patients with early and aggressive measures to improve oxygen delivery.

Animal and human studies suggest that although certain patients may tolerate very low hemoglobin levels, anemia in others may be harmful. However, it is not clear at what level of hemoglobin, and in what patients, transfusion is beneficial.

The notion that transfusing RBCs will acutely increase tissue oxygenation in sepsis is predicated on several assumptions: first, that tissue and cellular oxygenation are inadequate; second, that RBC transfusion improves tissue oxygen availability; third, that cells will be able to use the delivered oxygen; and lastly, that the benefit of transfusing the red cells outweighs the risk to the individual patient.[7]

[a] Department of Pulmonary and Critical Care Medicine, Oregon Health and Sciences University, OHSU-UHN-67, 3181 SW Sam Jackson Park Road, Portland, OR 97239, USA
[b] Department of Pulmonary and Critical Care Medicine Hemostasis & Thrombosis Service, Transfusion Medicine, Oregon Health & Sciences University, OHSU L471, 3181 SW Sam Jackson Park Road, Portland, OR 97239, USA
* Corresponding author.
E-mail address: harderl@ohsu.edu

Crit Care Clin 26 (2010) 335–354
doi:10.1016/j.ccc.2010.01.002
0749-0704/10/$ – see front matter © 2010 Elsevier Inc. All rights reserved.

criticalcare.theclinics.com

Increasing hemoglobin concentration by transfusion increases global oxygen delivery as measured by systemic variables, but little is known about whether transfusion provides an increase in the oxygen delivery to tissue at the microvascular level.[8]

PRINCIPLES OF OXYGEN TRANSPORT

All cells require oxygen for aerobic metabolism to maintain normal cellular function. Because oxygen cannot be stored in the cells, a constant supply that matches the metabolic needs of each cell is required.[9] Oxygen itself is poorly soluble in water and plasma, and is transported to tissues via hemoglobin.

There are four critical steps in the chain of oxygen transport: (1) delivery of oxygen to the lung; (2) diffusion into the blood, where it binds rapidly and reversibly to hemoglobin within the RBC; (3) transportation to the various tissues of the body by blood flow; and (4) diffusion down a concentration gradient into the tissue, and ultimately to the mitochondria of each cell.[9–11]

Oxygen demand differs markedly between and within specific organs.[12] Oxygen delivery is matched to local need by adjustments of vascular tone in the macro- and microcirculation,[13] which are under the control of autonomic signals and local metabolic stimuli.[11–13] These regulatory mechanisms are still not well understood, and even in the presence of regional cellular hypoxia, an increase in systemic oxygen delivery may not result in greater oxygen availability to the cell.[13] Once delivered, oxygen diffusion into the tissue is determined by the oxygen tension gradient between the blood and the tissue.[14,15]

Systemic oxygen delivery (DO_2) is dependent on cardiac output (CO) and arterial oxygen content (CaO_2)[10,13,14]:

$$DO_2 = CO \times CaO_2$$

Arterial oxygen content is the sum of hemoglobin-bound and dissolved oxygen.[10]

$$CaO_2 = (Hb)(1.34)(SaO_2) + (0.0031)(PaO_2)$$

where 1.34 is the amount of oxygen carried by 1 g of hemoglobin, Hb is the hemoglobin concentration (grams per 100 mL), SaO_2 is the arterial oxygen saturation, 0.0031 is the solubility of oxygen in the plasma, and PaO_2 is the partial pressure of oxygen in the blood.

Under normal physiologic conditions, dissolved oxygen in plasma and cells contributes minimally to the total oxygen content of the blood.[10,12] In nonanemic patients with a hemoglobin level of 14 g/dL and breathing room air, less than 2% of the arterial oxygen content is dissolved in the plasma. By contrast, in a severely anemic patient with a hemoglobin level of 5 g/dL and breathing 100% oxygen, 20% of the total arterial oxygen is dissolved in the plasma.[16,17]

At the cellular level tissue oxygenation is in part determined by the oxyhemoglobin dissociation curve.[12,18] The characteristic sigmoid shape of the oxyhemoglobin dissociation curve results from a complex interaction between hemoglobin subunits reflecting a nonlinear affinity for oxygen binding.[14] This binding affinity may be altered by pH, temperature, and RBC 2,3-diphosphoglycerate (2,3-DPG) levels.[17]

In health, the amount of oxygen delivered to the whole body exceeds resting oxygen requirements by a factor of two- to fourfold.[17] In a normal resting adult at sea level, DO_2 is approximately 1000 mL/min based on a cardiac output of 5 L/min, a hemoglobin level of 15 g/100 mL, and SaO_2 of 100%.[9] Under these conditions only about 25% (250 mL/min) of the oxygenated hemoglobin will be deoxygenated, providing a large physiologic reserve.[14,19] This ratio of oxygen consumption (VO_2) to DO_2 is termed the oxygen extraction ratio.[20]

As hemoglobin levels fall, oxygen consumption remains unchanged until a critical DO_2 ($DO_{2(crit)}$) is reached, where cardiac output and oxygen extraction compensation can increase no further, and oxygen consumption (VO_2) begins to drop.[21] In other words, VO_2 is limited by demand above critical DO_2 and by supply below it.[20,21]

In animal studies of euvolemic hemodilution, it has been shown that the hemoglobin level corresponding to $DO_{2(crit)}$ is approximately 3 to 3.5 g/dL.[22] This level is similar in healthy humans.[23] Of note, the microcirculation, where oxygen is delivered, is carefully regulated to a hematocrit of 12% to 15%, which corresponds to the above $DO_{2(crit)}$.[18]

CAUSES OF TISSUE HYPOXIA

Tissue hypoxia can be caused by decreased DO_2 from decreased hemoglobin concentrations (anemic hypoxia), decreased cardiac output (stagnant hypoxia), or low hemoglobin saturation (anoxic hypoxia).[11,17] A fourth term, cytopathic hypoxia, was coined by Fink.[24] Cytopathic hypoxia refers to a state of cellular hypoxia whereby generation of adenosine triphosphate (ATP) by means of aerobic metabolism is limited not by the availability of oxygen, but by alterations in the cellular elements needed to perform oxidative phosphorylation; this is believed to be the prevalent form of hypoxia in sepsis.[10] Anoxic hypoxia can also be related to abnormalities in oxyhemoglobin dissociation and the ability of the RBC to traverse the microcirculation.[10,17]

MEASUREMENT OF TISSUE OXYGENATION

Shock is the point at which $DO_{2(crit)}$ is reached and cellular respiration is compromised.[18] Clinical evaluation is frequently used at the bedside to assess shock. Commonly used markers include pulse rate, blood pressure, skin temperature, and urine output. These markers are unreliable, can be slow to change in the setting of acute shock, and may become apparent only in later stages of shock.[9,10,12] Laboratory markers such as base deficit, serum lactate, anion gap, and pH are also used to monitor impaired tissue oxygenation. Although these measurements have been shown to be predictive of poor outcome, increased mortality, and multiple organ failure, they are global measures that may obscure the presence of significant changes in oxygen uptake in individual organs.[9,10,12,25,26]

In sepsis there is marked variation in tissue oxygenation, and systemic oxygenation parameters often do not reflect local tissue oxygen levels.[27] Two recent studies in septic patients demonstrated that global parameters of hemodynamics and oxygenation had no correlation with measured changes in microvascular perfusion or tissue saturation.[26,28]

Determination of adequacy of tissue oxygenation ideally requires local organ measurements,[12] but at present there are few clinical techniques to directly monitor tissue oxygen levels or quantify tissue oxygen consumption[27] Methods such as gastric tonometry and near-infrared spectroscopy (NIRS) have been developed, and although promising, none has yet been validated for widespread clinical use.[9,16]

Measured CaO_2 and cardiac output are commonly used to assess global DO_2. Errors in measurements are common, especially in critically ill patients.[29] The accepted error of cardiac output measured by thermodilution is approximately 10%.[30] However, this error tends to be larger at extremely high or low values, such as those commonly observed in patients with septic or hypovolemic shock, respectively.[29] When pulmonary artery catheter-derived measured are used according to the inverse Fick method, both oxygen delivery and oxygen consumption use measurements of cardiac output and arterial oxygen content in their calculation. By a phenomenon known as mathematical coupling, this calculation may create the impression that cardiac output and oxygen consumption are positively correlated across a wide range of values.[10] Previous studies have suggested that in critically ill patients, interventions that increase DO_2 also appear to increase VO_2, creating a more linear relationship between DO_2 and VO_2 than that seen in healthy subjects. This "oxygen supply dependency," however, is highly artificial and confounded by mathematical coupling.[29,31] In studies in which VO_2 has been measured independently by indirect calorimetry, the apparent supply dependency is not seen.[10]

Mixed venous (or central venous) oxygen saturations are used clinically to monitor systemic DO_2, with the assumption that low levels imply inadequate oxygen supply. Central venous oxygen saturation is a recommended marker for evaluating adequacy of resuscitation in early sepsis.[5,6] Oxygen content in a mixed or central venous blood sample is a blood flow–weighted average of venous oxygen content of different organs,[9] making it an insensitive marker of tissue hypoxia in individual organs.[12] Blood transfusion increases mixed venous oxygen saturation, but may have no effect on tissue oxygenation. Stored erythrocytes tightly bind oxygen so mixed venous oxygen levels will be higher, even though tissue oxygenation may be unchanged.[18] Therefore, despite current recommendations,[5] mixed venous oxygen saturation is actually a poor indicator of tissue anoxia.[8]

Blood lactate levels are also commonly used clinically for monitoring systemic DO_2.[9,17] An elevated lactate implies inadequate tissue oxygenation and conversion to anaerobic metabolism. However, regional tissue hypoxia can be significant in the presence of normal lactate levels.[9]

PHYSIOLOGIC RESPONSE TO ACUTE ANEMIA

As long as euvolemia is maintained, normal physiologic compensatory mechanisms allow most critically ill patients to tolerate anemia surprisingly well.[14,18] There are few data regarding how the normal physiologic adaptive responses are affected by various disease states,[11] but presumably compensatory mechanisms are less effective in people who are ill or elderly.[16,20]

With acute normovolemic anemia, the reduction in arterial oxygen content is compensated for by (1) increasing the cardiac output, (2) altering the distribution of blood flow between and within organs, and (3) altering the amount of oxygen extracted from the blood.[16,18,21,32] When the capacity of these compensatory mechanisms is exhausted, tissue injury occurs.[12]

At first, compensation for the decreased oxygen content appears to be almost exclusively flow dependent. Cardiac output increases and systemic vascular resistance decreases.[33] The increase in cardiac output initially is mainly due to reduced blood viscosity, which improves the flow properties of blood.[11,14,21] Increased heart rate and contractility occur, but the exact mechanisms are unclear.[11]

As oxygen content decreases with progressive hemodilution, microcirculatory changes take place, leading to a recruitment of capillaries.[20] The red cell capillary transit time increases, allowing more time from gas exchange. In addition, anemia changes the oxygen extraction ratio from the erythrocyte itself by increasing red cell 2,3-DPG and shifting the oxyhemoglobin dissociation curve to the right, allowing increased oxygen release to the tissues.[10,11,18,20,21]

LIMITS OF ACUTE ANEMIA TOLERANCE

Animal studies have consistently demonstrated that healthy animals tolerate acute, isovolemic hemodilution to 5 g/dL without adverse consequences.[34–36] Further hemodilution results in cardiac ischemia and decreased oxygen uptake.[34,35] When hemoglobin levels drop below 3 g/dL there is increased lactate production, decreased left ventricular function and cardiac output, and increased risk of death.[32,36] In healthy humans, the critical hemoglobin level is unknown but is likely less than 5 g/dL.[16,33]

Young, healthy humans have consistently been shown to tolerate acute isovolemic hemodilution without symptoms until hemoglobin reaches 7 g/dL. Below that level subjects have demonstrated increases in heart rate and subjective decreased energy levels.[37] Subtle deficits in cognitive function begin to appear at a hemoglobin level of 6 g/dL; at 5 g/dL immediate and delayed memory are impaired,[38] heart rate and stroke volume increase, and systemic vascular resistance decreases. In one study, two of 32 healthy adults acutely hemodiluted to 5 g/dL developed asymptomatic, reversible ST changes on electrocardiography (ECG).[32] These nominal changes reversed immediately with transfusion to raise the hemoglobin level to 7 g/dL.[16,39]

Weiskopf and colleagues[39] made the interesting observation that the deterioration of neurocognitive function after isovolemic hemodilution from a hemoglobin of 12.7 $\pm$ 1.0 to 5.7 $\pm$ 0.3 was reversed by increasing PaO_2 from around 100 to 400 mm Hg. This value is equivalent to an increase in hemoglobin concentration of roughly 3 g/dL.[20] Similar results have been found in animal studies.[33]

Patients who refuse blood for religious reasons have given researchers the opportunity to observe outcomes in extreme anemia. In a case-control study of 125 such patients, postoperative mortality was inversely related to the preoperative hemoglobin level, rising from 7.1% for patients with levels above 10 g/dL to 61.5% for those with levels below 6 g/dL.[40] Viele and Weiskopf reviewed case reports of Jehovah's Witnesses who refused blood perioperatively, and found that all patients whose deaths were attributed to anemia had a hemoglobin level 5 g/dL or lower.[41]

Carson and colleagues, in a retrospective cohort study of surgical patients who refused blood, reported no deaths in patients, with nadir hemoglobin between 7.1 and 8.0 g/dL. Mortality for those with hemoglobin between 6.1 and 7.0 was 8.9%, and rose to 100% for patients with a hemoglobin level below 2.0 g/dL. Mortality rose sharply for those with hemoglobin less than 5.0 g/dL. Adjusted for age, cardiovascular disease and APACHE II score, the odds ratio for death for each gram decrease in hemoglobin below 7.0 was 2.1 (95% confidence interval, 1.7–2.6). The investigators reported increased morbidity for patients with hemoglobin below 7 g/dL, but this was not compared with patients with similar hemoglobin levels who received blood.[42]

ANEMIA AND THE HEART

Brain tissue and cardiac muscle extract much more oxygen from the blood than other tissues. Cerebral oxygen extraction can increase significantly in response to acute anemia.[11,20] The heart, on the other hand, is much more vulnerable to the effects of anemia.[20,34,43,44]

At rest the heart extracts 60% to 75% of all oxygen delivered to the coronary circulation.[11,20,34] Consequently, if oxygen delivery is decreased due to low arterial oxygen content, the only way for the myocardium to maintain adequate oxygen delivery is by increasing coronary artery flow.[20,33,34]

An early response to acute anemia is an increase in cardiac output, via both tachycardia and increased stroke volume, which increases myocardial oxygen requirements. Because the myocardium relies on increased coronary blood flow as a means to compensate for an acute decrease in CaO_2,[20] patients with coronary artery disease would seem to be at higher risks for adverse effects due to anemia. Indeed, studies in both animals and humans have suggested that individuals with cardiovascular disease are less tolerant of anemia.[45]

Animals with experimentally induced coronary stenosis demonstrate ST segment changes or locally depressed cardiac function at hemoglobin levels in the range of 7.0 to 10 g/dL, much higher than in animals with healthy coronary vessels.[20,35,46] In humans, the clinical data are inconclusive. Patients with coronary artery disease have tolerated mild to moderate normovolemic hemodilution without showing any increase in cardiac complications or silent ischemia during ECG monitoring.[43,47,48] However these subjects were otherwise stable patients undergoing elective hemodilution.

In a cohort study of critically ill patients, patients with cardiovascular disease had a trend toward an increased mortality when hemoglobin values were less than 9.5 g/dL (55% vs 42%, $P = .09$) compared with anemic patients with other diagnoses. Increasing hemoglobin values with transfusion of RBCs in these patients was associated with improved survival (odds ratio [OR] = 0.80 for each 1 g/dL increase, $P = .012$).[49] Rao and colleagues,[50] however, retrospectively pooled data from 3 large observational clinical trials on 24,112 patients with acute coronary syndromes. After adjustment for baseline characteristics and nadir hematocrit, these investigators found an increased risk of death in transfused patients. Gerber,[51] in a subgroup analysis of the TRICC trial, concluded that a restrictive RBC transfusion strategy is generally safe in most critically ill patients with cardiovascular disease, with the possible exception of patients with acute myocardial infarcts and unstable angina.

These studies were observational and retrospective, and in the Rau study the original trials from which the data was obtained were not designed to evaluate transfusion thresholds. While informative, these studies are hypothesis generating only.[50]

Anemic patients with coronary artery disease appear to be at increased risk of cardiac ischemia. However, with the exception of acute ST-elevation myocardial infarction, there are few data to show that transfusing RBCs improves outcomes.[52] Despite this, some investigators recommend maintaining higher hemoglobin levels in patients with cardiovascular disease.[14,52] Others recommend transfusing only when signs of inadequate myocardial oxygen supply start to develop.[20]

Two trials evaluating transfusion thresholds in patients with cardiovascular disease are currently ongoing. The FOCUS trial is a multicenter randomized trial of patients with cardiovascular disease undergoing hip surgery. Patients will either have postoperative hemoglobin levels kept above 10 g/dL, or be transfused only when symptomatic from anemia. Results are expected to be published next year.[53] The CRIT pilot trial will evaluate the effect of liberal versus restrictive transfusion strategy on outcome of anemic patients within 72 hours of myocardial infarction.[54]

RED CELL PHYSIOLOGY

RBCs are now considered as much more than just innocuous little packets of hemoglobin.[55] When oxygen content falls, red cells can regulate blood flow by releasing mediators like nitric oxide (NO)[56,57] and ATP, which can induce local vasodilation.[27,55,57,58] Hemoglobin itself may act as a tissue oxygen sensor.[27]

After a life span of 120 days, RBCs are removed from the circulation by macrophages, primarily in the spleen. This process may also occur in other microvascular networks that become obstructed by aged red cells.[59] Various signals can induce the exposure of epitopes on RBCs that indicate senescence; these epitopes are recognized by naturally occurring autoantibodies, initiating complement-dependent phagocytosis of aged or oxidatively stressed erythrocytes.[60]

Until recently, mature erythrocytes were not thought to be capable of undergoing apoptosis because the cells lack mitochondria and nuclei. However, it has now been shown that RBCs can undergo programmed cell death in response to oxidative stress. Therefore, oxidative stress due to critical illness may shorten RBC life span.[60]

RBCs are highly deformable, and as such are capable of passing through capillaries with diameters much smaller than their own.[55,59] This flexibility is a critical factor in ensuring microvascular function as well as ensuring efficient oxygen uploading in the lungs and offloading in the tissue.[59] Maintenance of red cell deformability depends on interactions between the outer plasma membrane and the underlying protein cytoskeleton.[60] Increases in intracellular hemoglobin, loss of biconcave shape, decreased erythrocyte ATP, or increased intracellular Ca^{2+} can all cause decreased RBC deformability.[60,61] The mechanisms are complex and only partially understood.[59–62]

The RBC membrane contains glycolytic enzymes, and is capable of synthesizing 2,3-DPG and ATP.[56] Alterations in the RBC membrane could therefore not only change cell shape and malleability but also alter RBC biochemistry.[55]

In critically ill patients, especially in sepsis, RBCs undergo structural and functional changes that are similar to those in naturally aged erythrocytes[55,60] RBC membrane components are modified, resulting in changed cell shape, decreased deformability,[63] and increased red cell aggregation.[17,55,62,64–66] These changes have been implicated in alteration of microvascular hemodynamics with a concomitant decrease in oxygen use and increased tissue ischemia.[59,62]

Inflammation may alter RBCs, and they in turn may affect the inflammatory response. Erythrocytes can bind opsonized immune complexes, restricting immune complex uptake and degranulation by macrophages. Oxidatively damaged RBCs can increase tumor necrosis factor (TNF)-α and interleukin (IL)-10 production by monocytes. Thus, inflammation appears to cause functional and structural changes in RBCs, but these altered RBCs can themselves modulate the immune response.[60]

BLOOD AND THE MICROCIRCULATION

The microcirculation is where oxygen diffusion takes place, and consists of all vessels smaller than 100 μm, including arterioles, capillaries, and venules.[27,55] Local microcirculatory control mechanisms, although poorly understood, are important in the maintenance and restoration of tissue oxygenation.[27]

Blood viscosity is an important regulator of blood flow.[18] Blood viscosity in turn depends on the concentration of cells, the ability of cells to aggregate and deform, and on plasma viscosity.[61] Of these, the hematocrit is the most important.[67] Blood viscosity is inversely related to flow, so that for a given vessel diameter an increase in hematocrit will reduce blood flow exponentially.[61] Very low hemoglobin concentrations impair the delivery of oxygen to tissues; paradoxically, a moderate decrease in hematocrit might improve oxygen transport by lowering blood viscosity.[33,60,61,68]

However, maintenance of blood viscosity is important in maintaining microvascular perfusion.[69] Increasing blood viscosity increases shear stress, which increases endothelial release of nitric oxide, resulting in local vasodilation. Experimentally, restoration of blood rheological properties improves resuscitation independently of any improvement in oxygen-carrying capacity.[70] Beneficial effects of blood transfusions may therefore be in part due to the increase or restoration of blood viscosity.[59]

THE STORAGE LESION

In the United States the average age of RBCs transfused in the critically ill is 21 days.[2,10,71,72] When stored, RBCs undergo several well-documented biologic and mechanical changes known as the "storage lesion." In 1997 Purdy and colleagues[73] first reported a correlation between increased age of transfused blood and increased mortality. Despite millions of transfusions since then, the clinical consequences of the storage lesion remain uncertain and controversial.[17,74]

A red cell normally contains 20 to 25 μmol of 2,3-DPG, which shifts the oxyhemo-globin dissociation curve to the right, allowing hemoglobin to release oxygen.[17,59] Erythrocyte 2,3-DPG levels begin to decline shortly after collection, and are near zero within 48 to 72 hours.[13,18,25,27,59,75] Therefore transfused cells are able to oxygenate well as they pass through the lungs, but in principle are unable to release oxygen to the tissue unless the tissue oxygen tension is very low.[8,10,18] Within several hours after transfusion 2,3-DPG levels begin to increase, and gradually return to normal by 24 hours after transfusion.[8,27,76]

Erythrocyte deformability is an energy-dependent process,[59] sustained by intracel-lular catabolism of glucose and generation of high-energy ATP.[17] RBC ATP levels drop with storage,[74,77] but it is not clear at what level RBC deformability is affected. Within the first 2 weeks after collection, erythrocytes begin to change shape and lose flexi-bility.[78] The RBC membrane loses proteins and phospholipids, and cells change from supple biconcave discs to stiff echinocytes and spherocytes.[17] When viewed under an electron microscope, these abnormal cells account for as much as 80% of the cell population at 3 weeks, and more than 95% by 35 days.[8,79] Such cells, when transfused, become trapped in the microvasculature[80,81] or are eliminated by the reticuloendothelial system.

In the normal erythrocyte, ATP stimulates NO production by endothelial cells. Trans-fusion of ATP-depleted RBCs may lead to decreased NO production and increased vascular resistance.[59] Similarly, erythrocyte S-nitrosohemoglobin concentrations have been noted to decline rapidly after red cell storage, decreasing the ability to locally control vasodilation.[82]

Within several hours of transfusion, ATP levels in viable cells are restored by uptake of adenosine from the plasma.[27] With prolonged storage time, however, a high percentage of cells will be irreversibly deformed and no longer viable.[17,79]

These misshapen cells exhibit increased osmotic fragility, releasing free hemoglobin into the plasma.[18,19,27,74,79] Free hemoglobin levels in stored cells increase signifi-cantly over time.[83] Free hemoglobin scavenges NO, even in very low concentrations, resulting in local and systemic vasoconstriction.[8,18,27,84]

Hemoglobin is a profound oxidizer and is highly toxic to endothelial cells. Endothelial cells pinocytose free hemoglobin, which leads to endothelial cell dysfunction exhibited as reperfusion injury and oxidative stress. Such cells, rather than being naturally anti-inflammatory, become proinflammatory and highly thrombotic.[18]

RBC storage increases RBC-endothelial interactions,[85] which are further increased by endotoxins and inflammatory cytokines.[17,86] A unique interaction between the RBC storage lesion and an injured microcirculation in sepsis might explain the inability to demonstrate improved tissue oxygenation after RBC transfusion in sepsis.[7]

Stored erythrocytes exhibit increased aggregation and adhesiveness,[74,79] and this increases with storage time.[18,79] The mechanism for this is unclear. Sialic acid main-tains a negative charge on the cell surface, and it has been hypothesized that decreased membrane sialic acid contributes to the aggregation.[74,79]

Storage Medium

In addition to alterations in the RBCs themselves, changes to the storage medium also occur. With time there is a progressive decrease in pH, increase in potassium, accumulation of cytokines (IL-1, IL-8, TNF),[72] and accumulation of other bioreactive substances such as histamine, soluble lipids, lysophosphatidylcholine.[74]

Studies

Together, the well-recognized changes to stored RBCs could decrease the benefit of transfusion, and possibly cause harm. Several animal studies have evaluated the clinical effect of red cell storage, with mixed results.[8,77,87,88]

Observational and retrospective studies in humans have shown age of transfused red cells to be associated with splanchnic ischemia,[25] increased risk of infection,[89–93] multiorgan failure,[94] increased hospital or ICU length of stay,[95,96] and mortality.[73,93,96] Weinberg and colleagues,[97] in their recently conducted retrospective cohort study to evaluate the association between the age of transfused blood and mortality among trauma patients, found that large volumes of transfused blood were associated with increased mortality and that the effect was potentiated with older blood. However, a large observational trial by van de Watering and colleagues[98] found no association between a prolonged storage time and increased mortality or longer stay in the ICU.

A recent literature review was inconclusive. The majority of studies analyzed were single-center with small sample size, and patient populations were heterogeneous, making it difficult to compare studies.[74]

There are limited randomized controlled trials evaluating the clinical effects of red cell storage. In mechanically ventilated, critically ill patients, Walsh and colleagues[99] compared packed RBCs of age 5 days or less versus 20 days or older, and found no difference in gastric pH or in global indices of tissue oxygenation. In a pilot trial to evaluate the feasibility of maintaining a supply of fresh blood, Hebert and colleagues[72] found no differences in major clinical outcomes between fresh and older blood.

At the microvascular level, Kiraly and colleagues,[100] using NIRS, found that transfusing old blood into trauma patients worsened microvascular oxygenation. Weiskopf and colleagues[101] showed that transfusion of "fresh" (mean age 3.5 ± 0.4 hours) and "old" (mean age 23 ± days) autologous erythrocytes to increase the hemoglobin level from 5 to 7 g/dL equally reversed neuropsychological deficits in acutely hemodiluted healthy volunteers.

Although theoretically and potentially harmful, it is difficult to determine from the currently available published data whether there is a relationship between the age of transfused RBCs and outcome in critically ill patients.[74]

TRANSFUSION-RELATED IMMUNOMODULATION

Although not definitively proven in randomized controlled trials, allogeneic blood transfusions have long been known to have immunosuppressive effects. Transfusion-related immunomodulation, or TRIM, refers to the proinflammatory and immunomodulatory laboratory findings and clinical effects of blood transfusion.[102,103]

In 1973 Opelz and colleagues showed improved survival in renal allograft recipients who had received blood. In the early 1980s, renal transplant recipients were often transfused prior to transplant to decrease rejection.[104] This practice fell out of favor with the recognition of AIDS as a significant risk of transfusion.[102]

Although TRIM is a widely acknowledged effect of blood transfusion, the exact clinical consequences remain uncertain. Observational studies show a strong correlation between blood transfusion and nosocomial infection,[4,14,105] but a causal effect has not yet been proven.[106] Other effects seen in observational studies include a reduced risk of Crohn's recurrence, decreased risk of spontaneous abortion in mothers who share human leukocyte antigen (HLA) antigens with the father, increased risk of activation of latent cytomegalovirus or human immunodeficiency virus infection, increased risk of cancer recurrence, and increased risk of multiple organ failure and all-cause mortality.[102]

Infection

Several observational studies in humans have linked packed red cell transfusion with nosocomial infection.[4,18,102,107–110] In a meta-analysis of such trials by Hill and colleagues,[111] the overall OR for transfusion and postoperative bacterial infection was 3.45 (range 1.43–15.15).

Recently, Taylor and colleagues[4] performed a large prospective, observational, cohort study of more than 2000 critically ill patients. Just over 21% received transfusions, with a mean pretransfusion hemoglobin level of 7.6 g/dL. The rate of nosocomial infection in transfused patients was 14.3%, significantly higher than the nosocomial infection rate of 5.8% in the nontransfused group ($P<.0001$). After multivariate logistic regression analysis of possible risk factors including patient age, the total units of RBCs transfused, or the maximum age of RBC units transfused, the number of RBC units transfused was the only significant, independent risk factor for nosocomial infection (OR 1.097, $P = .005$). That is, for every unit of packed cells transfused, the risk of infection increased 9.7%. Although the link appears strong, a definitive causal relationship between red cell transfusion and infection has not yet been established.[4]

Cancer

Animal data and observational studies have linked transfusion of RBCs to increased risk of cancer recurrence. To date there have been 3 randomized controlled trials of allogeneic blood transfusion and cancer recurrence, all in colorectal cancer patients after curative surgical resection, and the results are inconclusive.[102]

Heiss and colleagues[112] found significantly increased recurrent malignancy in colorectal cancer patients who received blood perioperatively at the time of resection. On the other hand, neither Busch and colleagues[113] nor Houbiers and Brand[114] noted increased cancer recurrence with transfusion in similar patient populations.

Vamvakas and Blajchman[102] have speculated that the negative results in the aforementioned studies are at least in part because colorectal cancer is not sufficiently antigenic to render an impairment of host immunity capable of facilitating tumor growth. To date, no randomized controlled trial has enrolled patients with tumors for which the immune response plays a major role, such as skin tumors and certain virus-induced tumors like Kaposi sarcoma and certain lymphomas.[109]

Leukocytes

Which component or components of blood mediates TRIM, and by what mechanism, are unknown.[20,115] Allogeneic blood transfusion has been shown to cause decreased helper T-cell count, decreased helper/suppressor T-lymphocyte ratio, decreased lymphocyte response to mitogens, decreased natural killer cell function, reduction in delayed-type hypersensitivity, defective antigen presentation, suppression of lymphocyte blastogenesis, decreased cytokine (IL-2, interferon-γ) production, decreased monocyte/macrophage phagocytic function, and increased production of anti-idiotypic and anticlonotypic antibodies.[109]

TRIM is thought by many to be mediated mainly by donor white blood cells.[116] Most transfusions currently administered in North America and Western Europe are leukoreduced red cells[117] Leukoreduction removes approximately 99% of the white blood cells present in whole blood, which still leaves approximately 10^6 – 10^9 white cells per unit.[18,118]

Animal models suggest leukocytes as probable causative agents of immunomodulation, but this has not been proven in humans.[103,104] Donor leukocytes may either directly downregulate the recipient's immune function, or indirectly mediate TRIM effects by releasing soluble mediators into the supernatant fluid of RBCs during storage.[109]

Leukocyte-derived soluble mediators are contained in intracellular white blood cell granules, and are released in a time-dependent manner as the leukocytes deteriorate during storage. Concentrations of histamine, eosinophil cationic protein, eosinophil protein X, myeloperoxidase, and plasminogen activator inhibitor-1 increase 3- to 25-fold in the supernatant fluid of packed reds cell between days 0 and 35 of storage.[109] Packed red cell supernatant induces regulatory T cells in recipients, but this is not altered by leukoreduction or prolonged storage. This induction seems to be independent of cytokines and is attenuated with washed red cells, implicating the plasma fraction.[105]

Frietsch and colleagues[106] recently conducted a multicenter, double-blind, randomized controlled trial comparing prestorage leukoreduced autologous blood to nonleukoreduced autologous blood in 1089 patients undergoing elective hip surgery. There was no difference between the 2 groups in postoperative infection rate or hospital length of stay, which argues against leukocyte-released biologic modifiers as a cause of the immunomodulatory effects of blood transfusion.

With the exception of cardiac surgery, the benefit of leukoreduction on overall mortality and on infectious complications is highly debated.[116] In 1998, van de Watering and colleagues[105] performed a randomized controlled trial comparing cardiac surgery patients receiving standard versus leukocyte-reduced allogeneic packed red cells, and found an association between the leukocyte-containing packed red cells and mortality from all causes. These results were confirmed in a repeat trial by the same investigators,[119] and in a similar randomized controlled trial by Boshkov and colleagues.[120]

A recent literature review[103] analyzed 19 randomized controlled trials on the effect of allogeneic leukocytes in transfusions. With the exception of the aforementioned cardiac surgery trials, the results were inconclusive. The mechanism of increased complications with cardiac surgery is uncertain, but the investigators suggest that leukocyte-containing transfusions during and after cardiac surgery add a second insult to the cardiopulmonary bypass procedure induced systemic inflammatory response.

Hebert and colleagues[121] retrospectively examined outcomes of critically ill patients in Canada before and after implementation of universal leukoreduction. These investigators found a small, but statistically significant, decrease in all-cause mortality (6.19% vs 7.03%; $P = .04$.) following universal leukoreduction. There was no significant decrease in infections.

Fergusson and colleagues[122] retrospectively compared outcomes of premature infants in Canada before and after implementation of universal leukoreduction. There was no difference in mortality or in the risk of bacteremia between the 2 study periods, but there was a reduction in bronchopulmonary dysplasia, retinopathy of prematurity, and necrotizing enterocolitis. This result would be consistent with a proinflammatory effect of allogeneic leukocytes.[109] Englehart and colleagues[123] recently performed a retrospective cohort analysis of trauma patients at a large level I trauma center that used only leukoreduced blood between 2002 and 2003. Before 2002, and after 2003, nonleukoreduced blood was standard. Englehart's group found no improvement in outcome in trauma patients receiving leukoreduced blood.

Transfusion-Related Lung Injury

Transfusion-related lung injury, or TRALI, is an increasingly recognized risk of blood transfusion. The estimated prevalence of TRALI is 1 in 5000 units of transfused RBCs.[124] TRALI is characterized by acute onset of severe hypoxemia, bilateral non-cardiogenic pulmonary edema, tachycardia, hypotension, and fever. With supportive care, most patients recover within 48 to 96 hours, but mortality can be as high as 25%.[125]

TRALI remains underrecognized, in part due to the lack of a standardized diagnostic criteria, possible confusion with other causes of acute respiratory failure, and lack of a definitive diagnostic test.[102,124] The National Heart, Lung and Blood Institute working group on TRALI recently presented a common definition of TRALI, and advised consideration of the diagnosis in any patient that develops acute lung injury within 6 hours of transfusion, with no preexisting acute lung injury before transfusion. Alternative causes of acute lung injury do not preclude a diagnosis of TRALI.[126]

The pathophysiology of TRALI is still being elucidated[125] and is likely multifactorial, involving both priming of recipient neutrophils by underlying condition[127] and biologic response modifiers with neutrophil-priming activity in the transfused blood product.[124,125] Most cases occur with blood products containing at least 50 mL of plasma, and TRALI is 17 times more likely with cellular blood products than with fresh frozen plasma. Anti-polymorphonuclear and anti-HLA class I antibodies in donor plasma have been strongly implicated in TRALI,[124] and exclusion of female donor plasma by the UK National Blood Services reduced the onset of acute lung injury from 36% to 21% ($P = .04$) in patients receiving multiple transfusions while undergoing elective repair of a ruptured abdominal aortic aneurysm.[128]

CLINICAL TRIALS

Despite the prevalent use of blood transfusion as a therapy, there have been surprisingly few randomized, controlled trials evaluating its effectiveness.[18]

Hebert's TRICC trial, published in 1999, was the sentinel study that changed transfusion practice. Hebert and colleagues[3] enrolled 838 critically ill patients in a multicenter, randomized controlled trial comparing a restrictive transfusion strategy (maintaining hemoglobin level between 7 and 9 g/dL) to a more liberal one (maintaining hemoglobin level between 10 and 12 g/dL). Not only was the restrictive strategy shown to be safe, but for younger (age <55 years) and less ill patients (APACHE II ≤20), mortality was lower in the restrictive group.

Based largely on the trial by Rivers and colleagues[6] of early goal-directed therapy (EGDT) in sepsis, current guidelines recommend a transfusion threshold of 10 g/dL in septic patients who are apparently oxygen dependent based on central venous oxygen saturation (ScvO$_2$). As pointed out by Jha and Gutierrez,[129] almost 65% of the EGDT subjects received transfusions, despite the fact that basal hematocrit was almost 35%. The intervention group received a large volume of intravenous fluids, resulting in greater hemodilution. According to the Fick principle, SvO$_2$ varies directly with arterial oxygen saturation, cardiac output, and hemoglobin concentration, and inversely with oxygen consumption. Hemodilution-induced decreases in hemoglobin concentration would depress SvO_2, regardless of whether the patients had entered an oxygen supply–dependent state. As discussed earlier in this article, transfusion of red cells could improve oxygen delivery systemically, without actually improving oxygen uptake by the tissues. Furthermore, central venous saturation has not been thoroughly validated as a measure of adequacy of DO_2 but was used in this study as a central end point for resuscitation.[10]

Numerous trials have demonstrated an association between red cell transfusions and infection,[71,107,110,130] multiple organ failure,[94,131] increased ICU and hospital length of stay,[71,95,132] and mortality.[71,73,97,132–134] Unfortunately most of these studies are observational, and cause and effect can only be proven by appropriately powered randomized controlled trials.[18] There are very few randomized controlled trials, other than the TRICC trial, comparing clinical outcomes between transfused and nontransfused patients. However, the sheer bulk of the data implicating transfusions in worsened clinical outcomes is compelling.

The primary goal of RBC transfusion is to improve oxygen delivery to tissues that are presumably oxygen dependent, or near their critical oxygen delivery threshold. Several clinical trials have examined the effect of RBC transfusion on oxygen consumption. In one of the few randomized controlled trials in septic patients, Fernandes and colleagues[135] determined that RBC transfusion did not increase oxygen use, whether indirectly calculated by the Fick method or directly measured by calorimetry. Shah and colleagues[136] found similar results in trauma patients. Suttner and colleagues[137] measured skeletal muscle oxygen tension in postoperative cardiac surgery patients. Transfusion improved systemic oxygen delivery, but had no effect on tissue oxygen tension. Conversely, inspiration of 100% oxygen improved both oxygen delivery and tissue oxygen tension. Walsh and colleagues[99] recently conducted a randomized trial to compare fresh with old blood. Although these investigators found no difference in oxygen uptake between the two, there was also no statistically or clinically significant improvement in any other oxygenation index for either group. In other words, even though the patients' attending physicians felt they would benefit from blood transfusion, objectively they showed no improvement after transfusion. Kiraly and colleagues,[100] using NIRS to measure tissue oxygen saturation in trauma patients, found no improvement with transfusion of fresh blood, and a deterioration of tissue oxygen saturation with blood older than 21 days.

SUMMARY

The concept of a universal transfusion threshold is very appealing. For years physicians used the "10/30" rule, but it is clear that this is no longer a clinically useful value. Most critically ill patients can tolerate much lower hemoglobin levels without adverse effects, but a safe threshold above which red cell transfusion is clearly unnecessary has not been established.[37,38] The ideal would be to identify a "critical hemoglobin concentration"—the point at which compensatory mechanisms for anemia have been maximized and further reduction in hemoglobin would result in compromised cellular metabolism—in individual patients.[21] At present clinicians have neither the technology to detect $DO_{2(crit)}$ nor the knowledge of how near to that level an individual patient might be.[18]

The goal of RBC transfusion is to improve tissue oxygenation; however, transfused red cells may increase oxygen delivery to the tissues without a corresponding increase in oxygen consumption.[118] First, most anemic patients do not have tissue hypoxia unless they also have acute circulatory failure.[13] Second, red cells may not be effective in their role as oxygen transporters, and they are now believed to pose additional risks for critically ill patients.[71]

The best available evidence does not support the use of a single criterion for transfusion. In the absence of acute cardiac ischemia or acute bleeding, hemoglobin levels of 7 to 9 g/dL are well tolerated in the critically ill.[118] The decision to transfuse should be based on thoughtful clinical judgment, on an individual basis.[135,138]

REFERENCES

1. National Blood Data Resource Center. The 2007 National Blood Collection and Utilization Survey Report. Available at: http://www.aabb.org/Content/Programs_and_Services/Data_Center/NBCUS/nbcus.htm. Accessed October 10, 2009.
2. Corwin H, Gettinger A, Pearl R, et al. The CRIT Study: anemia and blood transfusion in the critically ill—current clinical practice in the United States. Crit Care Med 2004;32(1):39–52.
3. Hebert P, Wells G, Blajchman M, et al. A multicenter, randomized, controlled clinical trial of transfusion requirements in critical care. N Engl J Med 1999; 340(6):409–17.
4. Taylor R, Manganero L, O'Brien J, et al. Impact of allogenic packed red blood cell transfusion on nosocomial infection rates in the critically ill patient. Crit Care Med 2002;30(10):2249–54.
5. Dellinger P, Levy M, Carlett J, et al. Surviving Sepsis Campaign: international guidelines for management of severe sepsis and septic shock: 2008. Crit Care Med 2008;36(1):296–327.
6. Rivers E, Nguyen B, Havstad S, et al. Early goal-directed therapy in the treatment of severe sepsis and septic shock. N Engl J Med 2001;345(19):1368–77.
7. Fitzgerald R, Martin C, Dietz G, et al. Transfusing red blood cells stored in citrate phosphate dextrose adenine-1 for 28 days fails to improve tissue oxygenation in rats. Crit Care Med 1997;25(5):726–32.
8. Tsai A, Cabrales P, Intaglietta M. Microvascular perfusion upon exchange transfusion with stored red blood cells in normovolemic anemic conditions. Transfusion 2004;44:1626–34.
9. Huang T. Monitoring oxygen delivery in the critically ill. Chest 2005;128: 554S–60S.
10. Hameed S, Aird W, Cohn S. Oxygen delivery. Crit Care Med 2003;31(Suppl 12): S658–67.
11. Hebert P, Van der Linden P, Biro G. Physiologic aspects of anemia. Crit Care Clin 2004;20:187–212.
12. Sibbald W, Messmer K, Fink M. Roundtable conference on tissue oxygenation in acute medicine, Brussels, Belgium 14-16 March 1998. Intensive Care Med 2000;26:780–91.
13. Van der Linden P, Vincent JL. Effects of blood transfusion on oxygen uptake: old concepts adapted to new therapeutic strategies? Crit Care Med 1997;25(5): 723–4.
14. Desai S, Manji M. Minimum haemoglobin in intensive care. Trauma 2004;6: 187–91.
15. Hsia D. Respiratory function of hemoglobin. N Engl J Med 1998;338(4):239–47.
16. Klein H, Spahn D, Carson J. Red blood cell transfusion in clinical practice. Lancet 2007;370:415–26.
17. Tinmouth A, Fergusson D, Yee I. Clinical consequences of red cell storage in the critically ill. Transfusion 2006;46:2014–27.

18. Spiess B. Red cell transfusions and guidelines: a work in progress. Hematol Oncol Clin North Am 2007;21:185–200.
19. Cabrales P, Tsai A, Intaglietta M. Modulation of perfusion and oxygenation by red blood cell oxygen affinity during acute anemia. Am J Respir Cell Mol Biol 2008;38:354–61.
20. Madjdpour C, Spahn D, Weiskopf R. Anemia and perioperative red blood cell transfusion: a matter of tolerance. Crit Care Med 2006;34(5):S102–8.
21. Morisaki H, Sibbald W. Tissue oxygen delivery and the microcirculation. Crit Care Clin 2004;20:213–23.
22. Torres Filho I, Spiess B, Pittman R, et al. Experimental analysis of critical oxygen delivery. Am J Physiol Heart Circ Physiol 2005;288:H1071–9.
23. Van Woerkens E, Trouwborst A, Lanschot J. Profound hemodilution: what is the critical level of hemodilution at which oxygen delivery-dependent oxygen consumption starts in an anesthetized human? Anesth Analg 1992;75:818–21.
24. Fink M. Cytopathic hypoxia in sepsis. Acta Anaesthesiol Scand Suppl 1997;110:87–95.
25. Marik P, Sibbald W. Effect of stored-blood transfusion on oxygen delivery in patients with sepsis. JAMA 1993;269(23):3024–9.
26. Sakr Y, Chierego M, Piagnerelli M, et al. Microvascular response to red blood cell transfusion in patients with severe sepsis. Crit Care Med 2007;35(7):1639–44.
27. Raat N, Ince C. Oxygenating the microcirculation: the perspective from blood transfusion and blood storage. Vox Sang 2007;93:12–8.
28. Leone M, Blidi S, Antonini F, et al. Oxygen tissue saturation is lower in nonsurvivors than in survivors after early resuscitation of septic shock. Anesthesiology 2009;111:366–71.
29. Walsh T. Recent advances in gas exchange measurement in intensive care patients. Br J Anaesth 2003;91:120–31.
30. Nishikawa T, Dohi H. Errors in the measurement of cardiac output by thermodilution. Journal Canadien d'anesthésie. Can J Anesth 2003;40:142–53.
31. Leach R, Treacher D. The pulmonary physician in critical care—2: oxygen delivery and consumption in the critically ill. Thorax 2002;57:170–7.
32. Weiskopf R, Viele M, Feiner J, et al. Human cardiovascular and metabolic response to acute, severe, isovolemic anemia. JAMA 1998;279:217–21.
33. Priebe H. Hemodilution and oxygenation. Int Anesthesiol Clin 1981;19:237–55.
34. Wilkerson D, Rosen A, Sehgal L, et al. Limits of cardiac compensation in anemic baboons. Surgery 1988;103(6):665–70.
35. Hagl S, Heimisch W, Meisner H, et al. The effect of hemodilution on regional myocardial function in the presence of coronary stenosis. Basic Res Cardiol 1977;72(4):344–64.
36. Neuhof H, Wolf H. Oxygen uptake during hemodilution. Bibl Haematol 1975;41:66–75.
37. Toy P, Feiner J, Viele M, et al. Fatigue during acute isovolemic anemia in healthy, resting humans. Transfusion 2000;40:457–60.
38. Weiskopf R, Kramer J, Viele M, et al. Acute severe isovolemic anemia impairs cognitive function and memory in humans. Anesthesiology 2000;92(6):1646–52.
39. Weiskopf R, Feiner J, Hopf H, et al. Oxygen reverses deficits of cognitive function and memory and increased heart rate induced by acute severe isovolemic anemia. Anesthesiology 2002;96:871–7.
40. Carson J, Spence R, Poses R, et al. Severity of anaemia and operative mortality and morbidity [abstract]. Lancet 1988;331(8588):727–9.

41. Viele M, Weiskopf R. What can we learn about the need for transfusion from patients who refuse blood? The experience with Jehovah's Witnesses [abstract]. Transfusion 2004;34(5):396–401.
42. Carson J, Noveck H, Berlin J, et al. Mortality and morbidity in patients with very low postoperative Hb levels who decline blood transfusion. Transfusion 2002;42:812–8.
43. Spahn D, Schmid E, Seifert B, et al. Hemodilution tolerance in patients with coronary artery disease who are receiving chronic p-adrenergic blocker therapy. Anesth Analg 1996;82:687–94.
44. Carson J, Reynolds R. In search of the transfusion threshold. Hematology 2005;10(Suppl 1):86–8.
45. Tobian A, Ness P, Noveck H, et al. Time course and etiology of death in patients with severe anemia. Transfusion 2009;49(7):1395–9.
46. Levy P, Kim S, Eckel P, et al. Limit to cardiac compensation during acute isovolemic hemodilution: influence of coronary stenosis. Am J Physiol Heart Circ Physiol 1993;265:H340–9.
47. Herregods L, Foubert L, Moerman A, et al. Comparative study of limited intentional normovolaemic haemodilution in patients with left main coronary artery stenosis. Anaesthesia 1995;50(11):950–3.
48. Catoire P, Saada M, Lui N, et al. Effect of preoperative normovolemic hemodilution on left ventricular segmental wall motion during abdominal aortic surgery. Anesth Analg 1992;75:654–9.
49. Hebert P, Wells G, Tweeddale M, et al. Does transfusion practice affect mortality in critically ill patients? Transfusion Requirements in Critical Care (TRICC) Investigators and the Canadian Critical Care Trials Group [abstract]. Am J Respir Crit Care Med 1997;155(5):1618–23.
50. Rao S, Jollis J, Harrington R, et al. Relationship of blood transfusion and clinical outcomes in patients with acute coronary syndromes. JAMA 2004;292(13):1555–62.
51. Gerber D. Transfusion of packed red blood cells in patients with ischemic heart disease. Crit Care Med 2008;36(4):1068–74.
52. Carson J, Terrin M, Magazine J, et al. Transfusion trigger trial for functional outcomes in cardiovascular patients undergoing surgical hip fracture repair (FOCUS). Transfusion 2006;46(12):2192–206.
53. Functional Outcomes in Cardiovascular Patients Undergoing Surgical Hip Fracture Repair (FOCUS). Available at: http://www.clinicaltrials.gov/ct2/show/NCT00071032?term=functional+outcomes+in+cardiovascular+patients&rank=1. Accessed November 3, 2009.
54. Conservative versus liberal red cell transfusion in myocardial infarction trial: the CRIT pilot. Available at: http://www.clinicaltrials.gov/ct2/show/NCT00126334?term=crit&rank=2. Accessed November 3, 2009.
55. Piagnerelli M. The red blood cell: an underestimated actor in alterations of the microcirculation. Crit Care Med 2009;37(3):1158–60.
56. Kleinbongard P, Schulz R, Rassaf T, et al. Red blood cells express a functional endothelial nitric oxide synthase. Blood 2006;107:2943–51.
57. Cao Z, Bell J, Mohanty J, et al. Nitrite enhances RBC hypoxic ATP synthesis and the release of ATP into the vasculature: a new mechanism for nitrite-induced vasodilation. Am J Physiol Heart Circ Physiol 2009;297:H1494–503.
58. Sprague R, Stephenson A, Ellsworth M. Red not dead: signaling in and from erythrocytes. Trends Endocrinol Metab 2007;18:350–5.
59. Cabrales P. Effects of erythrocyte flexibility on microvascular perfusion and oxygenation during acute anemia. Am J Physiol Heart Circ Physiol 2007;293:1206–15.

60. Scharte M, Fink M. Red blood cell physiology in critical illness. Crit Care Med 2003;31(12):S651–7.
61. Voerman H, Groeneveld A. Blood viscosity and circulatory shock. Intensive Care Med 1989;15:72–8.
62. Machiedo G, Zaets S, Berezina T. Trauma-hemorrhagic shock-induced red blood cell damage leads to decreased microcirculatory blood flow. Crit Care Med 2009;37(3):1000–10.
63. Boudjeltia Z, Piagnerelli M, Piro P. Decrease of red blood cell sialic acid membrane content in septic patients. Crit Care 2000;4(Suppl 1):P17.
64. Hurd T, Dasmahapatra K. Rush B: red blood cell deformability in human and experimental sepsis. Arch Surg 1988;123:217–20.
65. Powell R, Machiedo G, Rush B. Oxygen free radicals: effect on red cell deformability in sepsis. Crit Care Med 1991;19:732–5.
66. Hersch M, Bersten AD, Rutledge F, et al. Quantitative evidence of microcirculatory compromise in skeletal muscle of normotensive hyperdynamic septic sheep. Crit Care Med 1989;1:S60.
67. Salazar Vázquez B, Wettstein R, Cabrales P. Microvascular experimental evidence on the relative significance of restoring oxygen carrying capacity vs. blood viscosity in shock resuscitation. Biochim Biophys Acta 2008;1784: 1421–7.
68. Mirhashemi S, Ertefai S, Messmer K, et al. Model analysis of the enhancement of tissue oxygenation by hemodilution due to increased microvascular flow velocity. Microvasc Res 1987;34(3):290–301.
69. Tsai A, Acero C, Nance P, et al. Elevated plasma viscosity in extreme hemodilution increases perivascular nitric oxide concentration and microvascular perfusion. Am J Physiol Heart Circ Physiol 2005;288:H1730–9.
70. Cabrales P, Tsai A, Intaglietta M. Is resuscitation from hemorrhagic shock limited by blood oxygen-carrying capacity or blood viscosity? Shock 2007; 27(4):380–9.
71. Taylor R, O'Brien J, Trottier S, et al. Red blood cell transfusions and nosocomial infections in critically ill patients. Crit Care Med 2006;34:2302–8.
72. Hebert P, Chin-Yee I, Fergusson D, et al. A pilot trial evaluating the clinical effects of prolonged storage of red cells. Anesth Analg 2005;100:1433–8.
73. Purdy R, Tweeddale M, Merrick P. Association of mortality with age of blood transfused in septic ICU patients. Journal canadien d'anesthésie. Can J Anesth 1997;44:1256–61.
74. Lelubre C, Piagnerelli M, Vincent JL. Association between duration of storage of transfused red blood cells and morbidity and mortality in adult patients: myth or reality? Transfusion 2009;49:1384–94.
75. Haradin AR, Weed RI, Reed CF. Changes in physical properties of stored erythrocytes. Transfusion 1969;9:229–35.
76. Heaton A, Keegan T, Holme S. In vivo regeneration of red cell 2,3-diphosphoglycerate following transfusion of DPG-depleted AS-1, AS-3 and citrate phosphate dextrose adenine-1 red cells. Br J Haematol 1989;71:131–6.
77. Raat N, Verhoeven A, Mik E, et al. The effect of storage time of human red cells on intestinal microcirculatory oxygenation in a rat isovolemic exchange model. Crit Care Med 2005;33:39–45.
78. Berezina T, Zaets S, Morgan C. Influence of storage on red blood cell rheological properties. J Surg Res 2002;102:6–12.
79. Hovav T, Yedgar S, Manny N, et al. Alteration of red cell aggregability and shape during blood storage. Transfusion 1999;39:277–81.

80. Simchon S, Jan KM, Chien S. Influence of red cell deformability on regional flow. Am J Physiol 1987;253:H895–903.
81. Doyle M, Walker B. Stiffened erythrocytes augment the pulmonary hemodynamic response to hypoxia. J Appl Physiol 1990;69(4):1270–5.
82. Reynolds J, Ahearn G, Angelo M, et al. S-Nitrosohemoglobin deficiency: a mechanism for loss of physiological activity in banked blood. Proc Natl Acad Sci U S A 2007;104:17058–62.
83. Nishiyama T, Hanaoka K. Hemolysis in stored red blood cell concentrates: modulation by haptoglobin or ulinastatin, a protease inhibitor. Crit Care Med 2001;29:1979–82.
84. Semple J, Freedman J. Leukoreduction just doesn't take away immunogenic leukocytes, it creates an immunosuppressive leukocyte dose. Vox Sang 2002;83:425–7.
85. Luk C, Gray-Statchuk L, Cepinkas G, et al. WBC reduction reduces storage-associated RBC adhesion to human vascular endothelial cells under conditions of continuous flow in vitro. Transfusion 2003;43:151–6.
86. Chin-Yee I, Statchuk L, Milkovich S, et al. Transfusion of red blood cells under shock conditions in the rat microvasculature. Blood 2004;104:2713A.
87. Gonzalez A, Yazici I, Kusza K, et al. Effects of fresh versus banked blood transfusions on microcirculatory hemodynamics and tissue oxygenation in the rat cremaster model. Surgery 2007;141:630–9.
88. Van Bommel J, de Korte G, Lind A, et al. The effect of the transfusion of stored RBCs on intestinal microvascular oxygenation in the rat. Transfusion 2001;41:1515–23.
89. Vamvakas E, Carven J. Transfusion and postoperative pneumonia in coronary artery bypass graft surgery: effect of the length of storage of transfused red cells. Transfusion 1999;39:701–10.
90. Mynster T, Nielsen H. The impact of storage time of transfused blood on postoperative infectious complications in rectal cancer surgery. Scand J Gastroenterol 2000;35:212–7.
91. Offner P, Moore E, Biffl W, et al. Increased rate of infection associated with transfusion of old blood after severe injury. Arch Surg 2002;137:711–7.
92. Leal-Noval S, Jara-Lopez I, Garcia-Garmendia J, et al. Influence of erythrocyte concentrate storage time on postsurgical morbidity in cardiac surgery patients. Anesthesiology 2003;98:815–22.
93. Koch C, Li L, Sessler D, et al. Duration of red-cell storage and complications after cardiac surgery. N Engl J Med 2008;358:12291239.
94. Zallen G, Offner P, Moore E, et al. Age of transfused blood is an independent risk factor for postinjury multiple organ failure. Am J Surg 1999;178:570–2.
95. Keller M, Jean R, LaMorte W, et al. Effects of age of transfused blood on length of stay in trauma patients: a preliminary report. J Trauma 2002;53:1023–5.
96. Basran S, Frumento R, Cohen A, et al. The association between duration of storage of transfused red blood cells and morbidity and mortality after reoperative cardiac surgery. Anesth Analg 2006;103:15–20.
97. Weinberg J, McGwin G, Griffin R, et al. Age of transfused blood: an independent predictor of mortality despite universal leukoreduction. J Trauma 2008;65:279–82.
98. van de Watering L, Lorinser J, Versteegh M, et al. Effects of storage time of red blood cell transfusions on the prognosis of coronary artery bypass graft patients. Transfusion 2006;46:1712–8.
99. Walsh T, McArdle F, McLellan S, et al. Does the storage time of transfused red blood cells influence regional or global indexes of tissue oxygenation in anemic critically ill patients? Crit Care Med 2004;32:364–71.

100. Kiraly L, Underwood S, Differding J, et al. Transfusion of aged packed red blood cells results in decreased tissue oxygenation in critically injured trauma patients. J Trauma 2009;67:29–32.
101. Weiskopf R, Feiner J, Hopf H, et al. Fresh blood and aged stored blood are equally efficacious in immediately reversing anemia-induced brain oxygenation deficits in humans. Anesthesiology 2006;104:911–20.
102. Vamvakas E, Blajchman M. Transfusion-related immunomodulation (TRIM): an update. Blood Rev 2007;21:327–48.
103. Bilgin Y, Brand A. Transfusion-related immunomodulation: a second hit in an inflammatory cascade? Vox Sang 2008;95:261–71.
104. Blajchman M. Transfusion immunomodulation or TRIM: What does it mean clinically? Hematology 2005;10(Suppl 1):208–14.
105. van de Watering L, Hermans J, Houbiers J, et al. Beneficial effects of leukocyte depletion of transfused blood on postoperative complications in patients undergoing cardiac surgery: a randomized clinical trial. Circulation 1998;97:562–8.
106. Frietsch T, Karger R, Scholer M, et al. Leukodepletion of autologous whole blood has no impact on perioperative infection rate and length of hospital stay. Transfusion 2008;48:2133–42.
107. Landers D, Hill G, Wong K, et al. Blood transfusion-induced immunomodulation. Anesth Analg 1996;82:187–204.
108. Shorr A, Duh M, Kelly K, et al. Red blood cell transfusion and ventilator-associated pneumonia: a potential link? Crit Care Med 2004;32:666–74.
109. Vamvakas E, Carven J. RBC transfusion and postoperative length of stay in the hospital or the intensive care unit among patients undergoing coronary artery bypass graft surgery: the effects of confounding factors. Transfusion 2000;40: 832–9.
110. Carson J, Altman D, Duff A, et al. Risk of bacterial infection associated with allogeneic blood transfusion among patients undergoing hip fracture repair. Transfusion 1999;39:694–700.
111. Hill G, Frawley W, Griffith K, et al. Allogeneic blood transfusion increases the risk of postoperative bacterial infection: a meta-analysis. J Trauma 2003;54:908–14.
112. Heiss M, Mempel W, Delanoff C, et al. Blood transfusion-modulated tumor recurrence: first results of a randomized study of autologous versus allogeneic blood transfusion in colorectal cancer surgery. J Clin Oncol 1994;12:1859–67.
113. Busch OR, Hop WC, Hoynck van Papendrecht MA, et al. Blood transfusions and prognosis in colorectal cancer. N Engl J Med 1993;328(19):1372–6.
114. Houbiers J, Brand A. Randomised controlled trial comparing transfusion of leucocyte-depleted or buffy-coat-depleted blood in surgery for colorectal cancer. Lancet 1994;344(8922):573–8.
115. Baumgartner J, Silliman C, Moore E, et al. Stored red blood cell transfusion induces regulatory T cells. J Am Coll Surg 2009;208:110–9.
116. Buddeberg F, Beck Schimmer B, Spahn D. Transfusion-transmissible infections and transfusion-related immunomodulation. Best Pract Res Clin Anaesthesiol 2008;22(3):503–51.
117. Vamvakas E. White-blood-cell-containing allogeneic blood transfusion and postoperative infection or mortality: an updated meta-analysis. Vox Sang 2007;92:224–32.
118. Napolitano L, Corwin H. Efficacy of blood transfusion in the critically ill: does age of blood make a difference? Crit Care Med 2004;32(2):594–5.
119. Bilgin Y, van de Watering L, Eijsman L, et al. Double-blind, randomized controlled trial on the effect of leukocyte-depleted erythrocyte transfusions in cardiac valve surgery. Circulation 2004;109:2755–60.

120. Boshkov L, Furnary A, Morris C. Prestorage leukoreduction of red cells in elective cardiac surgery: results of a double blind randomized controlled trial [abstract 380]. (ASH Annual Meeting Abstracts). Blood 2004;104.

121. Hebert P, Fergusson D, Blajchman M, et al. Clinical outcomes following institution of the Canadian universal leukoreduction program for red blood cell transfusions. JAMA 2003;289:1941–9.

122. Fergusson D, Hebert P, Lee S, et al. Clinical outcomes following institution of universal leukoreduction of blood transfusions for premature infants. JAMA 2003;289:1950–6.

123. Englehart M, Cho S, Morris M, et al. Use of leukoreduced blood does not reduce infection, organ failure, or mortality following trauma. World J Surg 2009;33:1626–32.

124. Boshkov L. Transfusion-related acute lung injury and the ICU. Crit Care Clin 2005;21:479–95.

125. Despotis G, Zhang L, Lublin D. Transfusion risks and transfusion-related proinflammatory responses. Hematol Oncol Clin North Am 2007;21:147–61.

126. Toy P, Popovsky M, Abraham E, et al. Transfusion-related acute lung injury: definition and review. Crit Care Med 2005;33:721–6.

127. Silliman C. The two-event model of transfusion-related acute lung injury. Crit Care Med 2006;34:S124–31.

128. Wright S, Snowden C, Athey S, et al. Acute lung injury after ruptured abdominal aortic aneurysm repair: the effect of excluding donations from females from the production of fresh frozen plasma. Crit Care Med 2008;36:1796–802.

129. Jha V, Gutierrez G. Severe sepsis and septic shock should blood be transfused to raise mixed venous oxygen saturation? Chest 2007;131(4):1267–9.

130. Chang H, Hall G, Geerts W, et al. Allogeneic red blood cell transfusion is an independent risk factor for the development of postoperative bacterial infection. Vox Sang 2000;78:13–8.

131. Moore F, Moore E, Sauaia A. Blood transfusion: an independent risk factor for postinjury multiple organ failure. Arch Surg 1997;132:620–5.

132. Malone D, Dunne J, Tracy K, et al. Blood transfusion, independent of shock severity, is associated with worse outcome in trauma. J Trauma 2003;54: 898–907.

133. Engoren M, Habib R, Zacharias A, et al. Effect of blood transfusion on long-term survival after cardiac operation. Ann Thorac Surg 2002;74:1180–6.

134. Vincent J, Baron J, Reinhart K, et al. Anemia and blood transfusion in critically ill patients. JAMA 2002;288:1499–507.

135. Fernandes C, Akamine N, De Marco F, et al. Red blood cell transfusion does not increase oxygen consumption in critically ill septic patients. Crit Care 2001;5(6): 362–7.

136. Shah D, Gottlieb M, Rahm R, et al. Failure of red blood cell transfusion to increase oxygen transport or mixed venous PO_2 in injured patients. J Trauma 1982;22(9):741–6.

137. Suttner S, Piper S, Kumle B, et al. The influence of allogeneic red blood cell transfusion compared with 100% oxygen ventilation on systemic oxygen transport and skeletal muscle oxygen tension after cardiac surgery. Anesth Analg 2004;99:2–11.

138. Greenwalt T, Buckwalter J, Desforges J, et al. Consensus conference: perioperative red blood cell transfusion. JAMA 1988;260(18):2700–3.

Techniques for Determining Cardiac Output in the Intensive Care Unit

Imran Mohammed, MD, Charles Phillips, MD*

KEYWORDS

- Cardiac output • Intensive care unit • Resuscitation

Despite advances in cardiac monitoring, the thorough, focused physical examination remains an essential part of assessment of cardiovascular function. The physical examination is vital to the initial assessment and resuscitation of the patient and provides impetus for more advanced hemodynamic monitoring. All available data, including that from advanced hemodynamic monitoring, should be evaluated in the context of the physical examination. Serial examinations during treatment yield important information about the patient's cardiovascular state and the response to treatment.

The general appearance of the patient should be noted, to include mental status and level of consciousness before sedation. Vital signs should be reviewed, and trends noted (eg, increases or decreases in heart rate); these should be considered in light of the patient's current therapy. The respiratory examination may be particularly revealing. In the absence of sedation, metabolic acidosis may cause a compensatory tachypnea, which is frequently the first sign of hemodynamic compromise. Cheyne-Stokes pattern of respiration frequently is seen in heart failure (**Fig. 1**). Auscultation of the lungs can reveal rales, particularly at the lung bases, which may be indicative of congestive heart failure (CHF). Skin temperature, capillary refill time, and strength and quality of peripheral pulses can provide important information. Patients with cardiogenic, hypovolemic, or septic shock frequently will have reduced skin temperatures and delayed capillary refill, whereas those with neurogenic shock, or those being treated with vasodilators, frequently have brisk capillary refill.

The characteristics of the arterial pulse should be examined. A low-volume, rapid pulse signifies inadequate perfusion or low cardiac output. A rapid, bounding pulse in the presence of shock suggests vasodilatory shock, treatment with vasodilator chugs, or severe aortic regurgitation. The presence of pulsus paradoxus in

Division of Pulmonary and Critical Care Medicine, Oregon Health and Science University, UHN-67, 3181 Southwest Sam Jackson Park Road, Portland, OR, USA
* Corresponding author.
E-mail address: phillipc@ohsu.edu

Crit Care Clin 26 (2010) 355–364
doi:10.1016/j.ccc.2010.01.004
0749-0704/10/$ – see front matter © 2010 Published by Elsevier Inc.

criticalcare.theclinics.com

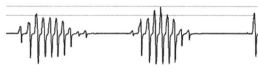

Alternating periods of shallow
and deep breathing.

Fig. 1. Cheyne-Stokes respiration. An abnormal type of breathing characterized by alternating periods of shallow and deep breathing.

a spontaneously breathing patient may be a reflection of severe obstructive lung disease or of cardiac tamponade. Diminished pulse volume and blood pressure after initiation of positive pressure ventilation may suggest hypovolemia. Water-hammer pulse (bounding and forceful) and Quincke' sign (pulsation of the capillary bed in the nail) can reveal the presence of severe aortic insufficiency.

Assessment of neck veins, while frequently confounded in severely ill patients can provide useful information. The height of neck veins and the qualities of the venous pulsations can provide information regarding ventricular function, intravascular volume status, pulmonary artery (PA) pressures, and right heart valvular function. Acutely distended neck veins may indicate intravascular volume overload, right or left ventricular failure, pulmonary hypertension with an incompetent pulmonic valve, noncompliance of the right ventricle, right ventricular outflow obstruction, or pericardial tamponade as examples. Abnormalities of the pulse contour can indicate abnormalities of valve or myocardial function. Cannon A waves are caused when the atrium contracts against a closed tricuspid valve and indicate atrio–ventricular dysynchrony. Kussmaul's sign is the observation of a jugular venous pressure that rises with inspiration and is seen with impediment to right heart filling. Abdomino–jugular reflux (increase in the jugular venous pulse with pressure on the abdomen) suggests the presence of right ventricular failure as the right ventricle is unable to accept the increased venous return.[1,2] Heart failure can lead to passive congestion of the liver, and assessing liver size while assessing for abdomino–jugular reflux can provide useful information. Assessment of heart rate and rhythm should be performed, keeping age-related norms and medications in mind. Auscultation of the heart sounds, noting the presence or quality of the first and second heart sounds, the presence or absence of third or fourth heart sounds, the presence and quality of murmurs, clicks, or friction rubs is important both during the initial assessment and as a means to assess response to therapy or changes in function. The development of a friction rub after cardiac surgery is not unexpected, but the development of such a rub during treatment for septic shock may indicate the presence of pericardial inflammation and effusion. Similarly, the development of an S3 gallop may be the first clear indication of worsening heart failure.

MEASURING CARDIAC OUTPUT

Means of measuring cardiac output include
Pulmonary artery catheter (PAC)
Transpulmonary thermodilution (TD)—PiCCO monitor (Pulsion Medical Systems, Munich, Germany)
Lithium dilution—LiDCO (LiDCO Group Plc, London UK)
Pulse contour analysis—calibrated (PiCCO, PulseCO system [LiDCO Ltd])—noncalibrated (Flo-trac Vigleo system [Edwards Life Sciences, Irvine California])
Mixed and central venous saturation.

PAC

The PAC first was introduced by Swan and Ganz in 1970.[3] The balloon-tipped, flow-directed catheter allowed clinicians for the first time to assess advanced parameters of hemodynamics and gas exchange at the bedside. It was widely adopted, so much so that it helped define the modern intensive care unit (ICU) in the coming years. But the PAC was introduced without any clinical trials establishing benefit in critically ill patients, and after several years of use concerns over its safety and efficacy were raised. The device never has been shown to improve major clinical outcomes,[3,4] and in fact might increase mortality and morbidity.[5,6] Furthermore, there is a growing body of evidence that the PAC adds little to information attainable by less invasive measures, and as such, it has been suggested that it no longer be used as part of routine management of the critically ill for conditions other than right heart failure, disorders causing abnormalities of pulmonary arterial pressure, and congenital heart disease.[7,8]

Cardiac output can be determined by different methods using the PAC. It can be measured using the Fick principle, which is a variation of the law of conservation and states that consumption of oxygen must equal the product of blood flow and the difference between the arterial and venous concentrations of the oxygen:

$$CO = (VO_2)/(Ca_{O2}) - (Cv_{O2})$$

where VO_2 is the oxygen consumption per minute; Ca_{O2} is the arterial oxygen content, and Cv_{O2} is the mixed venous oxygen content.

Systemic arterial and mixed venous blood samples are taken, and VO_2 is either measured using a calorimeter or is estimated. The Fick method is quite accurate for measuring CO when VO_2 is measured directly. it loses accuracy, however, if supplemental oxygen is given at FiO_2 greater than 0.6 or when there is significant oxygen consumption in the lung itself and VO_2 is estimated as, as is frequently the case in critically ill patients.

TD remains the most commonly used technique for obtaining cardiac output in critically ill patients. When using the PAC, 5 to 10 mL of cold saline ($\leq 25°C$) is injected through the catheter into the right atrium, where it mixes with venous blood, causing it to cool slightly. Cooled blood then passes through the right heart into the PA and by a thermistor near the tip of the PAC, and a TD curve is generated. CO then is calculated using the modified Stewart-Hamilton equation for TD.

$$Q = \frac{VI \times (TB - TI) \times SI \times CI \times 60 \times CT}{SB \times CB \times \int_0^\infty \Delta TB(t)dt}$$

where Q is the CO (L/min), VI is the volume of injectant (milliliters); TB is the blood temperature (°C). SI is the specific gravity of injectant; CI is the specific heat of injectate, and 60 is a constant for number of seconds per minute. CT is the correction factor, and SB is the specific gravity of blood, CB is the specific heat of blood, and $\int_0^\infty \Delta$ is the integral of blood temperature change (°C/sec) (area under the TD curve). The correction factor CT depends on the length from the proximal port of the PA catheter to the thermistor and the response time and sensitivity of the thermistor and electronic circuitry supplied by the manufacturer. Wide variation in CO occurs over the course of the respiratory cycle, and it is important to begin and complete each injection at the same time in the cycle. Injection is done in triplicate, and values are averaged. As the injections are being done, it is important to remember any loss of thermal indicator through right-to-left intracardiac shunts or remixing across incompetent pulmonary or tricuspid valves will cause erroneous increases in CO. Similarly, a large volume of injectate or too slow an injection can lead to a falsely low CO measurement. Temperature errors can occur with concomitant continuous intravenous infusions into the central veins. Thrombus or vessel wall impingement also can alter the thermistor function. Arrhythmias and atrial or ventricular ectopy can cause wide swings in preload and CO, confounding average CO determination. It is important to remember that even in the best circumstances, accuracy is only to 10% to 15% of the actual value, and any change in CO less then that should not be interpreted as significant.[3]

Complications of PAC are:

Line-related complications (pneumothorax, bleeding or infections)
Arrhythmias (benign and life-threatening ventricular arrhythmias and right bundle branch block)
PA-related complications (rupture, infarction, thrombi, hemorrhage, vegetations).

Transpulmonary TD

Whereas the PAC remains widely used, controversy surrounding its safety and efficacy has prompted development of newer less invasive techniques. For these purposes, the transpulmonary thermodilution technique (TPT) allows assessment of volumetric preload, cardiac output, and extravascular lung water without the need to pass a catheter through the right heart.

The PiCCO monitor is currently the only commercially available device that uses the TPT method to measure cardiac output. The device requires only central venous access and a specialized femoral or axillary arterial catheter with a thermistor at its tip. A known volume of thermal indicator (ice-cold saline) is injected via a central venous catheter. The resulting packet of cooler blood traverses the thorax and is sensed by a thermistor in the femoral or axillary position generating a TD dissipation curve. Cardiac output is then calculated from the curve using the modified Stewart-Hamilton equation for TD (as described in the PAC section). The average result from three consecutive bolus injections is recorded.

The technique is less invasive than the PAC, requiring only central venous and arterial lines, which many critically ill patients already will have required. Earlier studies[9] found the measurements of PiCCO are more consistent and are not influenced by respiratory cycle as compared with PAC. Its suitability to use in pediatric patients and reliability in cardiac unstable patients also are accepted.[10] TPT may give inaccurate measurements in patients with intracardiac shunt, aortic stenosis, aortic aneurysm, and extra corporeal circulation. Complications are all catheter-related to include infection (<0.3%) thrombosis, bleeding, and vascular injury resulting in limb ischemia or pseudoaneurysm (all combined approximately3%).

Lithium Dilution

Instead of using cold injectate indicator dilution, methods using intravenous lithium have been developed to determine CO (LiDCO). The advantage in doing this is that lithium can be injected via central or peripheral venous catheters and detected in a standard radial arterial line, negating the need to place a catheter across heart valves (PAC) or to place a femoral or axillary arterial catheter (TPT). Small amounts of lithium are injected intravenously and then detected in a specialized device attached to a standard radial artery catheter. A dye dissipation curve is generated, and cardiac output is determined using principles of Stewart-Hamilton similar to the special equation for TD. The technique has been found to provide accurate measurement of CO in critically ill patients.[11]

Pulse Contour Waveform Analysis

Pulse contour analysis uses pressure waveforms in arterial blood in the periphery to continuously calculate CO. Wesseling first described a clinically usable technique in 1983.[12] The arterial pressure waveform is obtained in the axillary or femoral arteries, and then assumptions are made to calculate predicted changes in pulse wave contour measured in the periphery in an attempt to estimate stroke volume (SV). The area under the systolic portion of the pressure waveform is proportional to the SV as the integral of the change in pressure from end diastole (t_0) to end systole (t_1) over time and inversely proportional to the impedence of the aorta (Z).

$$SV = \frac{\int_{t0}^{t1} dP/dt}{Z}$$

Sophisticated waveform analyses are employed, which account for finite pulse wave velocity and wave reflections. Accuracy then is enhanced further by calibration with an indicator dilution technique: transpulmonary TD for the PiCCO system and lithium chloride dilution for the PulseCO system (LiDCO Ltd). Studies comparing CO by pulse contour analysis techniques to the PA TD technique have found fairly good correlations with a correlation coefficient (r) ranging from 0.88 to 0.98 and precisions of ±0.3 to 1.26 L/min.[13,14] Variable results have been reported in studies involving patients with rapidly changing hemodynamics after initial calibration, but it is felt that the negative impact that hemodynamic instability has on this technique can be minimized by more frequent calibrations.[15]

Neither system requires right heart catheterization, making them less invasive than PACs, but they do require placement of both arterial and venous lines. Factors affecting accuracy include: nonlinearity of aortic compliance, differences in proximal aortic pressure to measure peripheral pressure, damped waveforms, variability of aortic diameter, aortic valve and vessel pathology, and body position.[16]

Pulse Contour Cardiac Output (Noncalibrated)—Flo-trac Vigleo System

The FloTrac system, comprised of the FloTrac sensor and Vigileo monitor, attempts to determine CO by pulse contour analysis without employing a second technique for calibration. Calibration allows a way to account for changes in vascular compliance, which cannot be easily measured clinically. The makers of the Flo-Trac device claim to have solved this problem using continuous self-calibration through an automatic vascular tone adjustment involving complex algorithms based on mean arterial pressure, age, height, weight, and gender of patients. Although accuracy of this system has been promising in limited studies involving fairly stable patients, further validation studies in severely ill patients are required.[17,18]

Mixed Venous Oxygen Saturation—Surrogate of CO

Mixed venous oxygen saturation requires sampling of blood in the pulmonary artery with a pulmonary artery catheter (PAC). A low mixed venous saturation (Svo2) in the absence of arterial hypoxemia is considered as a surrogate marker of poor cardiac output. Normal mixed venous saturation is approximately 70%. A very low mixed venous saturation (Svo2) is indicative of excessive extraction of oxygen per unit blood—under-resuscitation. A very high Svo2 value is difficult to interpret. It may represent the inability of the tissues to extract oxygen (cytopathic dysoxia seen in sepsis, mitochondrial poisoning and dysfunction seen in various conditions and exposures, or increased CO and oxygen delivery).

Because of the need to place a PAC to obtain mixed venous oxygen saturation, the use of central venous blood saturation has recently gained popularity. A study of 12 patients undergoing abdominal aortic surgery showed good correlation ($P<.001$) between Svo2 and CI measured by TD method (PAC). Another study of 18 severe heart failure patients[19] treated with milrinone and dobutamine showed excellent correlation of Svo2 and CI as measured by the PAC. Newer devices that can measure central venous blood saturation continuously, such as PiCCO and Swan-Ganz CCOmbo PAC (Edwards Life Sciences) have been developed and can measure CO by TD technique along with continuous measurement of mixed venous saturations.

NONINVASIVE TECHNIQUES

Noninvasive techniques include
   Thoracic bioimpedence (TEB)
   Electrical bioreactance cardiography
   Esophageal Doppler
   Transgastric Doppler
   Ultrasonic cardiac output monitor (USCOM, USCOM Pty Ltd, Coffs Harbour NSW Australia).

Echocardiography and carbon dioxide rebreathing method (non-invasive continuous cardiac output) are discussed in other articles in this issue.

TEB

TEB is a noninvasive technique developed by Kubicek[20] to measure cardiac output in astronauts. It involves delivery of low-amplitude high-frequency electrical current across the thorax (**Fig. 2**). A series of sensing electrodes measuring impedence are placed around the thorax. Hemodynamic measurements of CO using TEB devices relate to change in the thoracic electrical conductivity to changes in thoracic aortic blood volume and blood flow. This form of impedence cardiography has been proposed as a simple and readily reproducible noninvasive technique for the determination of CO, specifically, SV, contractility, systemic vascular resistance, and thoracic fluid content and filling index.[21] Proponents have claimed that TEB can measure CO with the same clinical accuracy as either the Fick or TD technique and that it offers the potential for sequential measurements of CO in patients for whom invasive measurements are impractical or contraindicated. Variations due to the heart beat in blood flow and volume in the ascending aorta cause a change in the total chest impedance, which, when continuously recorded, produces a dZ/dt wave (dZ = impedence change, dt = change in time).

Factors affecting measurement of impedance include height, weight, sex, circumference of chest, and hemoglobin. Models using algorithms based on these factors have been developed to improve accuracy of measurements. Newer technology uses chest baseline impedance-independent electrical impedance cardiography systems. This technique improves accuracy in those patients with large amounts of thoracic fluid that was a source of significant interference in older model measurements. This accuracy significantly increases the technique's usefulness in patients with pulmonary edema, chest trauma, congestive heart failure, and acute respiratory distress syndrome (ARDS). Meta-analysis, however, has shown a broad range of correlation to TD determinations of CO ($r = .44$ to $.74$).[22] Despite recent advances, the technique remains confounded by positive end-expiratory pressure (PEEP), chest wall edema, obesity, pleural fluid, and severe pulmonary edema.[23] One study has

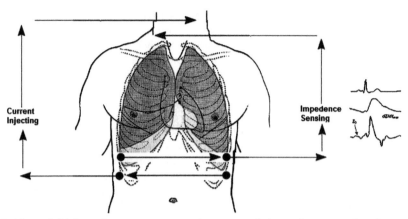

Fig. 2. Thoracic bioimpedence uses a tetrapolar system of electrodes, separating the current pathway from the sensing pathway. Current is injected, and the impendence against the flow of the current through the thorax along the path of least resistance is measured (ie, the great vessels).

shown that when patients with these confounders were excluded, correlation to TD determination of CO was improved to r = .93.[24]

Electrical Bioreactance Cardiography

To overcome some of the limitations and clinical confounders of bioimpedence, bioreactance recently has been employed as a means to measure CO noninvasively. Whereas bioimpedence is based on changes in amplitude of electrical resistivity as a function of CO, bioreactance is based on changes in frequency. Similar to FM radio, the signal is less susceptible to interference from chest wall movement, chest wall and lung edema, and pleural fluid (**Fig. 3**). Additionally, detection of frequency modulation is not as affected by the distance of electrode placement, so the electrodes can be placed anywhere on the chest.

The method used by the CheetahTM monitor (Cheetah Medical, Tel Aviv, Israel and Portland, Oregon) has shown good correlation with TD in several studies in critically ill patients.[25,26] A recent prospective pilot study between septic and nonseptic patients revealed significant differences in SV, cardiac index and peripheral vascular resistance, and predicted the need for hospitalization in sepsis.[27] Another study in

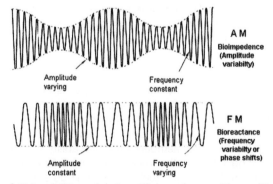

Fig. 3. Difference of AM and FM modulation. Bioimpedence with amplitude variability and Bioreactance with frequency variability or phase shift.

postoperative cardiac surgery patients compared bioreactance and pulse contour analysis (Flo-Trac Vigileo) with PAC TD and showed similar correlations of the two techniques to TD (0.77 and 0.69, respectively). Sensitivity and specificity for predicting trends in changes in cardiac output changes were 0.91 and 0.95, respectively, for the bioreactance and 0.86 and 0.92, respectively, for the FloTrac-Vigileo.[28]

Esophageal Doppler Technique

The esophageal Doppler technique measures blood flow velocity in descending aorta by a Doppler transducer (4 MHz continuous or 5 MHz pulsed wave) placed on the tip of an esophageal probe. The probe is introduced in the esophagus and rotated toward the descending aorta. The depth, rotation of the probe, and gain are adjusted to obtain an optimal aortic velocity signal. The positioning of probe is critical in estimating CO, as poor positioning can lead to underestimation of CO. It is operator-dependent and requires specialized training to use effectively. Studies have shown good correlation to TD (r = .95).[29] Advantages to its use are that it is relatively less invasive than a PAC, and it provides continuous flow information. Disadvantages are its initial cost, the need for sedation, and the need for a specialist trained in its use.

Transgastric Doppler Technique

Transgastric Doppler is a similar technique to esophageal Doppler with the probe positioned in the stomach instead of esophagus. In this technique, a thinner silicone probe (6 mm) is used, and its placement usually does not require sedation. The thinner probe can be more difficult to position, and it requires frequent repositioning. It has been shown to have acceptable correlation to TD in a study of 31 patients with 57 simultaneous TD and Doppler readings, which revealed a close correlation with r = .91, and $P<.001$, making it a promising new technique that may be used in selected patients for accurate measurement of cardiac output.[30]

USCOM

The USCOM ultrasonic cardiac output monitor is a noninvasive device that determines cardiac output by continuous-wave Doppler ultrasound. The flow profile is obtained using a transducer (2.0 or 3.3 MHz) placed on the chest in either the left parasternal position to measure transpulmonary blood flow or the suprasternal position to measure transaortic blood flow. This flow profile is presented as a time–velocity spectral display showing variations of blood flow velocity with time. Comparison of the technique with TD in one study of 22 cardiac patients showed a bias of 0.18 and limits of agreement of −1.43 to 1.78. The agreement was not as good between techniques at higher cardiac output values. Its suitability for use in high and low cardiac output states requires further validation.[31]

SUMMARY

Bedside determination of cardiac function and output is an evolving field. Several techniques are now available, each with their pros and cons. Clearly less invasive techniques are desired. Most lack clear clinical validation, however, and further study is required both in terms of determining accuracy and in demonstrating efficacy for improving outcome. It must be remembered that the ability to improve outcome will never rest solely on a device but rather on how it is used. New algorithmic strategies employing these various devices and techniques must be studied for their ability to improve outcome if bedside hemodynamic monitoring is to advance.

REFERENCES

1. Butman SM, Ewy GA, Standen JR, et al. Bedside cardiovascular examination in patients with severe chronic heart failure: importance of rest or inducible jugular venous distension. J Am Coll Cardiol 1993;22(4):968–74.
2. Garg N, Garg N. Jugular venous pulse: an appraisal. J Indian Acad Clin Med 2000;1(3):260–9.
3. Cook LB, Morgan M. Pulmonary artery catheterisation. Ann Acad Med Singapore 1994;23(4):519–30.
4. Guyatt G. A randomized control trial of right-heart catheterizationin critically ill patients. Ontario Intensive Care Study Group. J Intensive Care Med 1991;6:91–5.
5. Hayes MA, Timmins AC, Yau EH, et al. Elevation of systemic oxygen delivery in the treatment of critically ill patients. N Engl J Med 1994;330:1717–22.
6. Dalen JE, Bone RC. Is it time to pull the pulmonary artery catheter? JAMA 1996; 276:916–8.
7. Vernon C, Phillips CR. Pulmonary artery catheters in acute heart failure: end of an era? Crit Care 2009;13(6):1003.
8. Shure D. Pulmonary artery catheters—peace at last? N Engl J Med 2006;354(21): 2273–4.
9. Sakka SG, Rühl CC, Pfeiffer UJ, et al. Assessment of cardiac preload and extra-vascular lung water by single transpulmonary thermodilution. Intensive Care Med 2000;26(2):180–7.
10. Goedje O, Hoeke K, Lichtwarck-Aschoff M, et al. Continuous cardiac output by femoral arterial thermodilution calibrated pulse contour analysis: comparison with pulmonary arterial thermodilution. Crit Care Med 1999;27(11):2407–12.
11. Linton RA, Jonas MM, Tibby SM, et al. Cardiac output measured by lithium dilu-tion and transpulmonary thermodilution in patients in a paediatric intensive care unit. Intensive Care Med 2000;26(10):1507–11.
12. Wesseling KH, Dewitt B, Weber AP. A simple device for the continuous measure-ment of cardiac output. Adv Cardiovasc Phys 1983;5:1–52.
13. Buhre W, Weyland A, Kazmaier S, et al. Comparison of cardiac output assessed by pulse-contour analysis and thermodilution in patients undergoing minimally invasive direct coronary artery bypass grafting. J Cardiothorac Vasc Anesth 1999;13(4):437–40.
14. Zollner C, Haller M, Weis M, et al. Beat-to-beat measurement of cardiac output by intravascular pulse contour analysis: a prospective criterion standard study in patients after cardiac surgery. J Cardiothorac Vasc Anesth 2000;14(2):125–9.
15. Hamzaoui O, Monnet X, Richard C, et al. Effects of changes in vascular tone on the agreement between pulse contour and transpulmonary thermodilution cardiac output measurements within an up to 6-hour calibration-free period. Crit Care Med 2008;36(2):434–40.
16. van Lieshout JJ, Wesseling KH. Continuous cardiac output by pulse contour anal-ysis? Br J Anaesth 2001;86(4):467–9.
17. Marik PE, Baram M. Noninvasive hemodynamic monitoring in the intensive care unit. Crit Care Clin 2007;23(3):383–400.
18. Pestaña D, García de Lorenzo A, Madero R. Relationship between mixed venous saturation and cardiac index, hemoglobin and oxygen consumption in aortic surgery. Rev Esp Anestesiol Reanim 1998;45(4):136–40.
19. Nuñez S, Maisel A. Comparison between mixed venous oxygen saturation and thermodilution cardiac output in monitoring patients with severe heart failure treated with milrinone and dobutamine. Am Heart J 1998;135(3):383–8.

20. Kubicek WG, Karnegis JN, Patterson RP, et al. Development and evaluation of an impedence cardiac output system. Aerosp Med 1966;37(12):1208–12.
21. Summers RL, Shoemaker WC, Peacock WF, et al. Bench to bedside: electrophysiologic and clinical principles of noninvasive hemodynamic monitoring using impedence cardiography. Acad Emerg Med 2003;10(6):669–80.
22. Raaijmakers E, Faes TJ, Scholten RJ, et al. A meta-analysis of three decades of validating thoracic impedance cardiography. Crit Care Med 1999;27(6):1203–13.
23. Sageman WS, Amundson DE. Thoracic electrical bioimpedence measurement of cardiac output in postaortocoronary bypass patients. Crit Care Med 1993;21(8):1139–42.
24. Colombo J, Shoemaker WC, Belzberg H. Noninvasive monitoring of the autonomic nervous system and hemodynamics of patients with blunt and penetrating trauma. J Trauma 2008;65(6):1364–73.
25. Raval NY, Squara P, Cleman M, et al. Multicenter evaluation of noninvasive cardiac output measurement by bioreactance technique. J Clin Monit Comput 2008;22(2):113–9.
26. Squara P, Denjean D, Estagnasie P, et al. Noninvasive cardiac output monitoring (NICOM): a clinical validation. Intensive Care Med 2007;33(7):1191–4.
27. Hicks C. Hemodynamic changes in patients with sepsis. Acad Emerg Med 2009;16:397.
28. Marqué S, Cariou A, Chiche JD, et al. Comparison between Flotrac-Vigileo and Bioreactance, a totally noninvasive method for cardiac output monitoring. Crit Care 2009;13(3):R73.
29. Valtier B, Cholley BP, Belot JP, et al. Noninvasive monitoring of cardiac output in critically ill patients using transesophageal Doppler. Am J Respir Crit Care Med 1998;158(1):77–83.
30. Katz WE, Gasior TA, Quinlan JJ, et al. Transgastric continuous-wave Doppler to determine cardiac output. Am J Cardiol 1993;71(10):853–7.
31. Thom O, Taylor DM, Wolfe RE, et al. Comparison of a suprasternal cardiac output monitor (USCOM) with the pulmonary artery catheter. Br J Anaesth 2009;103(6):800–4.

The Role of Echocardiography in Hemodynamic Assessment of Septic Shock

Matthew J. Griffee, MD[a],*, Matthias J. Merkel, MD, PhD[a],
Kevin S. Wei, MD[b]

KEYWORDS

- Echocardiography • Septic shock • Resuscitation
- Fluid therapy • Cor pulmonale

Echocardiography was originally developed in the 1950s, but it was not until the late 1980s that a few pioneering intensivists advocated echocardiography as the preferred first-line technique for evaluation of patients with hemodynamic instability.[1] In the past decade, interest in applications of echocardiography in the intensive care unit (ICU) arena has greatly increased.[2] Clinical research questioning the diagnostic value of central venous and pulmonary artery (PA) pressure data, coupled with advances in portable ultrasound technology, have stimulated interest in echocardiography for hemodynamic assessment.[3] Experts in the United States, Canada, and Europe argue passionately for incorporating echo training into ICU fellowship requirements.[2,4,5] There are many strengths of echo for assessment of hemodynamic instability, including

- Speed: qualitative assessment of all chambers and the performance of both ventricles can be done within minutes
- Anatomic breadth: valves and pericardium are included in the echo assessment
- Noninvasive (transthoracic echocardiography [TTE] is completely noninvasive; transesophageal echocardiography [TEE] does require esophageal intubation)
- Intuitive: structure and function are assessed simultaneously, and many people prefer visual assessment to analysis of PA catheter numbers

---

[a] Department of Anesthesiology and Perioperative Medicine, Oregon Health and Science University, Mailstop UHS-2, 3181 SW Sam Jackson Park Road, Portland, OR 97239, USA
[b] Department of Medicine, Division of Cardiovascular Medicine, Oregon Health and Science University, UHN-62, 3181 SW Sam Jackson Park Road, Portland, OR 97239, USA
* Corresponding author.
E-mail address: griffeem@ohsu.edu

Crit Care Clin 26 (2010) 365–382
doi:10.1016/j.ccc.2010.01.001
0749-0704/10/$ – see front matter

- Diastolic dysfunction, hyperdynamic obstruction, and acute right heart failure can be diagnosed. These disorders may be difficult to diagnose using right heart catheterization alone, potentially leading to counterproductive treatment.[3,6]

Nevertheless, echo and central venous monitoring are complementary techniques. PA or transthoracic thermodilution catheters offer advantages compared with echo:

- Measurement of venous oxygen saturation (Sv_{O_2}), lung water, and continuous cardiac output
- Continuous monitoring.

This article introduces the techniques of hemodynamic assessment using echocardiography, highlights insights provided by echocardiography into the effects of sepsis on the heart, outlines credentialing and competency standards, and refers interested readers to resources for training and further education.

FUNDAMENTALS OF ECHOCARDIOGRAPHY

An ultrasound transducer contains crystals that emit sound waves when exposed to an electric field. The crystals are arranged in a matrix and send sound waves serially. Most of the time, the crystal is not vibrating; rather, it detects returning sound waves. These are produced when the sound waves moving through the patient encounter an interface between tissue layers with different acoustic properties or which block sound transmission altogether. Because the sound returns sooner if it is reflected from a more shallow source, the timing of reflected waves correlates with the depth of tissue interfaces. The returning sound causes the crystal to vibrate, which generates an electric signal. The pattern of returning sound impulses is processed electronically to provide a visual representation of the sonographic anatomy. Details can be found in a reference textbook.[7]

ECHOCARDIOGRAPHY EQUIPMENT

The ultrasound transducer for TTE has a square surface, rather than the elongated rectangle of the transducer used for vascular imaging (**Fig. 1**). There is an inverse relationship between sound wave frequency and depth of penetration, with an advantage in terms of better resolution with high frequency. Higher-frequency, lower-depth probes are used for vascular imaging with ultrasound. By contrast, an echocardiography transducer emits a variety of frequencies to provide optimal resolution at a range of depths. It also uses a high frame rate to capture cardiac motion and display it smoothly. By contrast, using the abdominal preset of the software menu produces blurred images of the beating heart. It is useful for an ICU to have a dedicated machine, available 24 hours per day, to make echocardiography a readily available diagnostic tool for unstable patients.[8]

EXAMPLE OF A FOCUSED ECHOCARDIOGRAPHY STUDY FOR HEMODYNAMIC ASSESSMENT

This section describes the cross-sectional anatomy revealed by standard transducer positions, or "echo windows," for hemodynamic evaluation of an ICU patient. Typical clinical scenarios for this application of ultrasound include patients who present with shock of unknown cause and patients who do not respond to standard resuscitation for presumed septic shock. The goal is to expeditiously rule in or rule out several potential causes of acute hemodynamic compromise.

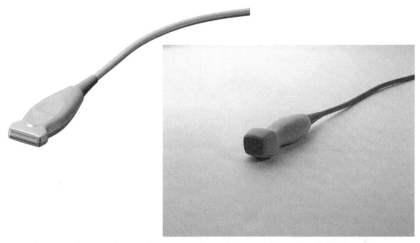

Fig. 1. Ultrasound transducers. The vascular ultrasound probe (*left*) has a rectangular profile. It is designed for high resolution of superficial structures and has a high-frequency ultrasound signal. The cardiac probe (*right*) has a square footprint. It is designed to send a range of frequencies into deeper depths, and has a high frame speed, when in the cardiac preset from the ultrasound menu. (*Courtesy of* SonoSite, Bothell, WA; with permission.)

The following example of an imaging sequence lists pertinent considerations for each window:

1. Parasternal long axis (**Fig. 2**)
   a. Evaluate global left ventricular (LV) systolic function. Does wall motion and thickening seem moderately or severely compromised?
   b. Evaluate mitral and aortic valves for gross anatomic abnormality, such as flail leaflet, vegetation, or severe restriction of movement.
   c. Evaluate right ventricular (RV) free wall for contractility and RV size relative to LV size. The right ventricle should appear smaller than the left ventricle.
   d. Evaluate for pericardial effusion. A pericardial effusion will appear as an echo-free space outside the epicardium, and will insinuate between the descending aorta in the far field and the posterior border of the left ventricle at the base of the heart. A pleural effusion will be located deep to the descending aorta.
2. Parasternal short-axis views (**Fig. 3**)
   a. Evaluate RV size and function. Watch septal motion in systole. Evaluate for increased RV systolic pressure, which may result in flattening of the interventricular septum, causing the left ventricle to have a D shape, instead of a circular cross section.
   b. Examine LV systolic function. Inspect inward excursion of the LV endocardium during systole, and note the thickening of the LV wall as it contracts. Evaluate for segments of the left ventricle that do not move as well as others. Categorize LV systolic function as normal, moderately impaired, or severely impaired.
3. Apical 4-chamber view (**Fig. 4**)
   a. Evaluate global LV systolic function. Does systolic function seem normal, or is it moderately or severely impaired? Observe LV cavity at end systole. Is there complete or near-complete obliteration, and extremely vigorous systolic wall excursion? This pattern is consistent with hyperdynamic function, low afterload, and inadequate preload.

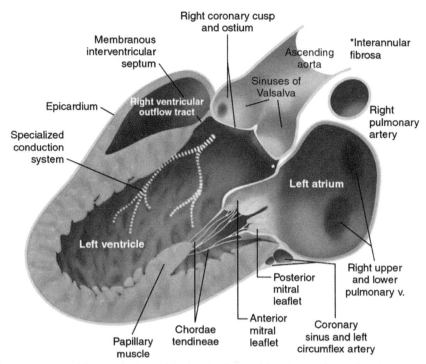

Fig. 2. Parasternal long-axis view. This view is obtained by placing the probe alongside the left upper sternal border, directing the marker to the patient's right shoulder. (*From* Otto CM. Textbook of clinical echocardiography. Philadelphia: Saunders Elsevier; 2009. p. 35; with permission. Original source credit [in caption of figure]: *From* Otto CM. Echocardiographic evaluation of valvular heart disease. In: Otto CM, Bonow R, editors. Valvular heart disease: a companion to Braunwald's heart disease. Philadelphia: Elsevier/Saunders; 2009; with permission, copyright Elsevier, 2009.)

    b. Inspect the mitral valve and tricuspid valve for any gross pathology (flail leaflet, vegetation).

    c. Evaluate RV size. Compare RV area with LV area. Estimate whether RV size is less than 60% of LV size (normal) vs between 60% and 90% of LV area (moderate dilation) or more than 90% of LV area (severe dilation).

    d. The degree of tricuspid annular systolic excursion correlates with RV ejection fraction (EF). If RV systolic function is normal, the plane of the tricuspid valve is expected to move toward the apex by 2 cm in systole.

4. Five-chamber view. Assess aortic valve for obvious structural abnormalities.

5. Returning to the apical 4-chamber view, the probe is rotated clockwise to obtain the apical 2- and 3-chamber views for evaluation of LV systolic function in additional cross-sectional planes.

6. Subcostal view (**Fig. 5**)

    a. Evaluate for pericardial effusion

    b. In suspected tamponade, evaluate for RV collapse in diastole and right atrial collapse in systole

    c. Compare size of right and left ventricles (see relative RV size assessment, discussed earlier).

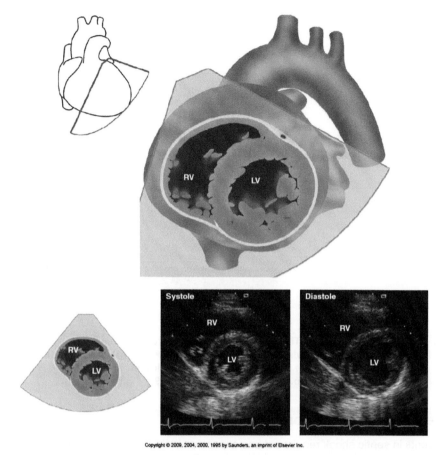

Fig. 3. Parasternal short axis. This view is obtained by rotating the transducer clockwise from the parasternal long-axis view, so that the ultrasound plane is now perpendicular to the long axis of the heart. LV systolic function and presence/absence of septal flattening are key observations to be obtained from this view. (*From* Otto CM. Textbook of clinical echocardiography. Philadelphia: Saunders Elsevier; 2009. p. 42, copyright Elsevier, 2009; with permission.)

7. Intrahepatic inferior vena cava (IVC) window. Assess volume status by measuring respiratory variation in IVC diameter (see section on volume responsiveness).
8. Lung bases. Image each lung base and diaphragm to evaluate for massive pleural effusion.[9]

Patient positioning is often adequate with the patient supine; however, poor views can often be improved with rotation of the patient 30% to 60% toward the left lateral position. If clinically safe, it may also improve acoustic windows to temporarily reduce positive expiratory end pressure (PEEP) during the examination.[10,11]

The examination sequence described here is an example of a focused echocardiographic evaluation. Detailed information with excellent illustrations is available from standard textbooks.[5,7]

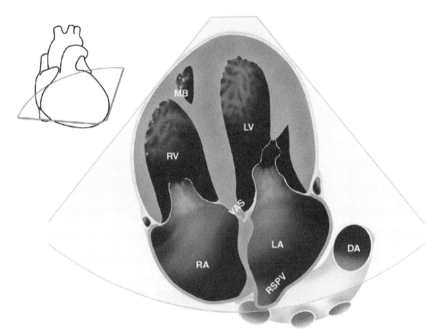

Fig. 4. Apical 4-chamber view. The transducer is moved laterally and caudally to the LV apex, at the point of maximum impulse. This view is useful for comparing the relative size of the right and left ventricles. (*From* Otto CM. Textbook of clinical echocardiography. Philadelphia: Saunders Elsevier; 2009. p. 43, copyright Elsevier, 2009; with permission.)

PRELOAD/PREDICTION OF VOLUME RESPONSIVENESS

Patients in septic shock require volume expansion in the initial phase of resuscitation to prevent hemodynamic collapse. However, after preload is optimized, further fluid loading may not only fail to increase oxygen delivery but may also cause harm (eg, it may lead to pulmonary edema [PE] and bacterial translocation across the gut).[12]

Traditional indices of preload, such as central venous pressure (CVP) and pulmonary artery pressure (PAP), have been found to be unreliable in predicting fluid responsiveness (defined as the potential to increase cardiac output significantly in response to a fluid challenge).[13] Because echocardiography is an alternative to invasive monitoring, there has been an interest in finding sonographic correlates of pulse pressure variation in patients with septic shock.[14]

The most useful echocardiographic parameters for assessment of fluid responsiveness are respiratory variation of vena cava diameter and of stroke volume.[14] As for any clinical prediction tool, it is important to understand the prerequisite criteria for applying these measurements, because there are multiple potential confounding factors. Patients must be in a controlled mode of ventilation, with a tidal volume of at least 8 mL/kg, and with no spontaneous respiratory effort. Similarly, patients must be in sinus rhythm. For indices of IVC size, patients must have normal intraabdominal pressure.[14] In addition, patients with acute cor pulmonale undergoing mechanical ventilation may have dynamic signs of fluid responsiveness (pronounced pulse pressure variation and IVC collapse) due to adverse effects of increased pleural and pulmonary pressure during inspiration on the dilated, failing right heart, but fluid challenge may worsen the RV failure and fail to increase cardiac output.[15]

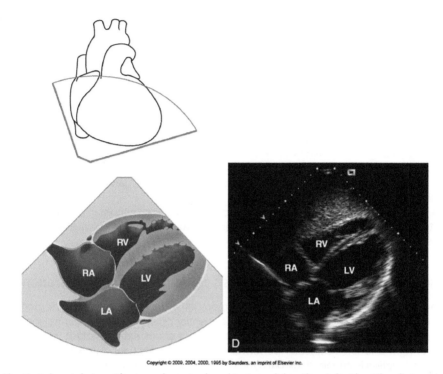

Fig. 5. Subcostal view. The transducer is placed just caudal to the xiphoid, with a flat angle, turned to scan into the left side of the thorax. The first structure encountered by the ultrasound from this view is the right ventricle. Sliding to the midline will reveal the inferior vena cava (IVC) and aorta. (*From* Otto CM. Textbook of clinical echocardiography. Philadelphia: Saunders Elsevier; 2009. p. 47, copyright Elsevier, 2009; with permission.)

In 2004, 2 groups reported a positive correlation between the magnitude of respiratory-induced changes in IVC diameter and volume responsiveness in patients requiring with septic shock.[16,17] Both groups measured fluctuations in IVC diameter associated with respiration before and after a fluid bolus and observed a highly significant correlation between variation in IVC diameter and the increase in cardiac output after the bolus.[16,17] Patients were categorized as responders if cardiac index increased by at least 15% after the bolus. An intriguing and potentially clinically useful finding was that there appeared to be a clear cutoff value for initial IVC size variation and the response to volume expansion. Feissel and colleagues[16] reported that using 12% as a threshold value for IVC size variability, responders to a fluid bolus could be predicted with positive and negative predictive values greater than 90%. Barbier and colleagues[17] found that a threshold variability in IVC size of 18% predicted the response to volume expansion with sensitivity and specificity of 90%.

Superior vena cava (SVC) diameter is also affected by the large fluctuations in intrathoracic pressure caused by positive pressure variation. A disadvantage of monitoring SVC caliber variation is that it requires TEE. However, because the SVC is intrathoracic, a potential advantage is less confounding from elevations of intraabdominal pressure. Vieillard-Baron and colleagues[18] noted a clustering of baseline SVC collapsibility between responders (with SVC collapse of 60% or more) and nonresponders (in whom SVC varied by 30% or less). This finding results in a specificity of 100% and a sensitivity of 90% for predicting a significant increase in cardiac output when the SVC collapsibility exceeds 36%.[18]

Another ultrasound technique for assessing volume responsiveness relies on Doppler measurements of stroke volume. Fluctuations in stroke volume associated with ventilator cycling are greater in the hypovolemic patient than in the completely resuscitated patient.[19]

Providing a temporary test dose of volume expansion can be accomplished with passive leg raising, which briefly redistributes blood pooled in the lower extremities to the central circulation. If stroke volume is measured before and after the position change, the intensivist can then evaluate the hemodynamic effect of increasing preload. Advantages of this technique are that it remains valid even if the patient is breathing spontaneously and even if the patient is not in sinus rhythm.[20]

A potential area for further research is to compare clinical outcomes of resuscitation protocols with versus without echocardiographic assessment of volume responsiveness to guide restoration of cardiac output.

ECHOCARDIOGRAPHIC DIAGNOSIS OF SEPSIS-INDUCED MYOCARDIAL DYSFUNCTION

Echocardiography provides a detailed, comprehensive evaluation of systolic performance and relies on pattern recognition to identify or exclude common categories of cardiac dysfunction (**Table 1**). The triage echo for shock should include interpretation of right and left ventricular performance (see later section). Furthermore, when systolic function is impaired, global hypokinesis should be distinguished from regional wall motion abnormalities. Echocardiography for patients who remain in shock despite volume expansion and norepinephrine is important because it may lead to changes in therapy.

Echocardiographic studies of cohorts of patients with septic shock and investigations with a longitudinal design have provided insight into the incidence, natural history, and mechanism of sepsis-induced cardiac dysfunction. Highlights include

1. Although cardiac output may be normal or even high in early septic shock, systolic function is often impaired. Furthermore, myocardial depression may only become apparent when afterload is restored with norepinephrine.[21,22] Impaired systolic function has been found in patients with low, normal, and even increased cardiac output.[23]
2. Approximately 20% of patients with septic shock have isolated diastolic dysfunction. Cardiac filling and relaxation are abnormal, whereas systolic function is preserved.[24,25]
3. Septic myocardial dysfunction may reflect impaired adrenergic responsiveness, rather than deranged myocyte contractile function.[26] Many clinical studies use the term contractility imprecisely, as a synonym for decreased EF. EF should not be confused with contractility, because EF is influenced by preload. When a more exacting, preload-independent index of contractility was measured in patients in septic shock, investigators noted preserved contractility. In contrast, most patients exhibited impaired adrenergic responsiveness, defined as a dose-dependent increase in cardiac output with escalating doses of dobutamine. In the course of 10 days, contractility changed little, whereas adrenergic responsiveness improved steadily.[26] The parallel in vitro finding of an impaired response to β-agonists despite normal intrinsic contractile function has been reported when cardiomyocytes have been exposed to sepsis serum.[27,28]

Table 1
Pattern recognition paradigms for evaluation of shock by ICU echocardiography

	Cardinal Findings	Clinical Scenario	Implications/Treatment
Hypovolemia	Significant collapse of IVC/SVC with respirations; obliteration of LV cavity at end systole	Prior to fluid challenge; ongoing volume losses; severe vasodilatation; internal bleeding	Volume expansion; reevaluate after volume challenges; consider vasoconstrictor for primary distributive problem
Impaired Systolic Function	Moderately to severely reduced LV systolic wall thickening and excursion; dilated IVC with no respiratory variation	Evidence of low cardiac output; low urine output; PE	Inotropic support; consider evaluation for myocardial ischemia; elicit history of heart failure or coronary artery disease (CAD)
RV failure	RV size equal to or larger than LV size; apex of heart dominated by right ventricle	Suspected PE; history of chronic obstructive pulmonary disease; acute respiratory distress syndrome (ARDS)/acute lung injury	Consider evaluation for PE; evaluate for excessive PEEP or airway pressure; consider measurement of PAP and maneuvers to reduce PAP; treat acidosis
Diastolic Dysfunction (not measured directly on basic ICU echo, but suspected by deduction given echo findings and clinical scenario)	Thick left ventricle with normal or hyperdynamic function; no evidence of systolic dysfunction; evidence of PE	History of hypertension; aortic stenosis	Consider decreasing β-agonists; consider β-blocker or milrinone
Tamponade	Pericardial effusion; right atrial or RV collapse; marked respiratory variation of pulse pressure, systolic pressure, and IVC size	Heart instrumentation; thoracic surgery; disease with possible pericardial manifestations; transient responses to fluid challenges	Pericardiocentesis. Tamponade may be suggested by echo, but remains a clinical diagnosis
Hyperdynamic Function	LV hypertrophy, vigorous systolic function, small LV cavity size, obliteration of LV cavity at end systole, tachycardia	Patient with poorly controlled hypertension, acute hypovolemia, and tachycardia	Stop inotropes, volume expansion, maintain afterload and coronary perfusion with vasoconstrictor, consider β-blockade

4. Sepsis-induced cardiac dysfunction seems to resolve completely, regardless of the severity of the dysfunction in the midst of the illness. The expected course is gradual improvement, with complete recovery within 4 weeks (among those who survive the episode of sepsis).[1]

PRACTICAL EVALUATION OF LV SYSTOLIC FUNCTION

The most common and important technique for evaluation of systolic function for ICU echocardiography is by visual estimate.[5] There are 2 components: amount of endocardial border excursion toward the center of the left ventricle and increasing wall thickness during contraction. Expert echocardiographers with extensive training and experience can accurately estimate small changes over time in estimated EF and have the ability to distinguish between normal and mildly impaired, or between mildly and moderately impaired systolic function by visual estimate. By contrast, competency in basic echocardiography is defined by the ability to categorize the systolic function as normal, moderate dysfunction, or severe systolic dysfunction.[5]

Classification of decreased systolic function as global versus regional can also be defined on expert and basic levels. The American Heart Association (AHA) defined standard views and segmental anatomy and nomenclature for the description of regional wall motion abnormalities.[29] The basic-level echocardiographer should distinguish between global and regional systolic dysfunction, but scoring and precise localization of regional dysfunction mandates expert consultation.

Two peculiar patterns of systolic function are of particular relevance in ICU echocardiography. In transient apical ballooning (also referred to as Takotsubo) there is hyperdynamic basal function with impaired midchamber function and aneurysmal dilation of the apex.[30] The distribution of dyskinesis does not follow the anatomic distribution associated with an episode of an acute coronary syndrome. Transient apical ballooning is often preceded by severe emotional stress (eg, loss of spouse, a life-threatening diagnosis) and presents with troponin elevation and ST-segment deviation. Epicardial coronary artery disease (CAD) is absent and the apical ballooning resolves in most cases.[30]

In dynamic left ventricular outflow tract (LVOT) obstruction, abnormally increased contractile function results in obliteration of the upper LV cavity before end systole, blocking further ejection, and thereby reducing stroke volume.[31] This may be associated with mitral regurgitation. Whereas systolic function is abnormally increased, diastolic performance of the hyperdynamic myocardium is reduced, resulting in reduced filling, especially in case of tachycardia. If hyperdynamic function with an underfilled ventricle is not recognized, counterproductive treatment may be used to treat presumed systolic dysfunction. Empiric administration of an inotrope results in worsening diastolic function, lower stroke volume, and LVOT obstruction earlier in systole, and may lead to myocardial ischemia. When dynamic obstruction is recognized, treatment includes stopping inotropes, administering volume, increasing afterload with phenylephrine, and, in some cases, administering β-blockers. Recognizing hyperdynamic LV function with end-systolic LV chamber obliteration will thus lead the intensivist to make dramatic changes in hemodynamic management.[31]

ECHOCARDIOGRAPHIC IDENTIFICATION OF ACUTE RV FAILURE

Echocardiography is essential to identify and monitor acute RV failure in bedside triage of the unstable patient. Discovery of RV failure may lead to significant changes in treatment. For example, the unexpected finding of severe, acute right heart dilation and failure may trigger an evaluation for thromboembolism, lead to changes of PEEP or other ventilator settings contributing to high airway pressure, or reverse a working diagnosis of hypovolemia.

The components of critical care echocardiography (CCE) to diagnose RV failure as a potential cause of shock are RV distention at end-diastole and the sign of RV pressure overload in systole. Because the right ventricle has a complex three-dimensional shape, its volume cannot be calculated accurately from cross-sectional diameter measurements using a simple geometric model. However, Jardin and colleagues[32] showed that the relative area of the right ventricle compared with the area of the left ventricle in the 4-chamber view can be used as a surrogate marker of RV dysfunction. The normal RV area/LV area is 0.36 to 0.6; moderate RV dilation corresponds to an RV/ LV ratio between 0.7 and 0.9, and severe RV dilation results in an area equal to or greater than that of the left ventricle. The relative areas of the right and left ventricles should be estimated or measured in an apical 4-chamber or subcostal view.

The sign of RV pressure overload, septal flattening or paradoxic septal motion, is also based on a comparison between the right and left ventricles. Because the interventricular septum is shared by both ventricles, its relative position (leftward or rightward) and shape (flattened or curved) are determined by the pressure difference between the left and right ventricles. Normally, systole and diastole occur in concert in the right and left ventricles, and the septum thickens toward the center of the left ventricle along with the LV free wall throughout systole. However, RV pressure overload results in prolongation of RV systole into the period of LV relaxation. The pressure gradient across the septum (with high pressure in the right ventricle at end systole and low pressure in the relaxing left ventricle) results in deviation of the septum toward the left ventricle, while the rest of the left ventricle is continuing to move outwards in diastole.[33] After RV systole is completed, and LV pressure exceeds RV pressure, the septum returns to its normal position, presenting a convex surface into the RV cavity. Septal dyssynergy, the abnormal alternating shift in septal position, can be identified visually from multiple windows, and it can be quantified using the eccentricity index, which is the ratio of anteroposterior diameter of the left ventricle (which is parallel to the septum and is not affected by septal shift) and the medial-lateral diameter of the left ventricle (which is perpendicular to the septum and is compressed during septal shift).[34]

Identifying RV failure by echo in an unstable patient may have prognostic and therapeutic implications. In a registry of 1416 patients with acute PE and overall mortality of 3.3%, the subset of patients with RV/LV area greater than 0.9 had a 6.6% mortality, compared with 1.9% for patients with RV/LV ratio less than 0.9.[35] If acute pulmonary hypertension is associated with RV dilation and failure, potentially modifiable factors include acidosis, PEEP, and hypoxemia. In a retrospective analysis of a database of 352 patients with acute respiratory distress syndrome (ARDS), Jardin and Vieillard-Baron[36] noted a higher frequency of acute cor pulmonale (defined by echo criteria) with higher plateau pressure (Ppl). There was no significant increase in mortality for the group with Ppl of 27 to 35 cm H_2O compared with the group with Ppl 18 to 26 cm H_2O when patients with acute cor pulmonale were excluded. Among patients with these ranges of Ppl who did manifest acute cor pulmonale, mortality was increased in the group with higher Ppl.

Sepsis-induced myocardial dysfunction can affect the right as well as the left ventricle. Just as LV dysfunction may be unmasked by starting a vasoconstrictor infusion, so too can RV failure become manifest only after institution of mechanical ventilation. Therefore, a cardinal virtue of a dedicated ICU echocardiography machine is the ability to repeat limited bedside evaluations after significant changes in support. Sepsis-induced RV dysfunction is expected to have the same natural history as LV failure, including reversibility to normal function within 10 days.[37] If the diagnosis of acute cor pulmonale is made in a patient in septic shock based on echo criteria (RV dilation and septal flattening), further volume expansion may serve only to exacerbate the RV dysfunction/dilatation, even though the left ventricle may appear empty. Expert opinion–level recommendations include fluid restriction, adjustment of ventilator settings to reduce airway pressure, correction of hypoxemia, and use of vasoconstrictors for maintaining coronary perfusion.[1] Volume expansion, on the other hand, proves detrimental by exacerbating RV dilation and failure. One pitfall of using dynamic indicators of fluid responsiveness without evaluation of right heart function is that positive pressure ventilation may exacerbate acute cor pulmonale during each inflation, yielding false positive pulse pressure variation and IVC collapsibility.

TAMPONADE, AN ALTERNATIVE DIAGNOSIS TO SEPSIS IN ACUTE HEMODYNAMIC INSTABILITY OF UNKNOWN CAUSE

Because pericardial tamponade is life-threatening and has been reported in 2% to 10% of ICU echo examinations, evaluation of the pericardium should be included in even a limited examination of patients in shock.[38] High-risk ICU populations include patients who have had cardiac surgery, coronary catheterization, PA catheter placement, and penetrating chest trauma.[39] Pericardial effusions appear as echo-free spaces surrounding the heart. Pericardial effusions can be distinguished from pleural effusions based on location and distribution: a pericardial effusion extends into the reflection of pericardium interposed between the descending aorta and the base of the left ventricle; the contour of a pleural effusion courses posterior to the descending aorta. In addition, a large pericardial effusion typically surrounds the heart, whereas a pleural effusion does not. However, in the case of heart surgery or recurrent pericardial effusion, a loculated effusion can form in a pocket, bordered by adhesions between the parietal and visceral pericardium. Such a loculated effusion can compress a single chamber, even at low volumes, because of the restricted volume within the pocket, and may require surgical treatment because adhesions may prevent percutaneous drainage.

Because the pericardium adapts to effusions that accumulate slowly by dilating, but develops sharp increases in pressure with rapidly expanding effusions (because it is inelastic), the absolute size of a pericardial effusion does not determine whether tamponade physiology is present. Instead, the diagnosis depends on evidence of increased intrapericardial pressure. Examples of this evidence include right atrial collapse occurring when the atrioventricular (AV) valves are closed and RV diastolic collapse. In addition, the finding of a fixed, engorged IVC caliber supports the clinical diagnosis.[40]

ECHO TRAINING FOR INTENSIVISTS

National board requirements, guidelines of national organizations, and international echo training pathway standards have been published. **Table 2** compares standards and guidelines. Recent trends in defining competency in ICU applications of echo include an emphasis on achieving competency, rather than specifying the duration of training or a precise number of studies, and interest in incorporating basic ICU echo into training requirements for fellows.[2,4,8,41]

A uniquely designed investigation regarding the rate of gaining proficiency in hand-held ultrasonography involved medical residents with less than 1 hour of formal teaching on principles of ultrasound followed by 1:1 bedside teaching by a sonographer.[42] Based on comparison with a comprehensive echocardiogram, the technical

Table 2
Comparison of guidelines or competency definitions for echocardiography

Organization and Reference	Duration of Training/Pathway Goal	Number of Examinations	Additional Requirement	Required Supervision
American Board of Echocardiography http://www.echoboards.org	12 mo/fellowship path for board certification	300	Written examination	Accredited fellowship
American College of Chest Physicians Chest 2009;135(4):1050–60	Basic CCE	Competency-based	"The goal of the statement is to describe the minimal standards for critical care ultrasound as a guide for the intensivist to achieve proficiency"	
	Advanced CCE	Competency-based		
American College of Cardiology/AHA J Am Coll Cardiol 2003;41 (4):687–708	Level 1 Level 2 Level 3	150 300 750	75 performed 150 performed 300 performed	
WINFOCUS Cardiovasc Ultrasound 2008;6:49	Emergency echo Level 1 Level 2 Level 3	Competency-based. Level 1 is all standard views and common abnormalities; level 3 is subspecialty echocardiographers		Level 1 staff Level 2 staff Level 3 staff Level 3 staff

quality of hand-held ultrasound and the interpretive skill were rated by a cardiologist. Residents performed examinations in the course of inpatient rotations. Performance improved as the number of supervised examinations increased, and linear regression of the adequacy of examinations suggested that between 20 and 30 examinations would be required for trainees to obtain studies with acceptable technical and interpretive accuracy.

TRAINING RESOURCES FOR INTENSIVISTS

The American College of Chest Physicians, the Society of Critical Care Medicine, the Society of Cardiovascular Anesthesiologists, and the American Society of Echocardiography have annual workshops with a focus on echocardiography training for noncardiologists, and upcoming conferences are listed on their respective websites. Contact information and additional resources are listed in Appendix 1.

RELIABILITY OF FOCUSED ICU ECHO USING HAND-HELD AND COMPACT PORTABLE DEVICES

The performance characteristics of focused echocardiography by nonspecialists using hand-held or limited ultrasound machines depends on multiple factors, including

- Amount of training in image acquisition and interpretation
- Sophistication of the device (eg, whether the device has harmonic imaging, controls for adjusting gain and focus, and color Doppler)
- Criteria for considering the examination successful (the definition of success covers a wide spectrum in the literature, from simply revealing diagnoses not found by physical examination alone, to finding all significant abnormalities from an 18-item list)
- Patient setting (ventilated vs not ventilated, surgical ICU vs medical ward).

Not surprisingly, the variety of reports of the diagnostic accuracy of portable ultrasound by beginners reflects the influence of the many variables involved. For example, if portable ultrasound is deemed successful simply by extending the physical examination, it has obvious relevance. Portable ultrasound reduces the number of major cardiac findings missed on physical examination from 43% to 21%.[43] By contrast, stringent comparison of beginner performance compared with that of experts reveals pitfalls of novice echocardiographic interpretation of potential clinical significance. After 20 hours of training and 20 supervised examinations, internal medicine residents and expert cardiologists used hand-held ultrasound to examine 300 patients who had undergone comprehensive echo studies.[44] From a list of 18 clinically significant findings, residents missed 23%, compared with 14% by experts ($P = .02$). Findings missed more often by trainees using portable echo included pericardial effusions, RV dysfunction, and regional wall motion abnormalities. The conclusion that the limited portable ultrasound in the hands of trainees is no substitute for a formal comprehensive echo is neither controversial nor surprising. However, it is notable that the residents' interpretations achieved the same specificity, positive predictive value, and negative predictive value as those of expert cardiologists.[44]

A far more practical study design limits the scope of the study and the modalities of the scanning, with the intention of using bedside ICU echo in goal-directed resuscitation. A proof-of-principle study by Manasia and colleagues[45] involved 6 intensivists using a hand-held device after only 10 hours of echo training. The intensivists limited the echo to two-dimensional views from 2 to 4 windows, and focused on LV function and size, volume status, and presence or absence of significant pericardial effusion. Using the comparison of a subsequent examination by an expert cardiologist, the intensivists' readings were correct in 84% of patients. Echo led to changes in treatment in 37% of the subjects and provided new diagnostic data (without changing treatment) in 48% of patients.[45] Similarly, Vignon and colleagues[46] described performance in ICU residents after an 8-hour training limited to two-dimensional imaging. Interpretation was limited to LV size and function, RV dilation, pericardial effusion, and pleural effusion. Residents were able to evaluate 93% of 366 clinical questions and showed close agreement with the interpretations of expert echocardiographers.

SUMMARY

The role of echocardiography in assessing unstable ICU patients with suspected, or known, septic shock has been discussed. The key points are

- Echocardiography is complementary to other monitors of hemodynamics. Positive aspects of echocardiography include noninvasiveness, rapid results, and the potential for comprehensive cardiac assessment.
- Dynamic signs of preload responsiveness, such as IVC collapse, are easily measured, and are more informative than filling pressures.
- Echocardiography can be used to identify and to follow the progress of sepsis-induced cardiac dysfunction, which is common. In addition, echocardiography may reveal isolated diastolic dysfunction. In some cases, unexpected echocardiographic findings lead to major changes in therapy.
- Consensus descriptions of competency in basic and advanced CCE have been published recently,[41] and CCE will likely be formally incorporated into ICU training programs soon.

REFERENCES

1. Vieillard-Baron A, Prin S, Chergui K, et al. Hemodynamic instability in sepsis. Am J Respir Crit Care Med 2003;168:1270–6.
2. Vieillard-Baron A, Slama M, Cholley B, et al. Echocardiography in the intensive care unit: from evolution to revolution? Intensive Care Med 2008;34:243–9.
3. Costachescu T, Denault A, Guimond JG. The hemodynamically unstable patient in the ICU: hemodynamic vs. transesophageal monitoring. Crit Care Med 2002; 30:1214–23.
4. Beaulieu Y. Bedside echocardiography in the assessment of the critically ill. Crit Care Med 2007;35(Suppl):S235–49.
5. Levitov A, Mayo PH, Slonim AD. Critical care ultrasonography. New York: McGraw Hill; 2009.
6. Swenson JD, Bull D, Stringham J. Subjective assessment of left ventricular preload using transesophageal echocardiography: corresponding pulmonary artery occlusion pressures. J Cardiothorac Vasc Anesth 2001;15(5):580–3.
7. Otto CM. Textbook of clinical echocardiography. Philadelphia: Elsevier; 2009.
8. Kaplan A, Mayo PH. Echocardiography performed by the pulmonary/critical care medicine physician. Chest 2009;135(2):529–35.
9. Jensen MB, Sloth E, Larsen KM, et al. Transthoracic echocardiography for cardiopulmonary monitoring in intensive care. Eur J Anaesthesiol 2004;21(9):700–7.
10. Cook CH, Praba AC, Beery PR, et al. Transthoracic echocardiography is not cost effective in critically ill surgical patients. J Trauma 2002;52:280–4.

11. Vignon P, Mentec H, Terre S, et al. Diagnostic accuracy and therapeutic impact of transthoracic and transesophageal echocardiography in mechanically ventilated patients in the ICU. Chest 1994;106:1829–34.

12. Grocott MP, Mythen MG, Gan TJ. Perioperative fluid management and clinical outcomes in adults. Anesth Analg 2005;100:1093–106.

13. Michard F, Teboul JL. Predicting fluid responsiveness in ICU patients. A critical analysis of the evidence. Chest 2002;121:2000–8.

14. Charon C, Caille V, Jardin F, et al. Echocardiographic measurement of fluid responsiveness. Curr Opin Crit Care 2006;12:249–54.

15. Mahjoub Y, Pila C, Friggeri A, et al. Assessing fluid responsiveness in critically ill patients: false positive pulse pressure variation is detected by Doppler echocardiographic evaluation of the right ventricle. Crit Care Med 2009;37(9):2570–5.

16. Feissel M, Michard F, Faller J-P, et al. The respiratory variation in inferior vena cava diameter as a guide to fluid therapy. Intensive Care Med 2004;30: 1834–7.

17. Barbier C, Loubieres Y, Schmit C, et al. Respiratory changes in inferior vena cava diameter are helpful in predicting fluid responsiveness in ventilated septic patients. Intensive Care Med 2004;30:1740–6.

18. Vieillard-Baron A, Chergui K, Rabiller A, et al. Superior vena cava collapsibility as a gauge of volume status in ventilated septic patients. Intensive Care Med 2004; 30:1734–9.

19. Feissel M, Ciahrd F, Mangin I. Respiratory changes in aortic blood velocity as an indicator of fluid responsiveness in ventilated patients with septic shock. Chest 2001;119:867–73.

20. Lamia B, Ochagavia A, Monnet X, et al. Echocardiographic prediction of volume responsiveness in critically ill patients with spontaneous breathing activity. Intensive Care Med 2007;33(7):1125–32.

21. Etchecopar-Chevreuil C, Francois B, Clavel M, et al. Cardiac morphological and functional changes during early septic shock: a transesophageal echocardiographic study. Intensive Care Med 2008;34:250–6.

22. Grocott-Mason RM, Shah AM. Cardiac dysfunction in sepsis: new theories and clinical implications. Intensive Care Med 1998;24:286–95.

23. Parker MM, Shelhamer JH, Bacharach SL, et al. Profound but reversible myocardial depression in patients with septic shock. Ann Intern Med 1984;100:483–90.

24. Bouhemad B, Nicolas-Robin A, Arbelot C, et al. Acute left ventricular dilatation and shock-induced myocardial dysfunction. Crit Care Med 2009;37:441–7.

25. Bouhemad B, Nicolas-Robin A, Arbelot C, et al. Isolated and reversible impairment of ventricular relaxation in patients with septic shock. Crit Care Med 2008;36:766–74.

26. Cariou A, Pinsky M, Monchi M, et al. Is myocardial adrenergic responsiveness depressed in human septic shock? Intensive Care Med 2008;34:917–22.

27. Silverman HJ, Penaranda R, Orens JB, et al. Impaired beta-adrenergic receptor stimulation of cyclic adenosine monophosphate in human septic shock: association with myocardial hyporesponsiveness to catecholamines. Crit Care Med 1993;21:31–9.

28. Bersten AD, Hersch M, Cheung H, et al. The effect of various sympathomimetics on the regional circulations (sic) in hyperdynamic sepsis. Surgery 1992;112: 549–61.

29. Cerqueira MD, Weissman NJ, Dilsizian V, et al. Standardized myocardial segmentation and nomenclature for tomographic imaging of the heart: a statement for healthcare professionals from the Cardiac Imaging Committee of the Council

on Clinical Cardiology of the American Heart Association. Circulation 2002;105: 539–42.

30. Antonopoulos A, Kyriacou C. Apical ballooning syndrome or Takotsubo cardio-myopathy: a new challenge in acute cardiac care. Cardiol J 2008;15(6):572–7.
31. Orpello JM, Manasia AR, Goldman M. Goal-directed echocardiography in the ICU. In: Levitov A, Mayo PH, Slonim AD, editors. Critical care ultrasonography. New York: McGraw Medical; 2009. p. 72–3.
32. Jardin F, Dubourg O, Bourdarias JP. Echocardiographic pattern of acute cor pul-monale. Chest 1997;111:209–17.
33. Kaplan A. Echocardiographic diagnosis and monitoring of RV function. In: Levitov A, Mayo PH, Slonim AD, editors. Critical care ultrasonography. New York: McGraw Medical; 2009. p. 125–34.
34. Ryan T, Petrovic O, Dillon JC, et al. An echocardiographic index for separation of right ventricular volume and pressure overload. J Am Coll Cardiol 1985;5:918–27.
35. Fremont B, Pacouret G, Jacobi D, et al. Prognostic value of echocardiographic right/left ventricular end-diastolic diameter ratio in patients with acute pulmonary embolism: results from a monocenter registry of 1,416 patients. Chest 2008;133: 358–62.
36. Jardin F, Vieillard-Baron A. Is there a safe plateau pressure in ARDS? The right heart only knows. Intensive Care Med 2007;33:444–7.
37. Rabeul C, Mebazaa A. Septic shock: a heart story since the 1960s. Intensive Care Med 2006;32:799–807.
38. Joseph MX, Disney PJ, Da Costa R, et al. Transthoracic echocardiography to identify or exclude cardiac cause of shock. Chest 2004;126:1592–7.
39. Sagrista-Sauleda J, Merce J, Permanyer-Miralda G, et al. Clinical clues to the causes of large pericardial effusions. Am J Med 2000;109:95–101.
40. Otto CM. Pericardial disease. In: Otto CM, editor. Textbook of clinical echocardi-ography. Philadelphia: Elsevier; 2009. p. 242–58.
41. Mayo PH, Beaulieu Y, Doelken P, et al. American College of Chest Physicians/La Societe de Reanimation de Langue Francaise statement on competence in crit-ical care ultrasonography. Chest 2009;135(4):1050–60.
42. Hellmann DB, Whiting-O'Keefe Q, Shapiro EP, et al. The rate at which residents learn to use hand-held echocardiography at the bedside. Am J Med 2005;118: 1010–8.
43. Spencer KT, Anderson AS, Bhargava A, et al. Physician-performed point-of-care echocardiography using a laptop platform compared with physical examination in the cardiovascular patient. J Am Coll Cardiol 2001;37(8):2013–8.
44. DeCara JM, Lang RM, Koch R, et al. The use of small personal ultrasound devices by internists without formal training in echocardiography. Eur J Echocar-diogr 2003;4:141–7.
45. Manasia AR, Nagaraj HM, Kodali RB, et al. Feasibility and potential clinical utility of goal-directed transthoracic echocardiography performed by noncardiologist intensivists. J Cardiothorac Vasc Anesth 2005;19(2):155–9.
46. Vignon P, Dugard A, Abraham J. Focused training for goal-oriented hand-held echocardiography performed by noncardiologist residents in the intensive care unit. Intensive Care Med 2007;33:1795–9.

APPENDIX 1: RESOURCES FOR ECHOCARDIOGRAPHY TRAINING FOR INTENSIVISTS

The American College of Chest Physicians holds annual national workshops in critical care ultrasonography, which includes echocardiography for diagnosis of the cause of shock. These workshops are open for members, nonmembers, and trainees, and involve small-group, hands-on teaching in ultrasonography. Web site: http://www.chestnet.org (accessed September 20, 2009).

The Society of Critical Care Medicine offered a workshop on echo and other applications of ultrasonography in July 2009, and may offer future similar workshops. Web site: http://www.sccm.org (accessed September 20, 2009).

Innovative Critical Care Ultrasonography is a company led by Yanick Beaulieu, MD, an intensivist-cardiologist in Montreal, which offers seminars on a regular basis and also offers on-site seminars (they travel to hospitals to train departments or practices). The Web site provides information on seminars, traveling seminars, and also on software for learning ICU echocardiography. Web site: http://www.iccuimaging.ca (accessed January 22, 2010).

The World Interactive Network Focused on Critical Ultrasound (WINFOCUS) has an annual congress, consensus documents, and Web-based ICU echocardiography teaching. Web site: http://www.winfocus.org (accessed September 20, 2009).

Noninvasive Monitoring Cardiac Output Using Partial CO_2 Rebreathing

Brian P. Young, MD[a],*, Lewis L. Low, MD[b]

KEYWORDS

- Cardiac output • Hemodynamic monitoring
- NICO • Partial CO_2 rebreathing

Proper management of critically ill patients requires the rapid and accurate assessment of cardiac function over a wide range of disease states. Hemodynamic assessment is essential for care of these patients and ideally would be accomplished with a minimally invasive device that can provide precise measurements with few risks to the patient. Advanced cardiovascular monitoring is a prerequisite to optimize hemodynamic treatment in critically ill patients who are commonly prone to cardiocirculatory failure.[1] Continuous measurement of cardiac output enables the early recognition of hemodynamic trends and allows for earlier therapeutic interventions. The most ideal cardiac output (CO) monitor should be reliable, continuous, noninvasive, operator-independent, cost-effective, and have a fast response time.[1] Technology should be applicable to both the ICU and the operating room monitoring for management of the patient. Moreover, cardiac output monitoring and early fluid management interventions may translate into better outcomes and cost savings through reduced length of ICU and hospital stay.[2]

Routine measurement of cardiac output has been available only since the 1970s, when Swan and colleagues[3] reported that pulmonary artery catheter (PAC) insertion could be performed at the bedside with a specially designed balloon tipped catheter. Cardiac output monitoring with a PAC using the bolus thermodilution method became the de facto gold standard shortly after its introduction. Continued questions about the PAC's effect on morbidity and mortality[4] have led to an increased interest in other methods, particularly noninvasive methods for cardiac output monitoring. In particular, noninvasive carbon dioxide (CO_2) Fick methods are seeing a resurgence in

---

[a] Kern Critical Care Unit, Good Samaritan Medical Center, Legacy Health, 2282 NW Northrup Street, Suite #42, Portland, OR 97210, USA
[b] Medical Specialties Division, Legacy Health, 2282 NW Northrup Street, Suite #41, Portland, OR 97210, USA
* Corresponding author.
E-mail address: byoung@lhs.org

Crit Care Clin 26 (2010) 383–392
doi:10.1016/j.ccc.2009.12.002
0749-0704/10/$ – see front matter © 2010 Published by Elsevier Inc.

research and clinical interest.[1,5–7] This article reviews one such device using partial CO_2 rebreathing to determine cardiac output and its application for hemodynamic monitoring in an ICU and the operating room setting.

THEORY OF OPERATION

Adolph Fick described the first method of cardiac output estimation in 1870.[7] This method remains the original reference standard by which all other means of determining cardiac output are evaluated. Fick postulated that oxygen uptake in the lungs is entirely transferred to the blood. Therefore, cardiac output can be calculated as the ratio between oxygen consumption (VO_2) and arteriovenous difference in oxygen ($AVDO_2$). The Fick principle allows substitution with a multitude of substitutes for oxygen consumption, including CO_2 clearance, and can be represented mathematically as shown in **Fig. 1**.

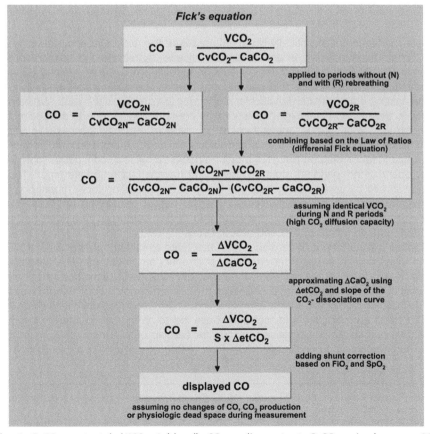

Fig. 1. $CaCO_2$ content (ml/100 mL blood); CO, cardiac output; $CvCO_2$, mixed venous CO_2 content (ml/100 mL blood); $etCO_2$, $etCO_2$ concentration (mmHg); FiO2, fraction of inspired oxygen; N, normal ventilation; R, rebreathing; S, slope of CO_2 dissociation curve; SpO_2, oxygen saturation obtained by pulse oximetry (%). (*From* Hofer CK, Ganter MT, Zollinger A. What technique should I use to measure cardiac output? Curr Opin Crit Care 2007;13(3):308–17; with permission.)

Venous CO_2 (VCO_2) can be calculated by the difference in CO_2 content between expired and inspired gases. The Fick equation can then be further modified by use of a partial CO_2 rebreathing technique. This involves a transitory interruption of CO_2 elimination by the addition of dead space to the ventilatory circuit, which leads to a progressive increase in end-tidal CO_2 ($etCO_2$) that approximates the mixed venous partial CO_2 value.[7–10] This eliminates the need for a direct measurement of $CvCO_2$ and, therefore, the need for a central venous catheter.[5,6,10] The change (delta) VCO_2 is then calculated by comparing normal and rebreathing values. The change (delta) in arterial CO_2 ($CaCO_2$) content can then be approximated by the change in $etCO_2$ multiplied by the slope of the CO_2 dissociation curve (S), which is linear between 15 and 70 mmHg of partial pressure of CO_2.[6,10] Because intrapulmonary shunts can affect estimates of CO with this technique, an arterial blood sample is required to enter arterial oxygen tension values for shunt estimation. This leaves the equation as follows:

$$CO = \Delta VCO_2 / S \times \Delta etCO_2$$

Combining measurements under normal and rebreathing conditions allow elimination of VCO_2 content from the Fick equation and, therefore, there is no requirement for a central venous access for data input in the calculations.[6,7,11]

COMMERCIAL SYSTEMS FOR HEMODYNAMIC MONITORING USING PARTIAL CO_2 REBREATHING

Of the partial CO_2 rebreathing cardiac output monitor systems that have been developed, the NICO (Noninvasive Cardiac Output) monitor (Novametrix Medical Systems, Inc, Wallingford, CT, USA) remains the most widely deployed and studied. This technology is essentially self-contained and requires little additional training for the clinician. The NICO monitor consists of a CO_2 sensor (infrared light absorption), a disposable airflow sensor (differential pressure pneumotachometer), a specific disposable rebreathing loop, and a pulse oximeter.[6,11] The production of CO_2 (VCO_2, mL/min) is calculated from minute ventilation and its instantaneous CO_2 content, whereas the $CaCO_2$ (mL/100 mL of blood) is estimated (**Fig. 2**) from $etCO_2$ (mmHg).

Kotake and colleagues[12] have subsequently demonstrated the improved performance of the NICO monitor equipped with updated software (version 5), improving correlation of the NICO monitor to the PAC over a range of cardiac outputs. Updates to version 5.0 attenuated the effects of rebreathing introduced by the NICO monitor without compromising the accuracy of the cardiac output measurement.

Taking advantage of modern sophisticated sensor and signal processing technology, NICO uses this ratio of the change in the change in the $etCO_2$ partial pressure, and CO_2 elimination to automatically derive cardiac output that is readily available for applications in the ICU and operating room settings. CO_2 production is calculated as the product of CO_2 concentration and air flow during a breathing cycle and $CaCO_2$ content is derived from $etCO_2$ and the CO_2 dissociation curve.[5,9–11] A disposable rebreathing loop allows an intermittent partial rebreathing state in cycles of 3 min. The rebreathing cycle induces an increase in $etCO_2$ and mimics a drop in CO_2 production. The obtained differences of these values are then used to calculate CO.

Good CO determination was observed as long as the NICO system was applied to intubated, mechanically ventilated patients with minor lung abnormalities and fixed ventilatory settings. Changes in VCO_2 and $etCO_2$ only reflect the amount of blood

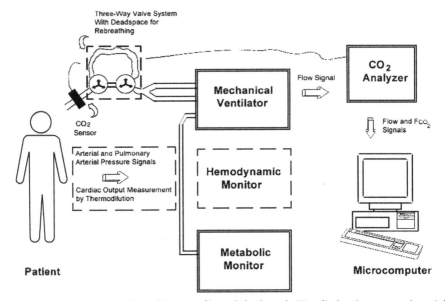

Fig. 2. Experimental setup for validation of breath-by-breath CO_2-elimination rate and partial CO_2 rebreathing measurements. The devices in the boxes marked with dashed lines were used for the partial CO_2 rebreathing experiments only. (*From* de Abreu MG, Quintel M, Ragaller M, et al. Partial CO_2 rebreathing: a reliable technique for noninvasive measurement of nonshunted pulmonary capillary blood flow. Critical Care Med 1997;25(4):675–83; with permission.)

flow that participates in gas exchange; hence, intrapulmonary shunt can affect the estimation of cardiac output by the NICO.[7]

NICO VALIDATION AND LIMITATIONS

Several animal and relatively small human subject trials have been conducted to evaluate the accuracy and precision of partial CO_2 rebreathing determined cardiac output compared with PAC-derived data. Early clinical human subject evaluations of the partial rebreathing technique[11,13–15] reported a relatively loose agreement (bias ± 1.8 l/min) between cardiac output measured using thermodilution and NICO. Cardiac output as determined by the NICO device in one study showed a 37% error compared with the PAC.[16] However, the investigators did note a better correlation between normal-to-low cardiac output values using the NICO monitor. Several studies have shown that the indirect Fick equation is only valid when the partial CO_2 is greater than 30 torr when the CO_2-hemoglobin dissociation curve is linear. Subsequent studies have shown better correlation with the PAC and, therefore, there are increasing applications for the NICO device.

The correlation between the NICO and standard thermodilution was shown to be severely adversely affected in spontaneously breathing patients.[17] The NICO value was inversely proportional to an etCO2 difference between pre-rebreathing and post-rebreathing. The large bias in spontaneously breathing patients is likely due to a small delta-etCO2 in spontaneously breathing patients and therefore the NICO tends to measure higher CO values in spontaneously breathing patients. To achieve optimal results with the NICO monitor, the patient should be maintained under fully controlled mechanical ventilation. Variations in ventilatory modalities, mechanically assisted spontaneous breathing, or use of this technique in patients with lung pathologies (increased shunt fraction) will, therefore, decrease accuracy of NICO-derived cardiac output readings.[5]

Odenstedt and colleagues[18] found a good correlation between NICO derived cardiac output, and cardiac output using the thermodilution technique with a pulmonary artery catheter (correlation coefficient, $r = 0.96$, within-subject correlation $r = 0.88$). They did identify a small underestimation of cardiac output by NICO of 0.04 L/min, with the limits of agreement (± 2 SD) being -1.68 and 1.76 L/min. They also found that in hemodynamically unstable patients the NICO method closely followed thermodilution derived cardiac output (TDCO) in tracking changes in CO. Pulmonary shunt was underestimated by approximately 11% compared with standard shunt calculations using arterial and mixed venous blood gases.

A case report[19] suggests that CO_2 insufflation during laparoscopic surgery does not affect the agreement between NICO and thermodilution.

AFFECT OF PULMONARY DISEASE

Increased intrapulmonary shunt and poor hemodynamic stability, common in critically ill patients, are likely to alter the precision of cardiac output estimation by the NICO monitor. Changes in VCO_2 and $etCO_2$ only reflect the amount of blood flow that participates in gas exchange; hence, intrapulmonary shunt can affect the estimation of cardiac output by the NICO.

Because noninvasive CO measurement depends on CO_2 rebreathing and assumes constant dead space and mixed venous CO_2 content through the CO_2 rebreathing procedure, Tachibana and colleagues[20] investigated in a prospective comparative study the effects of tidal volume (V_T), ventilatory mode, inspired oxygen fraction (FiO_2), and positive end-expiratory pressure (PEEP) on the accuracy of the measurement. They found that during mechanical ventilation with large constant V_T or during spontaneous breathing (PSV), CO measurements obtained by CO_2 rebreathing technique correlate with those obtained by thermodilution method and that, when minute ventilation is large, the accuracy of the CO_2 rebreathing technique is not affected by a selection of volume or pressure-controlled ventilation, or PSV, PEEP, or FiO_2. However, when V_T and minute ventilation are reduced, the CO_2 rebreathing technique underreports CO.

Neviere and colleagues[21] did find that in mechanically ventilated patients with chronic obstructive pulmonary disease, cardiac output measurements by the CO_2 rebreathing technique might correlate closely with thermodilution ($r2 = 0.92$, $P<.001$).

Increased intrapulmonary shunt and lack of hemodynamic stability, common in critically ill patients, may alter the precision of CO_2 estimation by the NICO. Patients with lung disease or postoperative atelectasis can contribute to decreased accuracy of the NICO measurements, a finding also experienced in a porcine model of trauma.[15]

Similarly, Nilsson and colleagues[14] found the reproducibility of thermodilution and CO_2-rebreathing cardiac output were excellent, with coefficients of reproducibility of 0.35 l/min and 0.60 l/min. They concluded the methods are not interchangeable with the present version of the NICO. The reproducibility of the partial CO_2-rebreathing technique holds promise that a sufficient accuracy may be obtained by suitable modifications of the monitor's algorithms.

CARDIOTHORACIC SURGERY PATIENTS

Several studies have evaluated the use of the NICO monitor for intraoperative monitoring during cardiothoracic surgery. Botero and colleagues[22] important study of patients undergoing cardiopulmonary bypass (CPB) conducted a unique evaluation of four simultaneous cardiac output measurements techniques, including ultrasound transit-time flowmetry, which may be considered the true gold standard for cardiac output measurement. Agreement with this reference method was best for NICO and worst for continuous thermodilution, with thermodilution bolus being intermediate, raising separate questions of the appropriate standard for comparison. NICO measurements seem to agree well with thermodilution before CPB but the tendency was for NICO to underestimate CO after CBP.[23] Crespo and colleagues[24] evaluated the NICO device in 25 patients undergoing elective cardiac surgery and found that the agreement between the NICO and continuous cardiac output is clinically acceptable and is unaffected by $etCO_2$. All these studies support the conclusion that the NICO monitor offers an appropriate alternative to invasive CO measurement.

Ng and colleagues[25] examined the use of the noninvasive partial CO_2 rebreathing system for cardiac output monitoring of patients undergoing thoracic surgery and one-lung ventilation. They found that the NICO device showed a tendency to underestimate CO compared with thermodilution CO at all measurement times. Although the study size was small, overall, the bias for the NICO was −0.29 L/min, and they concluded that the NICO device is still useful for monitoring during thoracic surgery. Gueret and colleagues[26] found that during off-pump cardiac surgery the noninvasive cardiac output reliably measures cardiac output and does it more rapidly than a PAC and may be more useful to detect rapid hemodynamic changes.

PARTIAL CO_2 REBREATHING MEASUREMENTS IN SEVERE LUNG INJURY

Neviere and colleagues[27] conducted a study to compare measurement of cardiac output by the CO_2 rebreathing method with the thermodilution cardiac output technique in mechanically ventilated patients with acute lung injury. This prospective study evaluated patients over a wide range of cardiac index for patients with acute lung injury. There was a significant correlation between thermodilution and CO_2 rebreathing methods (r2 = 0.82, $P<.01$) and the mean difference between the CO_2 rebreathing method and thermodilution was 0.05 l/min/m2, with a standard deviation for the bias of 0.38 l/min/m2. These results suggest that the CO_2 rebreathing method may be a reliable noninvasive technique to determine cardiac output in mechanically ventilated patients with acute lung injury.

This finding was contradicted in a more recent study evaluating patients with acute lung injury at two levels of severity (lung injury score <2.5, group A; and >2.5, group B).[28] Cardiac output was measured by thermodilution and partial CO_2 rebreathing (NICO). Patients with acute lung failure (partial O_2/FiO_2 < 300) showed a poor positive correlation between the methods for the patients from groups A (r = 0.52, $P<.001$) and B (r = 0.47, $P<.001$). Errors in estimating $CaCO_2$ content from $etCO_2$ and situations of hyperdynamic circulation associated with dead space or increased shunt may explain these results with a greater difference between NICO and TDCO the more critical the lung injury.

An animal study by Gama de Abreu and colleagues[29] looked at the performance of the partial CO_2 rebreathing technique with systematical modulation of cardiac output to achieve hypodynamic, normal, and hyperdynamic states. Their results showed that although pulmonary capillary blood flow is underestimated during hyperdynamic cardiac output states and high alveolar dead spaces, the performance of the partial CO_2 rebreathing technique was improved with arterial blood gas sampling and an algorithm that took into account the effects of nonequilibration of end-tidal partial pressure of CO_2 ($PetCO_2$). Such an algorithm may prove useful under moderately increased alveolar dead space and normal to hypodynamic cardiac output states.

Rocco and colleagues[30] conducted a small study investigating patients with high and low pulmonary shunt fractions. They found that the partial CO$_2$ rebreathing technique is reliable in measuring cardiac output in non-postoperative critically ill patients affected by diseases causing low levels of pulmonary shunt, but underestimates it in patients with shunt higher than 35%.

NICO IN PEDIATRIC AND GERIATRIC AGE GROUPS

Levy and colleagues[31] concluded that NICO is clinically acceptable in children with a body surface area of more than 0.6 m^2 and a tidal volume greater than 300 mL, whereas discrepancies with thermodilution were more important in smaller patients. Botte and colleagues[32] evaluated 21 mechanically ventilated children, weighing greater than 15 kg, in stable respiratory and hemodynamic condition. CO values obtained with this technique were in agreement with those obtained with Doppler echocardiography. Although NICO evaluation has yet to be completed in children in unstable respiratory and hemodynamic conditions, this would seem to be a reasonable endeavor for future investigations.

Yoshie[33] evaluated the NICO device in patients over 65 years of age scheduled for elective lower abdominal or surface surgery. They found that, although cardiac output measures were most reliable when the arterial pressure was above 100 mmHg, there was no statistical relationship between arterial pressure and cardiac output in all measurements. They found that age, blood pressure level, history of hypertension, and body structure affected cardiac output measurements, but that the NICO values were useful to monitor cardiac output in this age population cohort.

HIP SURGERY PATIENTS

Gueret and colleagues[34] specifically looked at the use of the partial CO$_2$ rebreathing monitor for monitoring patients undergoing repeat total hip replacements. They found a small perioperative bias with the NICO device and a slight underestimation of cardiac output when compared with the PAC. The bias was smaller when mean cardiac output was below 3L/min. An additional finding was that core temperature between 34.4°C and 37.6°C had no influence on the differences.

OTHER APPLICATIONS

Other investigators have proposed using noninvasive cardiac monitoring in the emergency department evaluation of patients for early identification of shock and the optimization of organ donation.[35] The NICO system seems well suited for such applications and these authors await further publication of such studies.

SUMMARY

Compared with conventional cardiac output methods, the partial CO$_2$ rebreathing technique is noninvasive, can easily be automated, and can provide real-time and continuous cardiac output monitoring.[10,36] Large outcome studies using monitoring devices such as the NICO for hemodynamic optimization are still lacking. The advantages and limitations of this technique is unique and may yet find a specific niche in which its advantages are be decisive. Partial CO$_2$ rebreathing derived cardiac output measurement does not seem ready to replace the PAC which remains unique in providing pressures (right atrial, pulmonary artery, and pulmonary "wedged"), and venous oxygen saturation in addition to cardiac output. These parameters are still extremely useful for the management of some of the most severely ill patients.[6] No single method stands out or renders the others obsolete. By making cardiac output easily measurable, however, these techniques should all contribute to improvement in hemodynamic management.[1]

REFERENCES

1. de Waal EE, Wappler F, Buhre WF. Cardiac output monitoring. Curr Opin Anaesthesiol 2009;22(1):71–7.
2. Venn R, Steele A, Richardson P, et al. Randomized controlled trial to investigate influence of the fluid challenge on duration of hospital stay and perioperative morbidity in patients with hip fractures. Br J Anaesth 2002;88(1):65–71.
3. Swan H, Ganz W, Forrester J, et al. Catheterization of the heart in man with use of a flow-directed balloon-tipped catheter. N Engl J Med 1970;283(9):447–51.
4. Harvey S, Harrison DA, Singer M, et al. Assessment of the clinical effectiveness of pulmonary artery catheters in management of patients in intensive care (PAC-Man): a randomized controlled trial. Lancet 2005;366(9484):472–7.
5. Hofer CK, Ganter MT, Zollinger A. What technique should I use to measure cardiac output? Curr Opin Crit Care 2007;13(3):308–17.
6. Cholley BP, Payen D. Noninvasive techniques for measurements of cardiac output. Curr Opin Crit Care 2005;11(5):424–9.
7. Chaney JC, Derdak S. Minimally invasive hemodynamic monitoring for the intensivist: current and emerging technology. Crit Care Med 2002;30(10):2338–45.
8. de Abreu MG, Quintel M, Ragaller M, et al. Partial carbon dioxide rebreathing: a reliable technique for noninvasive measurement of nonshunted pulmonary capillary blood flow. Crit Care Med 1997;25(4):675–83.
9. de Abreu MG, Geiger S, Winkler T, et al. Evaluation of a new device for noninvasive measurement of nonshunted pulmonary capillary blood flow in patients with acute lung injury. Intensive Care Med 2002;289(3):318–23.
10. Heigenhauser GJ, Jones NL. Measurement of cardiac output by carbon dioxide rebreathing methods. Clin Chest Med 1989;10(2):255–64.
11. Jaffe MB. Partial CO_2 rebreathing cardiac output—operating principles of the NICO system. J Clin Monit Comput 1999;15(6):387–401.
12. Kotake Y, Yamada T, Nagata H, et al. Improved accuracy of cardiac output estimation by the partial CO_2 rebreathing method. J Clin Monit Comput 2009;23(3):149–55.
13. van Heerden PV, Baker S, Lim SI, et al. Clinical evaluation of the non-invasive cardiac output (NICO) monitor in the intensive care unit. Anaesth Intensive Care 2000;28(4):427–30.
14. Nilsson LB, Eldrup N, Berthelsen PG. Lack of agreement between thermodilution and carbon dioxide-rebreathing cardiac output. Acta Anaesthesiol Scand 2001;45(6):680–5.
15. Maxwell RA, Gibson JB, Slade JB, et al. Noninvasive cardiac output by partial CO_2 rebreathing after severe chest trauma. J Trauma 2001;51(5):849–53.
16. Jover JL, Soro M, Belda FJ, et al. Measurement of cardiac output after cardiac surgery: validation fo a partial carbon dioxide rebreathing (NICO) system in comparison with continous thermodilution with a pulmonary artery catheter. Rev Esp Anestesiol Reanim 2005;52(5):256–62 [in Spanish].
17. Kimura C, Kunimoto F, Morishita Y. Cardiac output measurement using the non-invasive cardiac output (NICO) monitor: a comparative study with the standard thermodilution technique. Jpn J Thorac Cardiovasc Surg 2004;33(1):6–8.

18. Odenstedt H, Stenqvist O, Lundin S. Clinical evaluation of a partial CO$_2$ rebreathing technique for cardiac output monitoring in critically ill patients. Acta Anaesthesiol Scand 2002;46(2):152–9.
19. Suzuki M, Koda S, Nakamura Y, et al. The relationship between cardiac output measured by the thermodilution method and that measured by the carbon dioxide rebreathing technique during laparoscopic surgery. Anesth Analg 2005;100(5):1381–3.
20. Tachibana K, Imanaka H, Miyano H, et al. Effect of Ventilatory settings on accuracy of cardiac output measurement using partial CO$_2$ rebreathing. Anesthesiology 2002;96(1):96–102.
21. Neviere R, Mathieu D, Riou Y, et al. Carbon dioxide rebreathing method of cardiac output measurement during acute respiratory failure in patients with chronic obstructive pulmonary disease. Crit Care Med 1994;22(1):81–5.
22. Botero M, Kirby D, Lobato EB, et al. Measurement of cardiac output before and after cardiopulmonary bypass: comparison among aortic transit-time ultrasound, thermodilution, and noninvasive partial CO$_2$ rebreathing. J Cardiothorac Vasc Anesth 2004;18(5):563–72.
23. Neuhäuser C, Müller M, Bräu M, et al. Partial CO(2) rebreathing technique versus thermodilution: measurement of cardiac output before and after operations with extracorporeal circulation. Anaesthesist 2002;51(8):625–33 [in German].
24. Crespo AS, Galhardo C, Silveira CG, et al. Assessment of the agreement between cardiac output measured by thermal filament continuous thermodilution (CCO) and noninvasive partial CO$_2$ rebreathing (NICO) with particular reference to ETCO$_2$ levels. Crit Care 2002;6(Suppl 1):195.
25. Ng JM, Chow MY, Ip-Yam PC, et al. Evaluation of partial carbon dioxide rebreathing cardiac output measurement during thoracic surgery. J Cardiothorac Vasc Anesth. 2007;21(5):655–8.
26. Gueret G, Kiss G, Rossignol B, et al. Cardiac output measurements in off-pump coronary surgery: comparison between NICO and the Swan-Ganz catheter. Eur J Anaesthesiol 2006;23(10):848–54.
27. Neviere R, Mathieu D, Riou Y, et al. Non-invasive measurement of cardiac output in patients with acute lung injury using the carbon dioxide rebreathing method. Clin Intensive Care 1994;5(4):172–5.
28. Valiatti JL, Amaral JL. Comparison between cardiac output values measured by thermodilution and partial carbon dioxide rebreathing in patients with acute lung injury. Sao Paulo Med J 2004;122(6):233–8.
29. Gama de Abreu M, Winkler T, Pahlitzsch T, et al. Performance of the partial CO$_2$ rebreathing technique under different hemodynamic and ventilation/perfusion matching conditions. Crit Care Med 2003;31(2):543–51.
30. Rocco M, Spadetta G, Morelli A, et al. A comparative evaluation of thermodilution and partial CO$_2$ rebreathing techniques for cardiac output asessment in critically ill patients during assisted ventilation. Intensive Care Med 2004;30(1):82–7.
31. Levy RJ, Chiavacci RM, Nicolson SC, et al. An evaluation of a noninvasive cardiac output measurement using partial carbon dioxide rebreathing in children. Anesth Analg 2004;99(6):1642–7.
32. Botte A, Leclerc F, Riou Y, et al. Evaluation of noninvasive cardiac output in mechanically ventilated children. Pediatr Crit Care Med 2006;7(3):231–6.
33. Yoshie K. Comparison of three kinds of less invasive cardiac output measuring systems in aged patients. Masui 2008;57(12):1485–93 [in Japanese].

34. Gueret G, Kiss G, Khaldi S, et al. Comparision of cardiac output measurements between NICO and the pulmonary artery catherter during repeat surgery for total hip replacement. Eur J Anaesthesiol 2007;24(12):1028–33.

35. de la Torre AN, Fisher A, Wilson DJ, et al. Minimally invasive optimization of organ donor resuscitation: case reports. Prog Transplant 2005;15(1):27–32.

36. Haryadi DG, Orr JA, Kuck K, et al. Partial CO_2 rebreathing indirect Fick technique for non-invasive measurement of cardiac output. J Clin Monit Comput 2000; 16(5–6):361–74.

Mechanisms, Detection, and Potential Management of Microcirculatory Disturbances in Sepsis

Imran Mohammed, MD, Stephanie A. Nonas, MD*

KEYWORDS

- Sepsis • Microcirculatory disturbances
- Microvascular perfusion • Microvascular blood flow

Sepsis is a syndrome defined by the presence of systemic inflammation in the setting of known or presumed infection. Triggered by local or bloodstream infection, it is characterized by an exuberant and potentially harmful host response with widespread inflammation and circulatory disturbances, including systemic vasodilation and hypotension with heterogeneous microvascular blood flow and microvascular thrombosis, which are thought to contribute to tissue hypoxia and cellular injury. The magnitude of circulatory disturbance and extent of organ dysfunction are used to define severe sepsis and septic shock, in which end-organ damage is evident.[1] Together, severe sepsis and septic shock account for the majority of the more than 200,000 sepsis-related deaths occurring annually in the United States.[2]

The incidence of severe sepsis continues to grow yearly despite increasing research into the pathophysiology of sepsis and efforts to improve management. By now, most critical care physicians are well-versed in the principles of early goal-directed therapy, which have been incorporated into the Surviving Sepsis Guidelines and which strive to reverse hypotension and improve tissue perfusion in the first 6 hours of hospitalization.[3,4] This management protocol is based on global indices of perfusion, including mean arterial pressure (MAP), as well as lactate and mixed venous oxygen saturation

Division of Pulmonary and Critical Care, Oregon Health and Science University, 3181 SW Sam Jackson Park Road, UHN-67, Portland, OR 97239, USA
* Corresponding author.
E-mail address: nonas@ohsu.edu

Crit Care Clin 26 (2010) 393–408
doi:10.1016/j.ccc.2010.01.003
0749-0704/10/$ – see front matter © 2010 Published by Elsevier Inc.

(SvO$_2$) as markers of adequacy of tissue oxygenation. These global parameters indicate that tissue dysoxia and injury may continue at a local level even when central perfusion pressures and systemic oxygen delivery are restored.

In the past several years, there has been renewed interest in the abnormal behavior of the microcirculation in shock states and its possible contribution to disordered oxygen metabolism at the cellular level.[5,6] Indeed, recent clinical observations and animal studies have revealed marked alterations in the pattern and velocity of flow in microvessels during shock.[7–9]

AN OVERVIEW OF THE MICROCIRCULATION

The microcirculation is the site at which nutrient and gas exchange with the tissues occurs. It is defined by vessels less than 20 μm in diameter and includes capillaries and most small arterioles and venules. Once thought to act as a passive vascular conduit for the transport of cells and nutrients, the microvasculature is now understood to be a dynamic system that interacts with circulating and tissue-associated cells, elaborating mediators and contributing to local, downstream, and upstream vascular tone. An intact and properly functioning microcirculatory system is crucial for the efficient delivery of oxygen to the tissues. Under normal conditions, such as exercise, the microvasculature controls the distribution of blood flow within tissues by increasing the percentage of perfused capillaries in response to a sensed decrease in local oxygen tension.[10] In contrast, in shock states, injury to the microcirculatory system may affect all cellular components including endothelial cells and smooth muscle cells, as well as the constantly changing pool of circulating blood cells. Activation, dysfunction, and injury of endothelial cells may occur as a result of ischemia, inflammatory cell recruitment, and elaboration of inflammatory mediators and proteolytic enzymes. This can, in turn, lead to disruption of endothelial and epithelial barriers, microvascular thrombosis, and altered microvascular flow manifested by heterogeneous blood flow and disturbances in oxygen transport.[11,12] Microcirculatory dysfunction may therefore commonly occur despite preserved perfusion of larger vessels, and seems to be strongly associated with organ damage in animal models of sepsis as well as intensive care unit (ICU) patients with shock, as described in a later section.[13,14]

MECHANISMS OF MICROCIRCULATORY DYSFUNCTION IN SEPSIS

A variety of mechanisms have been suggested to contribute to impaired local oxygen delivery in sepsis, including alterations in vascular reactivity with development of functional arteriovenous shunts, local barrier disruption, thrombosis of microvessels, and perturbed rheologic properties of both red and white blood cells.[11,12] The area that has received the greatest attention in recent years involves impaired small vessel vasoreactivity and the more general concept of vasomotor paralysis. When vasomotor paralysis is present, vessels may exhibit both impaired constriction to exogenous or endogenous catecholamines and impaired dilation in response to an ischemic challenge—a response that may vary depending on tissue type and the caliber of vessel involved. Observations in humans, for example, have demonstrated a near doubling of skeletal muscle blood flow during septic shock, on the arteriolar level.[15] Because the skeletal microvascular volume is large, this may lead to overperfusion of low oxygen-consuming tissues and effective shunting of blood flow away from more vital areas, such as the intestinal microcirculation.[16]

Changes in the integrity of the microcirculation may also contribute to maldistribution of oxygen and nutrients in tissue beds by increasing the diffusion distance over which they must travel. These alterations in permeability occur because of breakdown of endothelial barrier function with loss of tight junctions between endothelial cells, release of vasoactive substances, and accumulation of neutrophils, macrophages, and mast cells. Increased permeability has been shown to occur in both pulmonary and systemic microvascular systems, and is distributed along the vessels nonhomogeneously. Because as much as 50% of the blood can be found in the microcirculation, at a given time, changes in permeability can lead to reductions in circulating volume and thereby contribute to perfusion abnormalities through diminished cardiac output until central volumes are restored.[11,12]

In addition to its function in gating blood flow, the microcirculation also plays a crucial role in the control and activation of coagulation and inflammatory processes, from overt disseminated intravascular coagulation (DIC) to more subtle microvascular thrombosis.[17] Nowhere is this more evident than in patients suffering from fulminant meningococcal sepsis. Extensive small-vessel thrombosis has been demonstrated in the limbs of these patients and has been shown to be associated with the loss of the endothelium-based anticoagulant, thrombomodulin.[18,19] With microvascular thrombosis as a target, multiple studies have looked at the potential therapeutic effects of tissue factor pathway inhibitor (TFPI), antithrombin (ATIII), heparin, and activated protein C (rAPC) in sepsis.[17] TFPI, ATIII, and rAPC were all shown to reduce organ dysfunction and mortality in animal models and phase 2 clinical trials of sepsis,[20] an effect that has been thought to be related to improvement in microvascular flow. However, only rAPC has been shown to have a proven benefit in phase 3 trials, and then only in a subset of patients.[21,22] With its wide range of actions, it remains unclear whether the beneficial effects of rAPC can be attributed to its anticoagulant properties alone, or other anti-inflammatory or antiapoptotic effects.[23]

Finally, abnormalities in blood cellular components are common in sepsis and contribute to impaired microvascular flow.[15] Normally, red blood cells (RBCs) must deform in order to squeeze through capillaries, which are smaller in diameter. In sepsis, changes in the dimension of small blood vessels as well as impaired endothelial structure and function can impair this transit. Perhaps as important are the biochemical and physiologic changes in the RBC membranes that reduce RBC deformability with resultant decreases in ability to traverse the microcirculation. Acidosis, hypothermia, and circulating cytokines can all contribute to changes in RBC membrane glycoproteins and resultant changes in geometry and loss of deformability.[24]

Likewise, there is ample evidence that white blood cell activation has profound effects on microcirculatory blood flow. Leukocytes are inherently less deformable than RBCs, and more likely to cause prolonged obstruction of the microcirculation than RBCs.[25] Adhesion of leukocytes to activated microvascular endothelium can increase flow resistance and impair RBC flow in microvessels, particularly in low-flow states such as sepsis, thus modulating oxygen delivery.[25] In addition, activation of leukocytes and accumulation in the microcirculation may increase microvascular permeability, further contributing to tissue edema and decreased circulating volume.[26]

MEASUREMENT OF MICROCIRCULATORY FUNCTION

Microcirculatory blood flow may be measured either directly, by use of microscopy and flowmetry techniques, or indirectly, using tissue oxygenation or carbon dioxide as markers for adequate tissue perfusion. This section reviews the different techniques and discusses the pros and cons of each technique used in measurement of microcirculatory dysfunction.

Microscopy/Videomicroscopy

Microcirculatory function has been measured by microscopy since the seventeenth century, when Malphigi and Leeuwenhoek first observed capillary blood flow in the tail of a tadpole. Using the principle that superficial tissues may be made translucent by reflected light, they demonstrated for the first time continuous single cell flow from artery through capillary to vein. In the twentieth century, this technique has been adapted to noninvasively study the microcirculation in the human nail fold, skin, and mucous membranes, including the lip and bulbar conjunctiva. Although this technique is limited in its ability to measure flow in only 2 dimensions, direct microscopy can nonetheless give a reasonable estimate of peripheral microvascular flow. Nail-fold microscopy, in particular, has been used in a variety of connective tissue diseases. For example, it can detect early changes in microvascular flow in systemic sclerosis identifying patients early in their disease course and those with limited skin involvement.[27] Nail-fold microscopy has the benefit of being easily accessed and noninvasive, and indeed is being used by many rheumatologists in the office setting. However, it is poorly suited for use in the ICU due to the difficulty of setup, and more importantly, due to the significant vasoconstriction response of the extremities to temperature changes and the heterogeneous effect of systemic diseases including peripheral vascular disease, diabetes, and hypertension.

Fluorescence Videomicroscopy

Fluorescence techniques, in which fluorescent dyes are injected into the bloodstream for deposition and washout studies, have long been used to measure blood flow distribution. Fluorescence videomicroscopy yields high-quality images of the microvasculature, and can be used to assess capillary permeability as well as capillary density and size. Unlike direct microscopy, which can measure individual capillary RBC flow, fluorescence microscopy gives an estimate of local blood flow over time—the greater the flow, the greater the accumulation of fluorescence in the tissues. Fluorescence microscopy can be used to measure capillary density and diameter, but is not well suited to measurement of acute changes in blood flow; it is relatively cumbersome and has been supplanted by newer techniques for clinical use.

Orthogonal Polarization Spectral Imaging

Orthogonal polarization spectral (OPS) imaging is an update of the standard videomicroscopy technique that makes use of polarized green light, which illuminates tissue to a maximal depth of 3 mm, and allows for the visualization of the microcirculation and specifically RBC transit.[28] This technique relies on cell transit to image the microvasculature; thus, vessels without cells will not light up. OPS imaging is noninvasive and can be used to visualize microcirculatory flow in a variety of mucosal surfaces, including the eyelids and rectal, vaginal, ileal, and colonic mucosa, but is most often used on the easily accessible sublingual mucosa. This technique has been shown to be comparable to the gold standard of fluorescence videomicroscopy in measuring vessel diameter, functional capillary density, and the proportion of perfused capillaries in animal models.[29] In addition to sepsis, OPS imaging has also been used to evaluate microvascular perfusion in transplanted organs, skin flaps, and even the cerebral microcirculation during aneurysm surgery.

However, the OPS technique also has some limitations, which include sensitivity to motion artifact and blurred images caused by secretions such as saliva and blood. In addition, measurements are subject to pressure artifact caused by the OPS system itself, and care must be taken when applying the OPS scope to the mucosa to minimize surface pressure that may alter the flow velocity in microcirculation. In addition, OPS has a maximum velocity resolution of approximately 1 mm per second with conventional illumination, which may limit its ability to measure arteriolar flow velocity and pulsatile flow patterns. Despite these limitations, the relative ease of use and portability of OPS makes it attractive for use in the ICU. OPS imaging has recently been used as a point-of-care assessment of microvascular dysfunction, and indeed may become the method of choice for ongoing clinical trials.[30]

Sidestream Dark-Field Imaging

Sidestream dark-field (SDF) imaging is new advancement to the basic OPS technique, in which a stroboscopic light-emitting diode (LED) ring provides sidestream illumination, minimizing signal degradation from tissue and surface reflection. SDF and standard OPS imaging provide similar quantitative data in terms of vessel diameters and RBC velocity; however, SDF provides a much higher image quality with more detail, capillary contrast and quality, and granularity of venular RBC columns.[28] SDF imaging also minimizes less motion blur by the use of stroboscopic LED ring-based SDF illumination. As with other microscopy techniques, SDF imaging has its limitations including sensitivity to secretions and pressure artifact, however, it is a powerful tool for the real-time assessment of microvascular flow and is being used to measure microcirculatory blood flow in sepsis, cardiac surgery, heart failure, and acute myocardial infarction.

Flowmetry

Laser Doppler flowmetry (LDF) is a noninvasive diagnostic method that uses the principle of Doppler flow to detect frequency shifts in laser light illuminating RBCs to measure microvascular blood flow. LDF measures perfusion in real time and is well suited to study the flow changes in response to acute stimuli. With LDF, the velocity measurement represents the average velocities in all the vessels comprised in this volume and hence gives a semiquantitative index of superficial tissue perfusion. Laser Doppler techniques can measure microcirculatory flow and velocity in very small tissue volumes, as small as 0.8 µL depending on the type of device used, in the skin and superficial mucosal surfaces (oral, rectal, vaginal), and can even be used to assess gastric or intestinal mucosal blood flow when mounted on a fiberoptic device.[31]

LDF is a simple and robust technique that has been adapted for a variety of clinical uses: for example, to measure retinal and optic nerve blood flow in glaucoma, diabetes, and optic neuritis, and to monitor cerebral blood flow during craniotomy and monitor for cerebral ischemia in comatose patients. LDF has the advantage of being noninvasive and adaptable to internal testing of the intestinal mucosa. LDF is also sensitive to acute changes in flow, making it especially well suited to studies that measure changes in flow in response to acute stimuli. However, LDF does have some disadvantages including sensitivity to motion artifact and the optical properties of the surrounding tissue. LDF does not give a truly quantitative measure of flow, but measures the average velocity in a given sample rather than the velocity through individual capillaries. Finally, other new techniques such as dynamic washout studies using microbubbles, as well as photoacoustic and optical coherence microscopy show promise in the in vivo measurement of the microvasculature.

Indirect Techniques

Because tissue ischemia and hypoxia are at the heart of sepsis and other shock states, another method of measuring the adequacy of microvascular perfusion is by estimating tissue oxygen and carbon dioxide. Direct measurement of tissue oxygenation can be performed by placing polarographic oxygen electrodes in the tissues; it can also be performed noninvasively using near-infrared spectrometry (NIRS), which uses multiple using near-infrared beams to detect the oxygenation of microvascular hemoglobin.

Similarly, tissue capnometry can be used to measure the partial pressure of carbon dioxide (PCO_2) as a marker of tissue perfusion. Impared microvascular perfusion leads to ischemia with resultant accumulation of protons (H+) and carbon dioxide (CO). Tissue pH and PCO_2 reflect anaerobic metabolism: inadequate perfusion leads to acid accumulation and a shift to increased PCO_2 by the Henderson-Hasselbach equation of acid-base homeostasis.

Tissue CO_2 correlates well with microvascular blood flow measured by the above techniques and can be thought of as a marker of local microvascular perfusion in the way that we now use lactate as a measure of global tissue perfusion and anaerobic metabolism.[32,33] Measurement of sublingual partial pressure of carbon dioxide ($P_{sl}CO_2$) is more technically simple and noninvasive than gastric measurement, and clinical studies have demonstrated a good correlation between gastric intramucosal carbon dioxide and sublingual mucosal carbon dioxide.[34]

TECHNICAL LIMITATIONS OF VARIOUS TECHNIQUES

The various indices, methods, and assessments mentioned earlier can be used to assess microcirculatory dysfunction as measured by blood flow and capillary distribution, blood velocity, tissue oxygenation, and tissue partial pressure of carbon dioxide (PCO_2). However, each method has some technical limitations, as outlined previously and in **Table 1**. For imaging techniques in particular, experts have recommended 5 key points to acquire optimal and reproducible images of the microvasculature: measurement of at least 5 sites per tissue, avoiding pressure artifact, eliminating secretions before measurement, ensuring adequate focus and contrast, and ensuring high recording quality.[35] These specialists further consolidated scoring systems to include an index of vascular density (total and perfused vessels), capillary perfusion, and a heterogeneity index, using venular perfusion, which should not be affected, as a control. With codification of methods and improvement in both image acquisition and analysis techniques, assessment of microcirculatory flow is becoming easier and more reproducible, and should be a powerful tool in the future.

PROGNOSTIC VALUE OF MEASURING MICROVASCULAR FLOW

Experimental evidence from animal models points to the widespread existence of microvascular dysfunction in sepsis. Using cecal ligation and puncture models, multiple investigators have shown decreased capillary flow and increased heterogeneity of microvascular blood flow in septic rats in skeletal muscle[36] and bowel.[37] To tease out the contributions of macro- and microcirculatory dysfunction in sepsis, Hiltebrand and colleagues[38,39] used LDF to measure central, regional, and microvascular flow in a swine fecal peritonitis model of severe septic shock both before and after resuscitation. Microcirculatory flow was significantly reduced (>40%) during septic shock in all abdominal tissues except for the jejunum. Aggressive fluid resuscitation restored systemic and regional blood flow to supranormal levels; however, the microvascular response was more heterogeneous with persistently decreased microvascular blood flow to the liver, pancreas, and kidneys. These investigators also showed that volume resuscitation increased cardiac output (CO) and superior mesenteric artery (SMA) flow and restored gastric mucosal blood, but did not restore local microvascular flow derangements in the muscularis layers of the jejunum and colon. Interestingly, this heterogeneity of microvascular blood flow is not limited to septic

Table 1
Techniques for assessing microvascular perfusion

Technique	Nail-Fold Videomicroscopy	Laser Doppler Flowmetry	Orthogonal Polarization Spectral Imaging (OPS)	Sidestream Dark-Field Imaging	Near-Infrared Spectroscopy	Tissue Capnometry
Direct or indirect measure of microvascular flow?	Direct	Direct	Direct	Direct	Indirect	Indirect
What is measured?	Capillary density Proportion of perfused vessels	Red blood cell velocity and flux	Capillary density Proportion of perfused vessels	Capillary density Proportion of perfused vessels	Tissue StO_2 as a marker for oxygen delivery and tissue perfusion	Tissue PCO_2 as a surrogate for tissue perfusion
Advantages	Conventional Simple Inexpensive	Easy to use at the bedside Noninvasive, but can be adapted for measurement of gastric blood flow Sensitive to acute changes in flow	Easy to use at the bedside Good reproducibility	Much higher image quality than OPS Less motion blur as compared with OPS	Noninvasive	Simple, noninvasive, instant, reproducible Easy to use at the bedside
Limitations	Limited areas visualized (ie, nails) Sensitive to temperature (peripheral vasoconstriction of the extremities) Common diseases like diabetes and vascular disease may hinder the measurements	Heterogeneity of flow is not measured Relative, rather than absolute, measure Subject to motion artifact	Sublingual measurements may not be representative of other capillary beds Semiquantitative Subject to pressure artifact and secretions	Sublingual measurements may not be representative of other capillary beds Semiquantitative Subject to pressure artifact and secretions	StO_2 may represent changes in oxygen utilization as well as oxygen delivery	Subject to technical limitations, ie, secretions, motion artifacts, etc Limited areas of use (typically mucosal surfaces)
Sites	Nail fold (can also be adapted for use on skin, lips)	Skin Intestinal and sublingual mucosa	Sublingual mucosa	Sublingual mucosa	Skin Muscle	Sublingual mucosa Gastric/intestinal mucosa

shock but is also seen in models of hemorrhagic and cardiogenic shock.[40,41,42] From these animal experiments, the authors may conclude that (1) microcirculatory derangements are common in sepsis as well as other shock states and (2) microvascular blood flow cannot be predicted from changes in systemic or regional hemodynamics. What about patients with sepsis or septic shock?

There is increasing evidence that microvascular blood flow is deranged in human patients and serves as an independent prognostic value with respect to morbidity and mortality in sepsis. Early studies using LDF demonstrated decreased basal microvascular flow and a reduction in the maximal flow that can be elicited in both skeletal muscle[43] and skin[44] of patients with severe sepsis and septic shock. In 2001, Marik[45] demonstrated that a higher sublingual to arterial PCO_2 gap ($P_{sl}CO_2$-P_aCO_2) was associated with increased mortality in ICU patients with septic or cardiogenic shock. Similarly, these investigators later showed that an elevated $P_{sl}CO_2$ on admission was a sensitive marker of poor tissue perfusion and that a high $P_{sl}CO_2$-P_aCO_2 gap was more predictive of mortality than $S_{cv}O_2$ or lactate (or APACHE II).[46]

In 2002, using sublingual OPS, De Backer and colleagues[47] demonstrated that decreased microvessel density and proportion of perfused vessels were common in sepsis and more severe in septic nonsurvivors compared with those patients who resolved. Likewise, Trzeciak and colleagues[8] demonstrated that microcirculatory dysfunction in the first 6 hours of diagnosis was more impaired in nonsurvivors than survivors. In 2004, Sakr and colleagues[7] further demonstrated that despite similar global oxygenation and hemodynamics with resuscitation, the persistence of microvascular dysfunction was associated with progression to multiorgan failure and death. Most recently, Creteur and colleagues[48] used NIRS to measure dynamic muscle tissue oxygenation (S_tO_2) and demonstrated that altered recovery of tissue oxygenation after a standardized ischemic occlusion period occurred more frequently in septic patients than in stable ICU patients and healthy volunteers. Also, the persistence of this altered vasoreactivity after 24 and 48 hours was associated with nonsurvival.

Thus, clinical studies have confirmed that microvascular dysfunction is common in sepsis and correlates with worst outcome. They also draw attention to the inadequacy of standard resuscitation techniques at restoring local tissue blood flow in sepsis. Can we then use these microvascular measures to predict outcome and, more importantly, to guide therapy?

RESUSCITATING THE MICROCIRCULATION IN SEPSIS

Standard resuscitative techniques for sepsis and septic shock include the use of antibiotics, fluids, vasopressors, and inotropes, with the use of adjunctive therapies such as steroids, blood transfusion, and activated protein C in appropriate subsets of patients. Vasopressors and inotropes have long been a mainstay of therapy in severe sepsis and septic shock. Microcirculatory disturbances are common in sepsis and may persist despite restoration of central perfusion pressures. What then are the effects of these therapies on microvascular flow?

Vasopressors and Inotropes

Early animal studies using a pig fecal peritonitis model demonstrated that although the adrenergic agents epinephrine, norepinephrine, and phenylephrine significantly increased MAP (by an average of 16 to 17 mm Hg), they failed to improve regional or microvascular blood flow.[13] In fact, both epinephrine and norepinephrine significantly reduced regional (SMA) and microcirculatory blood flow in the jejunal mucosa, decreasing mesenteric oxygen delivery, despite a marked increase in cardiac output and MAP. Similar findings were observed with the nonadrenergic agent vasopressin, which increased the MAP without increasing cardiac output, but again was unable to improve regional or microvascular flow to the abdominal organs–a finding that correlated with increased PCO_2 gap.[49,50]

Clinical studies in septic patients have been less clear and are complicated by the standard use of multiple vasoactive medications and adjunctive supportive therapies. One small study used LDF to evaluate gastric mucosal blood flow in 12 ICU patients with septic shock and showed that epinephrine increased gastric mucosal perfusion versus norepinephrine alone, but that the addition of dobutamine to norepinephrine significantly increased mucosal blood flow, often to even higher levels than epinephrine alone.[51] More recently, the effects of norepinephrine and epinephrine in 20 ICU patients with moderate and severe septic shock were compared using gastric tonometry.[52] In severe septic shock, despite an increase in cardiac index and MvO_2, neither drug was able to improve the gastric PCO_2 gap and epinephrine actually decreased splanchinic blood flow compared with norepinephrine. However, as this study did not control for the use of dobutamine, which was allowed as per the preference of the treating physician, it is difficult to draw strong conclusions about the specific effects of epinephrine versus norepinephrine. A more recent study looking specifically at the effects of increasing doses of norepinephrine on microcirculatory blood flow and oxygenation in 16 patients with septic shock showed no improvement in sublingual microvascular flow as measured by microvascular flow index, vessel density, or heterogeneity index despite increases in MAP, CI, and SvO_2.[53] With dopamine, the effects were even more mixed. In one study, low-dose (≤ 5 µg/kg/min) dopamine on regional and local blood flow demonstrated decreased gastric mucosal blood flow, measured by LDF, in patients with septic shock.[54] At higher doses (≥ 15 µg/kg/min), despite improving central blood flow, dopamine had unpredictable effects on regional muscle and splanchnic circulation.[55] Turning to vasopressin, although no clinical studies have studied the effects of vasopressin alone, the addition of vasopressin to norepinephrine has shown conflicting results, with one small study showing an increased gastric PCO_2 gap[56] and another larger study suggesting not only improved cardiac index and MAP but also improved gastric tonometry versus norepinephrine alone.[57] Despite the limitations of these small studies, it is clear that adrenergic and nonadrenergic vasopressors are unreliable in improving microvascular blood flow, and further studies are needed to define their precise role of in resuscitating the microcirculation during sepsis.

What, then, of the effects of inotropes on microcirculatory blood flow? Dobutamine is the most commonly studied inotrope in septic shock, either alone or in conjunction with vasopressors. In 1994, a small study of 21 septic patients[58] demonstrated a dose-dependent improvement in gastric tonometry with dobutamine, with a concomitant decrease in lactate in patients with hyperlactatemia. Two years later, the addition of low-dose dobutamine (5 µg/kg/min) to basal vasopressors was shown to increase gastric mucosal microvascular blood flow as measured by LDF, and improved the gastric PCO_2 difference in 10 patients with severe sepsis.[54] Although it is unclear whether these effects are governed in part by the vasodilatory as well as inotropic effects of dobutamine, these findings suggest a potential role for dobutamine in opening the microcirculation in sepsis, especially when vasopressors are required to maintain central perfusion pressures.

Vasodilators

If decreased microvascular perfusion is at the heart of sepsis, what then of treatment with direct vasodilators? Nitric oxide (NO), NO donors, and prostacyclin are commonly used to increase microvascular blood flow in myocardial ischemia and pulmonary hypertension, but their use in sepsis has been avoided due to concerns for systemic vasodilation and hypotension. Indeed, excessive NO production has been linked to the pathogenesis of systemic vasodilation in sepsis.[59] In an effort to combat this abnormal systemic vasodilation, several groups studied the effects of NO synthase (NOS) inhibition in sepsis, demonstrating that NOS inhibition can reliably increase central perfusion pressures, often as much as norepinephrine.[59,60] However, NOS inhibition did not improve gastric tonometry or improve mortality in sepsis and in fact one large randomized, placebo-controlled clinical trial of NOS inhibition in septic shock was stopped early because of increased mortality in the treated patients (59% vs 49%), seriously diminishing interest in NOS inhibition as a therapeutic approach in sepsis.[61] On the other side of the coin, several small studies have started to look at the microvascular effects of NO in sepsis, with mixed results. NO is a short-lived, highly reactive molecule (with a half-life of a few seconds); NO donors such as nitroglycerin and sodium nitroprusside are used to provide stable vasodilation in cardiac ischemia and hypertensive emergency. Several animal studies have suggested improved intestinal mucosal microvascular blood flow with nitroglycerin and nitroprusside during sepsis, with improved ileal and hepatic microvascular flow measured by intravital microscopy and SDF.[62,63] Likewise, in a small case-series of eight patients, infusion of nitroglycerin improved microvascular blood flow measured by sublingual OPS in patients resuscitated for septic shock.[64] However, in a larger recent clinical study, nitroglycerin did not improve microvascular flow index and demonstrated a trend towards increased mortality in patients with sepsis.[65]

Prostacyclin is a prostanoid released by endothelial cells that causes potent vasodilation as well as inhibition of platelet and leukocyte adhesion. Exogenous prostacyclin analogues, both intravenous and inhaled, are used in pulmonary hypertension to vasodilate constricted pulmonary microvessels. Animals models have demonstrated increased hepatic blood flow, oxygen delivery, and mesenteric perfusion and intramucosal pH with iloprost infusion, suggest a preferential role vasodilating the microcirculation (rassumsen). Early clinical studies with prostacyclin have delivered some encouraging results, showing that infusion of prostacyclin improved cardiac index, intestinal tonometry, and oxygen delivery in patients with sepsis.[66,67]

Other Therapies

Drotrecogin alfa (activated protein C, rAPC) has potent antithrombotic, fibrinolytic, and anti-inflammatory properties, and has been used to treat patients with sepsis since the early 2000s. Although initial enthusiasm has waned somewhat, due in part to significant risks of bleeding and other complications, drotrecogin alfa may have a role in treating patients with severe sepsis and septic shock in which its mortality benefits outweigh its risks.[21,22] Drotrecogin alfa may improve microvascular dysfunction in sepsis. De Backer and colleagues[23] demonstrated improvement in microcirculatory blood flow in 40 patients with severe sepsis as early as four hours into infusion of drotrecogin alfa—an effect that was associated with a faster resolution of hyperlactatemia. These results suggest that some of the improvements in mortality with drotrecogin alfa may be due to improved microcirculatory function.

Most intensivists are well-versed in the role of permissive hypercapnia in the setting of acute respiratory distress syndrome (ARDS)/acute lung injury (ALI), in which elevated PCO_2 and lower pH are tolerated to minimize further lung injury. Despite early concerns, a lung protective strategy that includes permissive hypercapnia is safe and improves outcomes in adults with ARDS, and is recommended in patients without cerebral dysfunction. Experimental evidence suggests that hypercapnia may be protective in sepsis and septic shock, decreasing proinflammatory cytokine production and improving mortality in animal models of endotoxin induced sepsis.[68–70] Unfortunately, clinical studies are lacking although recently Gnaegi and colleagues[71] showed that progressive hypercapnia (from 40 to 60 mm Hg) did not affect cardiac output, but did attenuate endotoxin-mediated decreases in adenosine triphosphate and accumulation of lactate in the splanchnic circulation, suggesting improved regional perfusion. In contrast, Taccone and colleagues showed[72] that impaired cerebral autoregulation is common in sepsis and worse during hypercapnia. Given the heterogeneous effects on different microvascular beds, further studies are needed before broadly recommending hypercapnia.

Although the routine use of blood transfusion in increasing oxygen delivery during sepsis has fallen out of general practice, clinical studies have suggested that transfusion may benefit those patients with the most severe microcirculatory dysfunction.[73,74] Similarly, in small studies, low-dose steroids increased microvessel density and proportion of perfused vessels in sepsis, mainly by recruitment of nonperfused vessels.[75] Medications such as pentoxifylline, a xanthine derivative sometimes used in the treatment of peripheral vascular disease, have been studied in animal models of sepsis with encouraging preliminary results, however have failed to translate into clinical trials.[76,77]

Perhaps the most promising medications being studied for the treatment of microvascular disturbances in sepsis are the endothelin receptor antagonists. Clinical studies have demonstrated elevated circulating endothelin-1 in human patients with sepsis and suggest a correlation between plasma endothelin levels and severity of illness.[78–80] The endothelin receptor antagonists bosentan and tezosentan have been shown to reverse the impaired blood flow seen in multiple animal models of sepsis and suggest that this class of drug holds promise as a new therapeutic for sepsis.[81–83]

SUMMARY

Microcirculatory dysfunction is common and plays a role in the pathogenesis of sepsis. Current therapeutic/resuscitative efforts often fail to correct microcirculatory disturbances. New techniques are available, and increasingly accessible, for the measurement of microvascular perfusion. With the aid of these new techniques, we may be able to better target our therapies toward restoring microcirculatory function in sepsis. Measurement of microvascular function may soon become a standard of care in the treatment of sepsis, providing prognostic value and allowing earlier identification of patients with worse outcomes, and may guide therapy in sepsis. Although it is clear that macrovascular end points are not sufficient in resuscitating the microcirculation, preliminary animal and early clinical studies have produced several new potential therapeutic agents that may play a key role in improving microvascular dysfunction in sepsis in the future.

REFERENCES

1. Matot I, Sprung CL. Definition of sepsis. Intensive Care Med 2001;27(Suppl 1): S3–9.
2. Angus DC, Linde-Zwirble WT, Lidicker J, et al. Epidemiology of severe sepsis in the United States: analysis of incidence, outcome, and associated costs of care. Crit Care Med 2001;29(7):1303–10.

3. Rivers E, Nguyen B, Havstad S, et al. Early goal-directed therapy in the treatment of severe sepsis and septic shock. N Engl J Med 2001;345(19):1368–77.

4. Dellinger RP, Levy MM, Carlet JM, et al. Surviving sepsis campaign: international guidelines for management of severe sepsis and septic shock: 2008. Crit Care Med 2008;36(1):296–327.

5. Ince C. The microcirculation is the motor of sepsis. Crit Care 2005;9(Suppl 4): S13–9.

6. Vincent JL, De Backer D. Microvascular dysfunction as a cause of organ dysfunction in severe sepsis. Crit Care 2005;9(Suppl 4):S9–12.

7. Sakr Y, Dubois MJ, De Backer D, et al. Persistent microcirculatory alterations are associated with organ failure and death in patients with septic shock. Crit Care Med 2004;32(9):1825–31.

8. Trzeciak S, Dellinger RP, Parrillo JE, et al. Early microcirculatory perfusion derangements in patients with severe sepsis and septic shock: relationship to hemodynamics, oxygen transport, and survival. Ann Emerg Med 2007;49(1): 88–98, 98 e1–2.

9. Trzeciak S, Rivers EP. Clinical manifestations of disordered microcirculatory perfusion in severe sepsis. Crit Care 2005;9(Suppl 4):S20–6.

10. Ellis CG, Jagger J, Sharpe M. The microcirculation as a functional system. Crit Care 2005;9(Suppl 4):S3–8.

11. Aird WC. The role of the endothelium in severe sepsis and multiple organ dysfunction syndrome. Blood 2003;101(10):3765–77.

12. Lush CW, Kvietys PR. Microvascular dysfunction in sepsis. Microcirculation 2000; 7(2):83–101.

13. Krejci V, Hiltebrand LB, Sigurdsson GH. Effects of epinephrine, norepinephrine, and phenylephrine on microcirculatory blood flow in the gastrointestinal tract in sepsis. Crit Care Med 2006;34(5):1456–63.

14. Trzeciak S, McCoy JV, Dellinger PR, et al. Early increases in microcirculatory perfusion during protocol-directed resuscitation are associated with reduced multi-organ failure at 24 h in patients with sepsis. Intensive Care Med 2008; 34(12):2210–7.

15. Astiz ME, DeGent GE, Lin RY, et al. Microvascular function and rheologic changes in hyperdynamic sepsis. Crit Care Med 1995;23(2):265–71.

16. Astiz ME, Rackow EC, Falk JL, et al. Oxygen delivery and consumption in patients with hyperdynamic septic shock. Crit Care Med 1987;15(1):26–8.

17. Schouten M, Wiersinga WJ, Levi M, et al. Inflammation, endothelium, and coagulation in sepsis. J Leukoc Biol 2008;83(3):536–45.

18. Diehl JL, Borgel D. Sepsis and coagulation. Curr Opin Crit Care 2005;11(5): 454–60.

19. Faust SN, Levin M, Harrison OB, et al. Dysfunction of endothelial protein C activation in severe meningococcal sepsis. N Engl J Med 2001;345(6): 408–16.

20. Looney MR, Matthay MA. Bench-to-bedside review: the role of activated protein C in maintaining endothelial tight junction function and its relationship to organ injury. Crit Care 2006;10(6):239.

21. Kanji S, Devlin JW, Piekos KA, et al. Recombinant human activated protein C, drotrecogin alfa (activated): a novel therapy for severe sepsis. Pharmacotherapy 2001;21(11):1389–402.

22. Martin G, Brunkhorst FM, Janes JM, et al. The international PROGRESS registry of patients with severe sepsis: drotrecogin alfa (activated) use and patient outcomes. Crit Care 2009;13(3):R103.

23. De Backer D, Verdant C, Chierego M, et al. Effects of drotrecogin alfa activated on microcirculatory alterations in patients with severe sepsis. Crit Care Med 2006; 34(7):1918–24.
24. Piagnerelli M, Boudjeltia KZ, Vanhaeverbeek M, et al. Red blood cell rheology in sepsis. Intensive Care Med 2003;29(7):1052–61.
25. Chien S. Rheology in the microcirculation in normal and low flow states. Adv Shock Res 1982;8:71–80.
26. Hinshaw LB. Sepsis/septic shock: participation of the microcirculation: an abbreviated review. Crit Care Med 1996;24(6):1072–8.
27. Secchi ME, Sulli A, Pizzorni C, et al. [Nailfold capillaroscopy and blood flow laser-Doppler analysis of the microvascular damage in systemic sclerosis: preliminary results]. Reumatismo 2009;61(1):34–40 [in Italian].
28. De Backer D. OPS techniques. Minerva Anestesiol 2003;69(5):388–91.
29. Harris AG, Sinitsina I, Messmer K. The cytoscan model E-II, a new reflectance microscope for intravital microscopy: comparison with the standard fluorescence method. J Vasc Res 2000;37(6):469–76.
30. Boerma EC, Mathura KR, van der Voort PH, et al. Quantifying bedside-derived imaging of microcirculatory abnormalities in septic patients: a prospective validation study. Crit Care 2005;9(6):R601–6.
31. Hiltebrand LB, Krejci V, Sigurdsson GH. Effects of dopamine, dobutamine, and dopexamine on microcirculatory blood flow in the gastrointestinal tract during sepsis and anesthesia. Anesthesiology 2004;100(5):1188–97.
32. Creteur J, De Backer D, Sakr Y, et al. Sublingual capnometry tracks microcirculatory changes in septic patients. Intensive Care Med 2006;32(4):516–23.
33. Fries M, Weil MH, Sun S, et al. Increases in tissue Pco2 during circulatory shock reflect selective decreases in capillary blood flow. Crit Care Med 2006;34(2): 446–52.
34. Marik PE. Regional carbon dioxide monitoring to assess the adequacy of tissue perfusion. Curr Opin Crit Care 2005;11(3):245–51.
35. De Backer D, Hollenberg S, Boerma C, et al. How to evaluate the microcirculation: report of a round table conference. Crit Care 2007;11(5):R101.
36. Piper RD, Pitt-Hyde M, Li F, et al. Microcirculatory changes in rat skeletal muscle in sepsis. Am J Respir Crit Care Med 1996;154(4 Pt 1):931–7.
37. Farquhar I, Martin CM, Lam C, et al. Decreased capillary density in vivo in bowel mucosa of rats with normotensive sepsis. J Surg Res 1996;61(1):190–6.
38. Hiltebrand LB, Krejci V, Banic A, et al. Dynamic study of the distribution of microcirculatory blood flow in multiple splanchnic organs in septic shock. Crit Care Med 2000;28(9):3233–41.
39. Hiltebrand LB, Krejci V, tenHoevel ME, et al. Redistribution of microcirculatory blood flow within the intestinal wall during sepsis and general anesthesia. Anesthesiology 2003;98(3):658–69.
40. Krejci V, Hiltebrand L, Banic A, et al. Continuous measurements of microcirculatory blood flow in gastrointestinal organs during acute haemorrhage. Br J Anaesth 2000;84(4):468–75.
41. Koo A, Tse TF, Yu DY. Hepatic microvascular effects of terbutaline in experimental cardiogenic shock in rats. Clin Exp Pharmacol Physiol 1979;6(5):495–506.
42. Fries M, Weil MH, Chang YT, et al. Microcirculation during cardiac arrest and resuscitation. Crit Care Med 2006;34(Suppl 12):S454–7.
43. Neviere R, Mathieu D, Chagnon JL, et al. Skeletal muscle microvascular blood flow and oxygen transport in patients with severe sepsis. Am J Respir Crit Care Med 1996;153(1):191–5.

44. Kubli S, Boegli Y, Ave AD, et al. Endothelium-dependent vasodilation in the skin microcirculation of patients with septic shock. Shock 2003;19(3):274–80.
45. Marik PE. Sublingual capnography: a clinical validation study. Chest 2001;120(3): 923–7.
46. Marik PE, Bankov A. Sublingual capnometry versus traditional markers of tissue oxygenation in critically ill patients. Crit Care Med 2003;31(3):818–22.
47. De Backer D, Creteur J, Preiser JC, et al. Microvascular blood flow is altered in patients with sepsis. Am J Respir Crit Care Med 2002;166(1):98–104.
48. Creteur J, Carollo T, Soldati G, et al. The prognostic value of muscle StO2 in septic patients. Intensive Care Med 2007;33(9):1549–56.
49. Krejci V, Hiltebrand LB, Jakob SM, et al. Vasopressin in septic shock: effects on pancreatic, renal, and hepatic blood flow. Crit Care 2007;11(6):R129.
50. Hiltebrand LB, Krejci V, Jakob SM, et al. Effects of vasopressin on microcirculatory blood flow in the gastrointestinal tract in anesthetized pigs in septic shock. Anesthesiology 2007;106(6):1156–67.
51. Duranteau J, Sitbon P, Teboul JL, et al. Effects of epinephrine, norepinephrine, or the combination of norepinephrine and dobutamine on gastric mucosa in septic shock. Crit Care Med 1999;27(5):893–900.
52. De Backer D, Creteur J, Silva E, et al. Effects of dopamine, norepinephrine, and epinephrine on the splanchnic circulation in septic shock: which is best? Crit Care Med 2003;31(6):1659–67.
53. Jhanji S, Stirling S, Patel N, et al. The effect of increasing doses of norepinephrine on tissue oxygenation and microvascular flow in patients with septic shock. Crit Care Med 2009;37(6):1961–6.
54. Neviere R, Mathieu D, Chagnon JL, et al. The contrasting effects of dobutamine and dopamine on gastric mucosal perfusion in septic patients. Am J Respir Crit Care Med 1996;154(6 Pt 1):1684–8.
55. Ruokonen E, Takala J, Kari A, et al. Regional blood flow and oxygen transport in septic shock. Crit Care Med 1993;21(9):1296–303.
56. van Haren FM, Rozendaal FW, van der Hoeven JG. The effect of vasopressin on gastric perfusion in catecholamine-dependent patients in septic shock. Chest 2003;124(6):2256–60.
57. Dunser MW, Mayr AJ, Ulmer H, et al. Arginine vasopressin in advanced vasodilatory shock: a prospective, randomized, controlled study. Circulation 2003; 107(18):2313–9.
58. Gutierrez G, Clark C, Brown SD, et al. Effect of dobutamine on oxygen consumption and gastric mucosal pH in septic patients. Am J Respir Crit Care Med 1994; 150(2):324–9.
59. Lange M, Enkhbaatar P, Nakano Y, et al. Role of nitric oxide in shock: the large animal perspective. Front Biosci 2009;14:1979–89.
60. Pullamsetti SS, Maring D, Ghofrani HA, et al. Effect of nitric oxide synthase (NOS) inhibition on macro- and microcirculation in a model of rat endotoxic shock. Thromb Haemost 2006;95(4):720–7.
61. Lopez A, Lorente JA, Steingrub J, et al. Multiple-center, randomized, placebo-controlled, double-blind study of the nitric oxide synthase inhibitor 546C88: effect on survival in patients with septic shock. Crit Care Med 2004;32(1):21–30.
62. Assadi A, Desebbe O, Kaminski C, et al. Effects of sodium nitroprusside on splanchnic microcirculation in a resuscitated porcine model of septic shock. Br J Anaesth 2008;100(1):55–65.

63. Gundersen Y, Corso CO, Leiderer R, et al. The nitric oxide donor sodium nitroprusside protects against hepatic microcirculatory dysfunction in early endotoxaemia. Intensive Care Med 1998;24(12):1257–63.
64. Spronk PE, Ince C, Gardien MJ, et al. Nitroglycerin in septic shock after intravascular volume resuscitation. Lancet 2002;360(9343):1395–6.
65. Boerma EC, Koopmans M, Konijn A, et al. Effects of nitroglycerin on sublingual microcirculatory blood flow in patients with severe sepsis/septic shock after a strict resuscitation protocol: a double-blind randomized placebo controlled trial. Crit Care Med 2009;38:93–100.
66. Radermacher P, Buhl R, Santak B, et al. The effects of prostacyclin on gastric intramucosal pH in patients with septic shock. Intensive Care Med 1995;21(5): 414–21.
67. Eichelbronner O, Reinelt H, Wiedeck H, et al. Aerosolized prostacyclin and inhaled nitric oxide in septic shock—different effects on splanchnic oxygenation? Intensive Care Med 1996;22(9):880–7.
68. Kimura D, Totapally BR, Raszynski A, et al. The effects of CO_2 on cytokine concentrations in endotoxin-stimulated human whole blood. Crit Care Med 2008;36(10):2823–7.
69. Hanly EJ, Fuentes JM, Aurora AR, et al. Carbon dioxide pneumoperitoneum prevents mortality from sepsis. Surg Endosc 2006;20(9):1482–7.
70. Hanly EJ, Bachman SL, Marohn MR, et al. Carbon dioxide pneumoperitoneum-mediated attenuation of the inflammatory response is independent of systemic acidosis. Surgery 2005;137(5):559–66.
71. Gnaegi A, Feihl F, Boulat O, et al. Moderate hypercapnia exerts beneficial effects on splanchnic energy metabolism during endotoxemia. Intensive Care Med 2009; 35(7):1297–304.
72. Taccone FS, Castanares-Zapatero D, Peres-Bota D, et al. Cerebral autoregulation is influenced by carbon dioxide levels in patients with septic shock. Neurocrit Care 2010;12(1):35–42.
73. Conrad SA, Dietrich KA, Hebert CA, et al. Effect of red cell transfusion on oxygen consumption following fluid resuscitation in septic shock. Circ Shock 1990;31(4): 419–29.
74. Sakr Y, Chierego M, Piagnerelli M, et al. Microvascular response to red blood cell transfusion in patients with severe sepsis. Crit Care Med 2007;35(7):1639–44.
75. Buchele GL, Silva E, Ospina-Tascon GA, et al. Effects of hydrocortisone on microcirculatory alterations in patients with septic shock. Crit Care Med 2009;37(4): 1341–7.
76. Krysztopik RJ, Bentley FR, Wilson MA, et al. Vasomotor response to pentoxifylline mediates improved renal blood flow to bacteremia. J Surg Res 1996;63(1):17–22.
77. Krysztopik RJ, Matheson PJ, Spain DA, et al. Lazaroid and pentoxifylline suppress sepsis-induced increases in renal vascular resistance via altered arachidonic acid metabolism. J Surg Res 2000;93(1):75–81.
78. Piechota M, Banach M, Irzmanski R, et al. Plasma endothelin-1 levels in septic patients. J Intensive Care Med 2007;22(4):232–9.
79. Sanai L, Haynes WG, MacKenzie A, et al. Endothelin production in sepsis and the adult respiratory distress syndrome. Intensive Care Med 1996;22(1):52–6.
80. Schuetz P, Christ-Crain M, Morgenthaler NG, et al. Circulating precursor levels of endothelin-1 and adrenomedullin, two endothelium-derived, counteracting substances, in sepsis. Endothelium 2007;14(6):345–51.

81. Krejci V, Hiltebrand LB, Erni D, et al. Endothelin receptor antagonist bosentan improves microcirculatory blood flow in splanchnic organs in septic shock. Crit Care Med 2003;31(1):203–10.
82. Andersson A, Fenhammar J, Frithiof R, et al. Mixed endothelin receptor antagonism with tezosentan improves intestinal microcirculation in endotoxemic shock. J Surg Res 2008;149(1):138–47.
83. Fenhammar J, Andersson A, Frithiof R, et al. The endothelin receptor antagonist tezosentan improves renal microcirculation in a porcine model of endotoxemic shock. Acta Anaesthesiol Scand 2008;52(10):1385–93.

Detection of Hypoxia at the Cellular Level

Laurie A. Loiacono, MD, FCCP[a,b,c,*], David S. Shapiro, MD[a,c]

KEYWORDS

- Sepsis • Tissue hypoxia • Cytopathic hypoxia • Mitochondria
- Multiple organ dysfunction syndrome • Biomarkers

Hypoxia (n.): a deficiency in the amount of oxygen that reaches the tissues of the body

As aerobic organisms, we have evolved the optimum function of our tissues and organ systems around the presence and effective use of oxygen as a substrate. When the use of oxygen by our cells is compromised, our intrinsic biologic processes become derailed. The definition of hypoxia at the start of this paragraph, therefore, describes only half of the dilemma that dysoxia creates. A more appropriate definition of hypoxia for the purpose of this article then becomes:

Hypoxia (n.): a deficiency in the bioavailability of oxygen to the tissues of the body

Connett and colleagues[1] define 3 theoretic thresholds of cell hypoxia:

1. The first is crossed when cellular oxygen decreases but adenosine triphosphate (ATP) production is maintained at a level sufficient to match ATP demand by metabolic adaptation (ie, redox recruitment, alteration of phosphorylation states, increased glycolysis). The critical level of mitochondrial Po_2 for oxidative phosphorylation depends on the ability of a cell to adapt the phosphorylation process metabolically, and the level of ATP demand.[2]
2. The second occurs when steady state ATP turnover can be maintained only by the production of ATP from anaerobic glycolysis by the Embden-Meyerhof pathway. This highly inefficient pathway generates only 2 molecules of ATP per 1 molecule of glucose metabolized. For highly metabolic tissues such as the brain, kidney, and liver, anaerobic glycolysis is too cumbersome to be effective and these organs

[a] Saint Francis Hospital and Medical Center, Department of Surgery, 114 Woodland Street, Hartford, CT 06105, USA
[b] Department of Surgery, Saint Francis Hospital and Medical Center, 114 Woodland Street, Hartford, CT 06105, USA
[c] University of Connecticut School of Medicine, Department of Surgery, 263 Farmington Avenue, Farmington, CT 06030, USA
* Corresponding author. Saint Francis Hospital and Medical Center, Department of Surgery, 114 Woodland Street, Hartford, CT 06105.
E-mail address: lloiacon@stranciscare.org

Crit Care Clin 26 (2010) 409–421
doi:10.1016/j.ccc.2009.12.001
0749-0704/10/$ – see front matter © 2010 Published by Elsevier Inc.

criticalcare.theclinics.com

develop ATP depletion rapidly under hypoxic conditions.[2] Dysoxia can be defined below this threshold.
3. The third threshold is crossed when glycolysis becomes insufficient to produce enough ATP to maintain cell function and structural integrity.

In severe sepsis and septic shock, the cause of tissue dysoxia is multifactorial and is commonly believed to affect patient outcome directly and negatively via the development of multiorgan system dysfunction (MOSD). Most data on hypoxia-related cell dysfunction are from in vitro studies; mechanisms are complex and poorly understood, and the application to clinical pathophysiology is speculative. How sepsis-associated dysoxia relates to the development of and mortality from MOSD is controversial.

Straightforward tissue ischemia resulting from anoxia leads to cell death and tissue necrosis. However, histologic examination of patients who have succumbed to sepsis, shock, and MOSD reveals that with the exception of generally small focal areas of sold organ tissue injury, major regional anatomic abnormalities tend to be conspicuously absent,[3] lending credence to the concept that the MOSD seen in these septic patients tends to be more metabolic than anatomic.

Clinically, organ performance is linked to tissue integrity. Tissue integrity is linked to cellular function and homeostasis. Cellular function and homeostasis are linked to oxygen and almost countless enzymatic reactions (aerobic and anaerobic). In stress and sepsis these processes are also influenced by mediators of inflammation (cytokines). The cause and perpetuation of organ dysfunction in sepsis are increasingly linked to this relationship between tissue dysoxia and inflammation.

To best understand the pathology related to cellular hypoxia in sepsis, the physiology should first be reviewed.

EFFECTIVE TISSUE OXYGENATION
Basics

Overall tissue performance depends on effective tissue oxygenation, particularly in highly metabolic tissues such as skeletal muscle, cardiac muscle, and liver. Normally, the Po_2 of dry air at sea level is 159 mm Hg, alveolar Po_2 is about 100 mm Hg, and mean capillary Po_2 is about 50 mm Hg. Hemoglobin normally delivers oxygen to transcapillary tissues at partial pressures between 20 and 40 mm Hg. From capillaries O_2 diffuses down further concentration gradients from 1 cell to another, and within cells, such that normal mitochondrial Po_2 ranges from 4 to 20 mm Hg.[4] This transcapillary diffusion gradient distance becomes particularly problematic for tissues such as the liver in which the centrilobular cells are so far away from the capillaries that they are particularly susceptible to hypoxia and undergo necrosis early under hypoxic conditions.

The normal utilization coefficient (the fraction of blood that gives up its oxygen as it passes through the tissue capillaries) is 25% under basal metabolic conditions but can increase to 75% to 85% with strenuous exercise, stress, or metabolic right-shifts of the oxyhemoglobin dissociation curve. Across most tissues, under normal physiologic conditions, only a minute level of intracellular cytosolic oxygen pressure ($Po_2 > 3$–5 mm Hg) is required for normal intracellular chemical reactions to take place.[5] The mitochondria then use this oxygen to produce ATP from adenosine diphosphate (ADP) through the process of oxidative phosphorylation when the Po_2 within the mitochondrion is above a critical threshold, believed to be in the order of 1 mm Hg.[2]

Tissues that are more highly metabolic have slightly higher baseline cellular Po_2, for example intracellular Po_2 in skeletal and cardiac muscle average 5 to 6 mm Hg[5,6] and in liver measure 0 to 10 mm Hg.[7] Normal tissue Po_2 levels in the brain are difficult to assess but are slightly higher. So, theoretically, under poor Vo_2 conditions and maximal metabolic stress (85% O_2 extraction), a baseline transcapillary Po_2 of 20 mm Hg can be diminished to at least as low as 3 mm Hg by the time O_2 equilibrates with the cytosol. Chance and colleagues[8] indicate that O_2 use in mitochondria under conditions of tight respiratory coupling and in the presence of ADP is inhibited 50% at Po_2 of 0.01 to 0.05 mm Hg, suggesting that the Po_2 in mitochondrial cristae can be as low as 0.01 mm Hg and still demonstrate some function.

So, generally, whenever the partial pressure of intracellular oxygen is more than 3 to 5 mm Hg, oxygen availability is not a limiting factor in the rate of oxidative cellular chemical reactions. Instead, the concentration of other substrates such as cellular ADP and pyruvate become the rate-limiting elements. If the availability of substrates required for oxidative phosphorylation is altered, the rate of oxygen use changes in proportion to the change in oxidative substrate concentration. For example, if ADP concentration is low, less O_2 is used to make ATP and the Po_2 level in the cytosol increases. As intracellular ATP is used to provide energy, it is converted into ADP. Increasing ADP concentration increases the metabolic usage of oxygen and the essential nutrients that combine with oxygen to release energy. Cytosolic O_2 then decreases because of O_2 use by mitochondria to reform ATP. Therefore, under normal physiologic conditions the rate of oxygen use by cells is controlled by the rate of energy expenditure within the cells (the rate at which ADP is formed from ATP) and not by the availability of oxygen to the cells.[5]

INEFFECTIVE TISSUE OXYGENATION
Basics

Three predominant scenarios pose barriers to effective tissue oxygenation.

- Inadequate O_2 content (Vo_2), that is, hypoxic environment, severe anemia, O_2 displacement toxicity (ie, carbon monoxide)
- Inadequate O_2 transport (Do_2), that is, low-flow shock states: obstructive/cardiogenic/hypovolemic/distributive shock, organ-specific emboli, or focal hypoperfusion secondary to arteriosclerotic cardiovascular disease
- Ineffective use of O_2 at the cellular level, that is, altered cellular energy metabolism.

The first 2 predominate in low-flow or hypodynamic shock states in which O_2 delivery to tissues is poor and global tissue hypoperfusion that is O_2 dependent occurs. This global tissue hypoxia triggers or exacerbates preexisting sepsis-related inflammatory cascades.[9–11]

With aggressive resuscitative measures targeting Vo_2 and Do_2 deficits, and sepsis source control, low-flow hypodynamic shock can be converted to a more hemodynamically compensated, hyperdynamic state that becomes O_2 independent. Once this relative compensation occurs, however, microcirculatory dysfunction and tissue dysoxia often persist to progress to MOSD,[9,10] and evidence suggests that the explanation for this relates to cellular metabolic dysfunction.[12–17]

Management of Hypodynamic State in Sepsis

Characterized by O_2-dependent global tissue hypoxia, this uncompensated shock state quickly triggers systemic inflammatory responses that are linked to early and late sepsis-related hospital mortality.[18,19] Rivers and colleagues[20] demonstrated the physiologic value of early goal directed therapy (EGDT) in the management of severe sepsis and septic shock and subsequently noted several biomarkers that can be identified early in these patients within the first 3 hours of hospital presentation. They then tracked these biomarkers to assess the efficacy of early hemodynamic optimization.[11]

The biomarkers in the study by Rivers and colleagues[11] represented proinflammatory, antiinflammatory, endothelial, and apoptotic aspects of systemic inflammation: interleukin 1 receptor antagonist (IL-1ra), intercellular adhesion molecule 1 (ICAM-1), tumor necrosis factor α (TNF-α), caspase-3, and IL-8. These markers were studied on hospital presentation and throughout the first 72 hours of resuscitation using EGDT compared with controls. Each of the 2 groups was stratified into severe global tissue hypoxia (lactate $\geq$ 4 mmol/L and $ScVo_2 < 70\%$), moderate global tissue hypoxia (lactate $\geq$ 2, but <4 mmol/L and $ScVo_2 < 70\%$), and resolved global tissue hypoxia (lactate < 2 and mmol/l and $ScVo_2 \geq 70\%$). This study showed that peak biomarker concentrations during 72 hours were directly related to severity of sepsis as defined by lactate level and $ScVo_2$. Peak concentration for IL-1ra occurred at 12 hours, peak concentration for TNF-α, caspase-3, and IL-8 occurred at 24 hours, and peak concentration for ICAM-1 occurred at 36 hours. Each biomarker peak concentration during 72 hours of initial treatment was lower in the EGDT group compared with controls, and significant direct relationships were noted between biomarker concentrations and organ dysfunction scores at each time point.

The study by Rivers and colleagues[11] demonstrates the value of early (within the first 72 hours) aggressive hemodynamic optimization in attenuating the early inflammatory response trigger related to low-flow tissue hypoxia in sepsis. So, early in severe sepsis/septic shock the degree of cellular hypoxia can be indirectly assessed by the level of associated early inflammatory response, and the efficacy of resuscitation strategies can be monitored. Attenuation of this initial inflammatory response may have implications for moderation of the later cytopathic component of high-flow sepsis-related MOSD.

Hyperdynamic Sepsis and Cytopathic Hypoxia

Commonly, following and despite effective compensation for Vo_2 and Do_2 abnormalities, organ dysfunction continues to progress. This MOSD progression occurs in the face of an O_2-independent, high-flow, hyperdynamic state. Evolving evidence suggests that the third scenario, cellular metabolic derangement or cytopathic hypoxia,[12] plays a key role in this sepsis-associated organ dysfunction. Mitochondrial dysfunction occurs despite adequate Po_2 in the cytosol. Fink[12] defines cytopathic hypoxia as sepsis-induced alterations in cellular energy metabolism caused by acquired intrinsic derangements in cellular respiration.[6]

To better understand the potential derangements discussed later, some basic concepts of energy metabolism are now reviewed.

ATP can be generated in cells as a result of aerobic or anaerobic processes. Virtually all cellular processes are driven by energy released when ATP is hydrolyzed to ADP and inorganic phosphate (Pi).

$$ATP \leftrightarrow ADP + Pi + H^+$$
yielding 7.3 kcal/mol.

Aerobic generation of ATP occurs in the mitochondria via oxidative phosphorylation along the electron transport chain in which nicotine adenine dinucleotide (NADH) and flavin adenine dinucleotide ($FADH_2$) are reduction-oxidized (redox) by molecular oxygen,

$$NADH + \tfrac{1}{2} O_2 + H^+ \leftrightarrow H_2O + NAD^+$$

yielding 52.6 kcal/mol, which is used in the electron transport chain to create ATP from $ADP + Pi + H^+$.

Anaerobic generation of ATP occurs in the cytosol and in the mitochondria via ATP-generating reactions that catalyze the following substrates with ADP into ATP:

1,3-Diphosphoglycerate + ADP <———————————>3-diphosphoglycerate + ATP
Phosphoglycerate
kinase

Phosphoenolpyruvate + ADP <———————————> pyruvate + ATP
Pyruvate
kinase

1,3-Succinyl CoA + ADP <———————————> succinate + ATP
Succinyl CoA
Synthase

Oxidative phosphorylation is a more efficient process than substrate level phosphorylation, yielding up to 8 times more ATP than the anaerobic pathway per mole of glucose.

Potential Mechanisms to Explain Cytopathic Metabolic Dysfunction in Sepsis

Inactivation of pyruvate dehydrogenase
Pyruvate dehydrogenase (PDH) activity in the mitochondria is compromised, leading to decreased use of glucose through the mitochondrial tricarboxylic acid cycle and increased accumulation of pyruvate in the cytoplasm of cells. This process results in the production of lactate in sepsis even in the absence of hypoxia.[21-23]

Inhibition of mitochondrial respiration by nitric oxide
Sepsis-associated increased production of nitric oxide (NO) has been noted throughout the literature as the result of nitric oxide synthase (NOS) induction. NO is a reversible inhibitor of cytochrome oxidase, the terminal step in the mitochondrial electron transport chain, by competing with O_2 for the same binding site on the enzyme complex.[24,25] The effect is exacerbated during low Po_2.[25]

Evidence to support this mechanism was reported by Piel and colleagues,[26] who showed that administration of exogenous cytochrome c was not only taken up by the cardiomyocytes from septic rats but was also stored in the cardiac mitochondria and improved myocardial contractility in sepsis-induced myocardial dysfunction as 1 possibility.

Inhibition of mitochondrial respiration by peroxynitrite
NO can interact with superoxide (O_2^-) to form peroxynitrite ($ONOO^-$), which is a potent oxidizing agent. $ONOO^-$ causes irreversible inhibition of mitochondrial respiration via several mechanisms.

Uncoupling of oxidative phosphorylation
This concept implies that oxygen becomes unlinked as the final proton acceptor for the oxidation of NADH and $FADH_2$, thus derailing the electron transport chain.

Activation of poly-(ADP-ribose) polymerase

Poly-(ADP-ribose) polymerase (PARP) is a nuclear enzyme that is activated by single strand breaks in nuclear DNA and leads to decreased ATP production caused by depletion of NAD^+/NADH.

THE ROLE OF LACTATE IN SEPSIS

Traditionally, increased lactate has been considered a marker of tissue hypoxia and anaerobic glycolysis in critically ill patients, particularly those in shock states. In the past decade, numerous investigators have questioned the reliability of lactate as an indicator of tissue hypoxia because increased serum lactate levels are often present in certain patient populations in the absence of clear signs of tissue hypoperfusion or significant hypoxemia, leading to the proposal that in certain patient populations this increased lactate level is related to metabolic processes other than primary hypoxemia,[27] such as overproduction of pyruvate.

Under normal physiologic conditions, lactate is produced in the cytosol of highly metabolic tissues such as muscle, skin, brain, intestine, liver, red blood cells, and many other tissues, including inflammatory cells, by the following equation. Pyruvate is a by-product of glucose/glycogen metabolism, or muscle catabolism via the deamination of alanine. Pyruvate is then either used by the mitochondria in the Krebs cycle or converted to lactate anaerobically via:

$$Pyruvate + NADH + H^+ \leftrightarrow lactate + NAD$$

This reaction favors lactate formation, yielding a 10-fold lactate/pyruvate ratio. Lactate is then metabolized predominantly by the liver and kidney. In physiologic steady state, normal serum lactate levels remain less than 2 mmol/L.

Once produced, lactate readily moves between lactate-producing and lactate-consuming sites via intracellular and extracellular lactate shuttles.[28] These shuttles are facilitated by concentration and hydrogen ion gradients and lactate transport proteins called monocarboxyate transporters.[28] Lactate is cleared predominantly via 3 paths: oxidation, gluconeogenesis/glyconeogenesis, and transamination. Lactate accumulates when production exceeds clearance.

Type A and Type B Lactic Acidosis

Type A lactic acidosis occurs when there is clinical evidence of tissue hypoxia, and is seen most commonly in low cardiac output shock states such as[29]:

- Cardiogenic shock
- Hypovolemic shock
- Low-flow septic shock (catecholamine resistant circulatory failure)[20,30,31]
- Septic shock before volume expansion.[11,29]

Existing Do_2 or Vo_2 deficits can be clear in these scenarios.

Type B lactic acidosis occurs when there is no clinical evidence of tissue hypoxia and increased lactate levels are attributed to stress-related metabolic imbalances. Sepsis is accompanied by a characteristic hypermetabolic state in which increased pyruvate production results from catecholamine-induced accelerated aerobic glycolysis, muscle protein catabolism, and inflammation.[32,33] When pyruvate production exceeds the capacity of the mitochondria to metabolize this substrate because of substrate overload or mitochondrial dysfunction, hyperlactatemia can occur in the presence of adequate tissue oxygenation.

The theory of sepsis-related metabolic adjustment resulting in hyperlactacidemia is supported by the following:

- Hyperlactacidemic septic patients do not consistently demonstrate inadequate Do_2
- Tissue Po_2 in septic patients is often within normal limits or increased[34]
- Muscle ATP levels are normal in septic human muscle[35]
- Numerous animal models and several human studies have shown that dichloroacetate, a PDH activator that converts pyruvate into acetyl-CoA via the respiratory chain, significantly decreases lactatemia in septic states[36,37]
- Lactate can originate from a regional source, ie, from infiltrating inflammatory cells in lungs during acute respiratory distress syndrome.[38–41]

Other causes of aerobic hyperlactatemia can include reduction of lactate clearance by the liver or kidneys and PDH dysfunction.

What is the Metabolic Value of Aerobic Hyperlactatemia?

Hyperlactatemia in shock states may reflect an adaptive protective mechanism by favoring oxidation of lactate rather than glucose in tissues in which oxygen is available, thus preserving glucose in tissues in which oxygen content is rare.[30,33] For example, brain[42] and heart[43–46] can use lactate as a preferred source of energy in certain situations of physiologic stress.

TISSUE-SPECIFIC CONSIDERATIONS

The lungs, liver, and kidneys are the organs most commonly affected by the dysoxia in severe sepsis; however, the function of other tissues such as the heart, skeletal muscle, brain, microcirculation, and thyroid can be just as severely affected.

Lung

The intricacy of distal respiratory anatomy is a testament to the fragile nature of the integrity of lung tissue. Distal to the respiratory bronchioles lie the alveolar ducts, then the alveolar sacs and alveoli.[8]

Alveolar ducts are minute aggregates of smooth muscle cells with associated collagen and elastic fibers that form rings around the openings of the alveolar sacs and alveoli. Cytoplasm of alveolar duct smooth muscle is composed of parallel myofilaments that occupy most of the cytoplasm and are powered by energy released from mitochondria and glycogen granules diffusely interspersed throughout the cytosol.[8] Intercellular contact areas facilitate spread of excitation throughout the smooth muscle. These alveolar ducts regulate alveolar air movement and this function can be easily derailed by mitochondrial dysfunction.

The alveolar ducts lead to the alveolar sacs, which structurally give rise to clusters of alveoli. Each alveolus is lined with 2 types of epithelial cells (type I and type II pneumocytes) and surrounded by connective tissue with its associated cell types and blood vessels with their associated cell types. These tissue components are responsible for the structural and functional integrity of the alveoli. Type I pneumocytes are large flattened cells with large cell membranes that line most of the alveolar surface area (about 97%) and are predominantly responsible for gaseous diffusion. Type II pneumocytes are round cells present in larger numbers than type I cells but occupying much smaller (about 3%) alveolar surface area and are responsible for surfactant secretion. Highly energy-dependent active transport of solutes and fluid across the alveolar epithelium occurs under normal physiologic and pathologic conditions.[47]

Surrounding the alveoli and within the attenuated, fine-reticular collagen connective tissue are elastic fibers, fibroblasts, a rich plexus of capillaries, and alveolar macrophages. In most of the alveolar wall, the basement membrane that supports the capillary endothelium is directly applied to the basement membrane supporting the surface epithelium and is devoid of connective tissue to maximize the air-blood interface to facilitate diffusion.

Hypoxia induces pulmonary vascular smooth muscle proliferation and vascular remodeling by affecting cell adhesion and migration, and secretion of extracellular matrix proteins.[48] This smooth muscle proliferation can contribute to pulmonary hypertension. Negash and colleagues[48] recently demonstrated that decreased cyclic guanosine monophosphate (cGMP)-dependent protein kinase (PKG) activity noted in acute hypoxia may play a significant role in this process.

Local macrophage and fibroblast activation in addition to systemic sepsis-triggered cytokine release that compromises mitochondrial energy production make this tissue a prime target for organ failure. Alveolar macrophages derived from circulating blood monocytes reside in the alveolar walls and alveolar spaces to promote phagocytic function for particulate matter in the alveoli. These alveolar macrophages in addition to connective tissue fibroblasts and systemic inflammatory cells can all be major contributing factors to the IL-1β and TNF-α inflammatory acute lung injury (ALI)[49,50] noted in sepsis. Loss of type I pneumocyte cellular membrane integrity leads to compromised alveolar diffusion and exacerbating deficits in Vo_2. Compromised surfactant production from type II pneumocytes can lead to alveolar collapse, also compromising Vo_2. Compromised monocytes and fibroblast function related to impaired cellular respiration can affect clearance of intra-alveolar debris and connective tissue remodeling following ALI.

Liver

The high metabolic demands of the liver are explained by the numerous concurrent metabolic and biosynthetic functions it provides, such as detoxification of metabolic waste products, destruction and recycling of spent red blood cells (alone or in combination with the spleen), synthesis and secretion of bile into the duodenum via the biliary system, synthesis of plasma proteins including clotting factors, and synthesis of plasma lipoproteins.

The liver is unique in that it has a dual blood supply. Most metabolic substrates for hepatic metabolism are provided by the portal circulation and are codependent on the functional integrity of the gastrointestinal tract, whereas oxygen required to support the intense metabolic activity is predominantly supplied in arterial blood by the hepatic artery.

Hepatocyte cytoplasm is crowded with energy- and oxygen-dependent organelles such as smooth and rough endoplasmic reticulum, mitochondria, and lysosomes. In addition, lobular sinusoids are populated with aggressive phagocytic monocyte-macrophage defense system cells called Kupffer cells that can augment the intense inflammatory response that occurs in sepsis.

The large size of the liver and complex nature of the hepatic lobular structure predispose to cardiopulmonary hypoperfusion and hypoxia-related tissue injury based on the distance between the afferent arteriole network and the capillary bed at the center of the hepatic lobules. Hepatic injury resulting from hypoperfusion of hypoxemia, or dysoxia from cytokine-mediated mitochondrial injury/dysfunction in sepsis, has been demonstrated recently by Struck and colleagues,[51] who discovered that septic patients consistently exhibited increased levels of carbamoyl phosphate synthetase (CPS-1), an enzyme primarily confined to hepatic mitochondria that catalyzes the first step in the urea cycle.[51] CPS-1 release can be considered a marker of mitochondrial damage that is prevalent in the context of liver sepsis.[51] Subsequent study by Crouser and colleagues[52–54] confirmed that increased CPS-1 levels occurred in a septic animal model of oxidative stress, and that these increased CPS-1 levels were associated with significant depletion of mitochondrial mass in the liver but suggested that accelerated mitochondrial clearance from the cell (ie, autophagy) not cell death accounted for mitochondrial depletion during the subacute phase of sepsis.

Kidney

Nephrons are the functional units of the urinary system. There are approximately 1 million nephrons per kidney and they are responsible for osmoregulation and excretion via filtration of most small molecules from blood plasma followed by selective reabsorption of most of the water and other molecules from this filtrate and the secretion of some excretory products directly from the blood into the filtrate to be eliminated in the urine.

Additional renal functions include support of blood pressure homeostatic mechanisms mediated by the renin-angiotensin-aldosterone mechanism and erythrocyte production in the bone marrow stimulated by erythropoietin production. Both functions contribute to the oxygen-carrying capacity of the blood.

The 2 major components of the nephron are the renal corpuscle (Bowman capsule and the glomerulus) and the renal convoluted tubules (proximal convoluted tubule [PCT], loop of Henle, distal convoluted tubule [DCT], and collecting ducts). The corpuscle creates a filtrate from the blood plasma and these tubules selectively reabsorb water, inorganic ions, and other molecules from the glomerular filtrate, and actively secrete some organic ions directly from the blood into the lumina of the tubule. The PCT actively reabsorbs about 75% of the glomerular filtrate and has a cytosol packed principally with mitochondria, reflecting the high-energy demands of this process.

The bulk of the renal cortex is composed of corpuscles and PCTs. The loop of Henle is located closest to the tip of the renal medulla and the collecting tubules in the medulla permit production of an increasing osmotic gradient from the cortex to the medulla by osmosis in the presence of ADH. This is a less energy-dependent process than PCT reabsorption. The DCTs are shorter than and located adjacent to the PCTs, have fewer cellular organelles than PCTs, and are mainly involved in aldosterone-mediated active reabsorption of sodium ions from the tubular fluid.

Total renal blood flow normally exceeds the oxygen requirements of the organ but the renal medulla receives only about 10% to 15% of renal blood flow, and the Pao_2 of the renal medulla is about 8 to 25 mm Hg under normoxic conditions.[55] Although this tissue oxygenation is acceptable under compensated physiologic conditions, this anatomy combined with the metabolic activity of the medulla and subcortical region make the nephron in this region particularly susceptible to hypoperfusion or hypoxemia. Hypoperfusion from hypovolemia can be temporarily and partially compensated for via afferent arteriolar vasodilatation and efferent arteriolar vasoconstriction to maintain glomerular filtration rate until neuron-hormonal mechanisms facilitate the recovery of intravascular volume and vasomotor tone.

Acute renal failure (ARF) is described as a sudden and sustained decrease in glomerular filtration associated with accumulation of metabolic waste products and water. If sepsis then cytokine-related ARF develop and proceed uncorrected, a cycle of renal-associated metabolic dysfunction, cytokine release, and multiorgan dysfunction occurs; such pathophysiology is associated with 10% to 95% mortality even when hemodynamic dysfunction is corrected. It is unclear whether hypoxia per se or reperfusion causes the renal injury but the confirmed absence of devastating anatomic injury on autopsy specimens refocuses the literature on the concept of cytopathic hypoxia.

What is the Next Best Thing to Detection of Hypoxia at the Cellular Level?

Somewhere between direct detection of hypoxia at the cellular level (ie, biomarkers, enzyme assays, complex histopathologic analyses) and indices of global hypoperfusion (ie, lactate, $ScVo_2$, urine output) lies a potentially more practical and economical method of tissue oxygenation assessment: near-infrared spectroscopy (NIRS).

NIRS is an evolving technology that uses near-infrared light to provide a continuous assessment of regional, microvascular blood flow and is measured as the quantitative clinical variable tissue-oxygen saturation (Sto_2). Biologic tissues are transparent to light in the near-infrared spectrum, whereas oxyhemoglobin (Hbo_2) and deoxyhemoglobin (Hb) have significantly different spectra[56] ($Sto_2 = Hbo_2/[Hbo_2 + Hb]$). This technology can be used invasively via transcranial or percutaneous catheters, or noninvasively using cutaneously applied probes.

In the past decade, this technology has been validated in several studies, including various tissue oxygenation assessments of healthy human subjects,[57,58] and studied in selected populations of critically ill trauma patients,[59,60] several animal models,[61,62] and selected populations of septic human patients.[63–65] However, strong data validating the efficacy of NIRS in patients with severe sepsis and septic shock are lacking.

A multicenter clinical trial is under way to study NIRS in severe sepsis (OTO-STS). This study was set to conclude in December 2009 and it is hoped that it will shed much anticipated light on the value of NIRS as a tool in the resuscitation management of septic patients.

SUMMARY

- Organ function is critically linked to the way tissues use available oxygen.
- In sepsis, tissue-related hypoxic injury is the result of hypoxemia and hypoperfusion and cytokine-mediated mitochondrial dysfunction termed cytopathic hypoxia
- Organ dysfunction in sepsis is more likely related to derailment of the metabolic processes of cells to use available oxygen.
- Cellular dysoxia rather than hypoxia may be the most appropriate way of describing sepsis-related tissue injury
- Lactate is a marker of aerobic mitochondrial dysfunction and anaerobic tissue metabolism and in some circumstances is considered the fuel of choice for certain tissues
- The concept of cellular metabolic derangement or cytopathic hypoxia as a potential cause for MOSD in sepsis may direct efforts to optimize outcome in septic patients from the classic targets of CO, tissue perfusion, DVo_2, and Vo_2 toward moderating sepsis-related early cytokine response, maximizing mitochondrial function, and using biomarkers to monitor treatment response.

REFERENCES

1. Connett RJ, Honig CR, Gayeski EJ, et al. Defining hypoxia: a systems view of VO2, glycolysis, energetics, and intracellular PO2. J Appl Phys 1990;68:833–42.
2. Duke T. Dysoxia and lactate. Arch Dis Child 1999;81:343–50.
3. Hotchkiss RS, Swanson PE, Freeman BD, et al. Apoptotic cell death in patients with sepsis, shock, and multiple organ dysfunction. Crit Care Med 1999;27: 1230–51.
4. Nunn JF. Oxygen. In: Nunn JF, editor. Nunn's applied respiratory physiology. Oxford: Butterworth-Heinemann Ltd; 1993. p. 247–305.

5. Guyton AC. Transport of oxygen and carbon dioxide in the blood and body fluids. In: Textbook of medical physiology. 5th edition. Philadelphia: WB Saunders; 1976. p. 543–71.

6. Whalen WJ. Intracellular PO_2 in heart and skeletal muscle. Physiologist 1971;14: 69–82.

7. Kessler MH, Lang H, Sinagowitz R, et al. Homeostasis of oxygen supply in liver and kidney. In: Bicher HI, Bruely DF, editors, Oxygen transport to tissue. Instrumentation, methods and physiology. Advances in experimental medicine and biology, vol. 37A. New York: Plenum Press; 1973. p. 351–60.

8. Chance B, Oshino N, Sugano T, et al. Basic principles of tissue oxygenation determination from mitochondrial signals. In: Bicher HI, Bruely DF, editors, Oxygen transport to tissue. Instrumentation, methods and physiology. Advances in experimental medicine and biology, vol. 37A. New York: Plenum Press; 1973. p. 277–92.

9. Treciak S, Dellinger RP, Abate NL, et al. Translating research to clinical practice: a 1-year experience with implementing early goal-directed therapy for septic shock in the emergency department. Chest 2006;129:225–32.

10. Boulos M, Astiz ME, Barua RS, et al. Impaired mitochondrial function induced by serum from septic shock patients is attenuated by inhibition of nitric oxide synthase and poly (ADP-ribose) synthase. Crit Care Med 2003;31:353–8.

11. Rivers EP, Kruse JA, Jacobson G, et al. The influence of early hemodynamic optimization on biomarker patterns of severe sepsis and septic shock. Crit Care Med 2007;35(9):2016–24.

12. Fink M. Cytopathic hypoxia in sepsis. Acta Anaesthesiol Scand Suppl 1997;110: 87–95.

13. Fink MP. Cytopathic hypoxia. A concept to explain organ dysfunction in sepsis. Minerva Anestesiol 2000;66(5):337–42.

14. Fink MP. Cytopathic hypoxia in sepsis: a true problem? Minerva Anestesiol 2001; 67(4):290–1.

15. Fink M. Cytopathic hypoxia. Is oxygen use impaired in sepsis as a result of an acquired intrinsic derangement in cellular respiration? Crit Care Clin 2002; 18(1):165–75.

16. Fink MP. Research: advances in cell biology relevant to critical illness. Curr Opin Crit Care 2004;10:279–91.

17. Fink MP. Administration of exogenous cytochrome c as a novel approach for the treatment of cytopathic hypoxia. Crit Care Med 2007;35(9):2224–5.

18. Gogos CA, Drosou E, Bassaris HP, et al. Pro- versus anti-inflammatory cytokine profile in patients with severe sepsis: a marker for prognosis and future therapeutic options. J Infect Dis 2000;181:176–80.

19. Osuchowski MF, Welch K, Siddiqui J, et al. Circulating cytokine/inhibitor profiles reshape the understanding of the SIRS/CARS continuum in sepsis and predict mortality. J Immunol 2006;177:1967–74.

20. Rivers E, Nguyen B, Havstad S, et al. Early goal-directed therapy in the treatment of severe sepsis and septic shock. N Engl J Med 2001;345: 1368–77.

21. Fink MP. Cytopathic hypoxia. Mitochondrial dysfunction as mechanism contributing to organ dysfunction in sepsis. Crit Care Clin 2001;17(1):219–37.

22. Vary TC. Sepsis-induced alterations in pyruvate dehydrogenase complex activity in rat skeletal muscle: effects on plasma lactate. Shock 1996;8:89.

23. Vary TC, Hazen S. Sepsis alters pyruvate dehydrogenase kinase activity in skeletal muscle. Mol Cell Biochem 1999;198:113.

24. Borutaite V, Brown GC. Rapid reduction of nitric oxide by mitochondria, and reversible inhibition of mitochondrial respiration by nitric oxide. Biochem J 1996;315:295.

25. Cassina A, Radi R. Differential inhibitory action of nitric oxide and peroxynitrite on mitochondrial electron transport. Arch Biochem Biophys 1996;328:309.

26. Piel DA, Gruber PJ, Weinheimer CJ, et al. Mitochondrial resuscitation with exogenous cytochrome c in the septic heart. Crit Care Med 2007;35:2120–7.

27. Gladden LB. Lactate metabolism – a new paradigm for the third millennium. J Physiol 2004;558:5–30.

28. Brooks GA. Intra- and extra-cellular lactate shuttles. Med Sci Sports Exerc 2000; 32(4):790–800.

29. Cohen RD, Woods HF. Clinical and biochemical aspects of lactic acidosis. Boston: Blackwell Scientific Publications; 1976.

30. Levy B, Sadoune LO, Gelot AM, et al. Evolution of lactate/pyruvate and arterial ketone body ratios in the early course of catecholamine-treated septic shock. Crit Care Med 2000;28:114–9.

31. Gilbert EM, Haupt MT, Mandanas RY, et al. The effect of liquid loading, blood transfusion, and catecholamine infusion on oxygen delivery and consumption in patients with sepsis. Am Rev Respir Dis 1986;134:873–8.

32. Gore DC, Jahoor F, Hibbert JM, et al. Lactic acidosis during sepsis is related to increased pyruvate production, not deficits in tissue oxygen availability. Ann Surg 1996;224:97–102.

33. Levy B. Lactate and shock state: the metabolic review. Curr Opin Crit Care 2006; 12:315–21.

34. Boeksteggers P, Weidenhofer S, Kapsner T, et al. Skeletal muscle partial pressure of oxygen in patients with sepsis. Crit Care Med 1994;22:640–50.

35. Hotchkiss RS, Karl IE. Reevaluation of the role of cellular hypoxia and bioenergetic failure in sepsis. JAMA 1992;267:1503–10.

36. Stacpoole PW, Harman EM, Curry SH, et al. Treatment of lactic acidosis with dichloroacetate. N Engl J Med 1983;309:390–6.

37. De Baker D, Creteur J, Silva E, et al. The hepatosplanchnic area is not a common source of lactate in patients with severe sepsis. Crit Care Med 2001;29:256–61.

38. Iscra F, Gullo A, Biolo G. Bench-to-bedside review: lactate and the lung. Crit Care 2002;6:327–9.

39. Zeller WP, The SM, Sweet M, et al. Altered glucose transporter mRNA abundance in the rat model of endotoxemic shock. Biochem Biophys Res Commun 1991; 176:535–40.

40. Karimova A, Pinsky DJ. The endothelial response to oxygen deprivation: biology and clinical implications. Intensive Care Med 2001;27:19–31.

41. Wheater PR, Burkitt HG, Daniels VG, et al. Functional histology: a text and colour atlas. New York: Churchill Livingstone; 1979.

42. Schurr A, Payne RS, Miller JJ, et al. Brain lactate is an obligatory aerobic energy substrate for functional recovery after hypoxia: further in vitro validation. J Neurochem 1997;69:423–6.

43. Kline JA, Thronton LR, Lopaschuk GD, et al. Lactate improves cardiac efficiency after hemorrhagic shock. Shock 2000;14:215–21.

44. Levraut J, Ciebiera JP, Chasve S, et al. Mild hyperlactatemia in stable septic patients is due to impaired lactate clearance rather than overproduction. Am J Respir Crit Care Med 1998;157:1021–6.

45. Revelly JP, Tappy L, Martinez A, et al. Lactate and glucose metabolism in severe sepsis and septic shock. Crit Care Med 2005;33:2235–40.

46. Stacpoole PW, Nagaraja NV, Hutson AD. Efficacy of dichloroacetate as a lactate-lowering drug. J Clin Pharmacol 2003;43:683–91.
47. Guidot DM, Folkesson HG, Jain L, et al. Integrating acute lung injury and regulation of alveolar fluid clearance. Am J Physiol Lung Cell Mol Physiol 2006;291: L301–6.
48. Negash S, Narasimhan SR, Zhou W, et al. Role of cGMP-dependent protein kinase in regulation of pulmonary vascular smooth muscle cell adhesion and migration: effect of hypoxia. Am J Physiol Heart Circ Physiol 2009;297(1):H304–12.
49. Baboolal HA, Ichinose F, Ullrich R, et al. Reactive oxygen species scavengers attenuate endotoxin-induced impairment of hypoxic pulmonary vasoconstriction in mice. Anesthesiology 2002;97(5):1227–33.
50. Liang W, Ray JB, He JZ, et al. Regulation of proliferation and membrane potential by chloride currents in rat pulmonary artery smooth muscle cells. Hypertension 2009;54:286–93.
51. Struck J, Uhlein M, Mortgenthaler NG, et al. Release of mitochondrial enzyme carbamoyl phosphate synthase under septic conditions. Shock 2005;23:533–8.
52. Crouser ED, Julian MW, Huff JE, et al. Carbamoyl phosphate synthase-1: a marker of mitochondrial damage and depletion in the liver during sepsis. Crit Care Med 2006;34(9):2439–46.
53. Sykes E, Cosgrove JF. Acute renal failure and the critically ill surgical patient. Ann R Coll Surg Engl 2007;89(1):22–9.
54. Rosenberger C, Rosen S, Heyman SN. Renal parenchymal oxygenation and hypoxia adaptation in acute kidney injury. Clin Exp Pharmacol Physiol 2006;33:980–8.
55. Tillyard A, Keays R, Soni N. The diagnosis of acute renal failure in intensive care: mongrel or pedigree? Anaesthesia 2005;60:903–14.
56. Jobsis FF. Noninvasive, infrared monitoring of cerebral oxygen sufficiency and circulation parameters. Science 1977;198(4323):1264–7.
57. Mancini DM, Bolinger L, Li H, et al. Validation of near-infrared spectroscopy in humans. J Appl Physiol 1994;776:2740–7.
58. Colier WNJM. Near-infrared spectroscopy: toy or tool? An investigation on the clinical applicability of near-infrared spectroscopy. Thesis, University of Nijmegen. The Netherlands; 1995. p. 9–106.
59. Cairns CB, Moore FA, Haenel JB, et al. Evidence for early supply independent mitochondrial dysfunction in patients developing multiple organ failure after trauma. J Trauma 1997;423:532–6.
60. McKinley BA, Marvin RG, Cocanour CS, et al. Tissue hemoglobin O2 saturation during resuscitation of traumatic shock monitored using near-infrared spectrometry. J Trauma 2000;48:637–42.
61. Ince C, Sinaasappel M. Microcirculatory oxygen and shunting in sepsis and shock. Crit Care Med 1999;27:1369–77.
62. Nahum E, Skippen PW, Gagnon RE. Correlation of transhepatic near-infrared spectroscopy readings with liver surface readings and perfusion parameters in a piglet endotoxemic shock model. Liver Int 2006;26(10):1277–82.
63. Mesquida J, Masip J, Gili G, et al. Thenar oxygen saturation measured by near-infrared spectroscopy as a noninvasive predictor of low central venous oxygenation in septic patients. Intensive Care Med 2009;35(6):1106–9.
64. Poeze M. Tissue-oxygenation assessment using near-infrared spectroscopy during severe sepsis: confounding effects of tissue edema on StO2 values. Intensive Care Med 2006;32:788–9.
65. Fredrich O. Critical illness myopathy: sepsis-mediated failure of the peripheral nervous system. Eur J Anaesthesiol Suppl 2008;42:73–82.

Index

A

Acetaminophen, lactic acidosis due to, 265
Acidosis, lactic, **255–283.** See also Lactic acidosis.
Acute hemodynamic instability of unknown cause, tamponade vs. sepsis in, 376
β_2-Adrenergic agents, lactic acidosis due to, 268
Alcohol(s)
    sugar, lactic acidosis due to, 270
    toxic, lactic acidosis due to, 265–266
Aliphatic nitriles, lactic acidosis due to, 271
Anemia
    acute
        physiologic response to, 338
        tolerance to, limits of, 339
    cardiac effects of, 339–340
    RBCs transfusion for, 329
Anesthetics, general, lactic acidosis due to, 271
Arterial lactate, venous lactate vs., 261–262

B

Biotin, lactic acidosis due to, 269–270
Bleeding, $SCVO_2$ monitoring as indicator of, 329
Blood, microcirculation and, 341

C

Cancer(s), transfusion-related immunomodulation and, 344
Cardiac cycle, effects of, 298
Cardiac output
    estimation of, methods of, history of, 384–385
    in ICU, techniques for determination of, **355–364**
        electrical bioreactance cardiography, 363
        esophageal Doppler technique, 363
        FloTrac Vigleo system, 359
        lithium dilution, 358
        measurement in, 356–360
        mixed venous oxygen saturation, 359–360
        noninvasive techniques, 360–362
        pulmonary artery catheter, 357–358
        pulse contour waveform analysis, 359
        TEB, 360

Crit Care Clin 26 (2010) 423–432
doi:10.1016/S0749-0704(10)00014-X
0749-0704/10/$ – see front matter © 2010 Elsevier Inc. All rights reserved.

criticalcare.theclinics.com

Cardiac output (*continued*)
    transgastric Doppler technique, 363
    transpulmonary thermodilution, 358
    USCOM, 363
  noninvasive monitoring of, partial CO_2 rebreathing in, **383–392.** See also *Partial CO_2 rebreathing, noninvasive monitoring cardiac output using.*
Cardiothoracic surgery patients, NICO monitor in partial CO_2 rebreathing evaluation effects on, 387–388
Cheyne-Stokes respiration, 356
Children, NICO monitor in, 389
Cocaine, lactic acidosis due to, 270
Continuous RVEDV, 301–303
Convective transport, delivered oxygen–oxygen consumption and, relationship between, 241–242
"Critical" DO_2, 243–245
CVP, 296
Cyanide, lactic acidosis due to, 271
Cyanogenic compounds, lactic acidosis due to, 271
Cytopathic metabolic dysfunction, in sepsis, mechanisms of, 413–414

D

Delivered oxygen–oxygen consumption, convective transport and, relationship between, 241–242
Diethyl ether, lactic acidosis due to, 271
DO_2, "critical," 243–245
Do_2–VO_2, dobutamine and, 247–248
Do_2–VO_2–guided therapy, trials of, 245–247
Dobutamine, Do_2–VO_2 and, 247–248
Dopamine, in pharmacologic support of MAP in sepsis, 292
Drotrecogin alfa, in resuscitation of microcirculation in sepsis, 402

E

Early goal-directed therapy (EGRT), 248–249
Echocardiography
  described, 365
  in hemodynamic assessment of septic shock, **365–382**
    acute right ventricular failure, 374–376
    equipment for, 366
    focused study of, 366–369
    fundamentals of, 366
    hand-held and compact portable devices in, reliability of, 378–379
    left ventricular systolic function, 374
    strengths of, 365–366
    training related to, for intensivists, 376–378
    volume responsiveness in, preload/prediction of, 370–372
  in sepsis-induced myocardial dysfunction diagnosis, 372–374
EEO pressure. See *End-expiratory occlusion (EEO) pressure.*
EGRT. See *Early goal-directed therapy (EGRT).*
Elderly, NICO monitor in, 389

Electrical bioreactance cardiography, in determination of cardiac output in ICU, 361–362
End-expiratory occlusion (EEO) pressure, 316–317
Epinephrine, in pharmacologic support of MAP in sepsis, 291
Esophageal Doppler technique, in cardiac output determination in ICU, 363
External reference landmark, 296–297

F

Fick, Adolph, in cardiac output estimation, 384–385
FloTrac Vigleo system, in determination of cardiac output in ICU, 359
Flowmetry, in microcirculatory dysfunction measurement, 397
Fluorescence videomicroscopy, in microcirculatory dysfunction measurement, 396
5-Fluorouracil (5-FU), lactic acidosis due to, 271
Fructose, lactic acidosis due to, 270
5-FU. See *5-Fluorouracil (5-FU)*.

G

GEDV, 301–303
General anesthetics, lactic acidosis due to, 271

H

Halothane, lactic acidosis due to, 271
Heart
    anemia effects on, 339–340
    physiologic and anatomic properties of, 298–301
Hematocrit, optimal, **335–354**
    clinical trials related to, 346–347
Hemodynamic support, optimization of, in septic shock, central and mixed venous
    oxygen saturation in, **323–333.** See also *Septic shock, hemodynamic support in,
    optimization of, central and mixed venous oxygen saturation in.*
Hepatic failure, lactic acidosis and, 265
Hip surgery patients, NICO monitor in, 389
Hyperlactatemia
    aerobic, metabolic value of, 415
    drugs causing, 265–269
Hypoxia
    at cellular level, detection of, **409–421**
        described, 409–410
        tissue-specific considerations in, 415–418
    cytodynamic, hyperdynamic sepsis and, 412–413
    defined, 409
    tissue, causes of, 337

I

Immunomodulation, transfusion-related, 343–346
    cancer and, 344
    infection and, 344
    leukocytes, 344–346

Inborn errors of metabolism, lactic acidosis and, 271–272

Infection(s), transfusion-related immunomodulation and, 344

Inferior vena cava, respiratory variability of, 312–313

Inotropes, in resuscitation of microcirculation in sepsis, 400–401

Intensive care unit (ICU), cardiac output determination in, techniques for, **355–364.**
    See also *Cardiac output, in ICU, techniques for determination of.*

Intensivists, echocardiography training for, 376–378

Iron, lactic acidosis due to, 269–270

K

Kidney(ies), in detection of hypoxia at cellular level, 417

L

Lactate
    arterial, vs. venous lactate, 261–262
    as prognostic marker in critically ill patients, 258–259
    clearance of, 260–261
    formation of, 256
    history of, 255–256
    in sepsis, 414–415
    metabolism of, 256–258
    venous, vs. arterial lactate, 261–262

Lactated Ringer solution, 262

Lactate:pyruvate ratios, 259–260

Lactic acidosis, **255–283**
    D-, 272
    described, 255–256
    diseases underlying, 262–265
    hepatic failure and, 265
    malignancy-associated, 262–265
    SIRS and, 265
    thiamine deficiency and, 269–270
    type B, 262, 414–415
        causes of, 264
    type B2
        aliphatic nitriles and, 271
        biotin and, 269–270
        cocaine and, 270
        cyanide and, 271
        cyanogenic compounds and, 271
        diethyl ether and, 271
        drugs causing, 265–271
            acetaminophen, 265
            β_2-adrenergic agents, 268
            general anesthetics, 271
            halothane, 271
            linezolid, 268
            metformin, 267
            methamphetamine, 270–271
            nitroprusside, 271

NRTIs, 266–267
    propofol, 267–268
    salicylates, 268
    sulfasalazine, 269
    toxic alcohols, 265–266
  fructose and, 270
  5-FU and, 271
  iron and, 269–270
  malaria and, 270
  sorbitol and, 270
  strychnine and, 270
  sugar alcohols and, 270
  valproic acid and, 270
  xylitol and, 270
 type B3, 271–272
 types A and B, 414–415
D-Lactic acidosis, 272
Left ventricular systolic function, evaluation of, echocardiography in, 374
Lesion(s), storage, 342–343
Leukocyte(s), transfusion-related immunomodulation and, 344–346
Linezolid, lactic acidosis due to, 268
Lithium dilution, in cardiac output determination in ICU, 358
Liver, in detection of hypoxia at cellular level, 416–417
Liver failure, lactic acidosis and, 265
Lung(s), in detection of hypoxia at cellular level, 415–416
Lung injury(ies)
 severe, partial CO_2 rebreathing measurements in, 388–389
 transfusion-related, 346

M

Malaria, lactic acidosis due to, 270
Malignancy, lactic acidosis and, 262–265
MAP. See Mean arterial pressure (MAP).
Mathematical coupling, 242–243
Mean arterial pressure (MAP), **285–293**
 defined, 286–287
 monitoring of, 287–289
  invasive, 288–289
  noninvasive, 287–288
 pharmacologic support of, in sepsis, 289–292
 physiology of sepsis and, 289
Metabolism, inborn errors of, lactic acidosis and, 271–272
Metformin, lactic acidosis due to, 267
Methamphetamine, lactic acidosis due to, 270–271
Microcirculation
 blood and, 341
 in sepsis
  disturbances in, **393–408.** See also Sepsis, microcirculatory disturbances in.
  resuscitation of, 400–403
 overview of, 394

Microscopy, in microcirculatory dysfunction measurement, 396

Microvascular flow, measuring of, prognostic value of, 398–400

Mixed venous oxygen saturation, in cardiac output determination in ICU, 359–360

Myocardial dysfunction, sepsis-induced, diagnosis of, echocardiography in, 372–374

N

NICO (Noninvasive Cardiac Output) monitor, in partial CO_2 rebreathing evaluation, 385–388

   described, 385–386

   in cardiothoracic surgery patients, 387–388

   in children, 389

   in hip surgery patients, 389

   in the elderly, 389

   limitations of, 386–387

   pulmonary disease effects on, 387

   validation of, 386–387

Nitric oxide, inhibition of mitochondrial respiration by, cytopathic metabolic dysfunction in sepsis related to, 413

Nitriles, aliphatic, lactic acidosis due to, 271

Nitroprusside, lactic acidosis due to, 271

Noninvasive Cardiac Output (NICO) monitor, 385–388. See also *NICO (Noninvasive Cardiac Output) monitor.*

Norepinephrine, in pharmacologic support of MAP in sepsis, 290–291

NRTIs. See *Nucleoside/tide reverse transcriptase inhibitors (NRTIs).*

Nucleoside/tide reverse transcriptase inhibitors (NRTIs), lactic acidosis due to, 266–267

O

OPS imaging. See *Orthogonal polarization spectral (OPS) imaging.*

Orthogonal polarization spectral (OPS) imaging, in microcirculatory dysfunction measurement, 396–397

Oxidative phosphorylation, uncoupling of, cytopathic metabolic dysfunction in sepsis related to, 413

Oxygen consumption, macrocirculatory perspective of, **237–253**

Oxygen delivery, macrocirculatory perspective of, **237–253**

Oxygen transport, principles of, 336–337

Oxygenation, tissue

   effective, 410–411

   ineffective, 411

   measurement of, 337–338

Oxyge–oxygen consumption, delivered, convective transport and, relationship between, 241–242

P

Partial CO_2 rebreathing, noninvasive monitoring cardiac output using, **383–392**

   in severe lung injury, 388–389

   NICO monitor in, 385–388. See also *NICO (Noninvasive Cardiac Output) monitor, in partial CO_2 rebreathing evaluation.*

Passive leg raising (PLR), 314–315

Peroxynitrite, inhibition of mitochondrial respiration by, cytopathic metabolic dysfunction in sepsis related to, 413

Phenylephrine, in pharmacologic support of MAP in sepsis, 291–292

Plethmysography, 311–312

PLR. See *Passive leg raising (PLR)*.

Poly-(ADP-ribose) polymerase, activation of, cytopathic metabolic dysfunction in sepsis related to, 414

P_{pao}, 296

PPV. See *Pulse pressure variation (PPV)*.

Preload

  assessment of, static measures of, **295–305**

    pressure measurements, 296–301

    volumetric measurements, 301–303

  dynamic indices of, **307–321**

    Cavallaro group A and B indices, cautions regarding, 313–314

    EEO pressure, 316–317

    physiologic rationale of, 308–309

    plethmysography, 311–312

    PLR, 314–315

    PPV, 310–313

    RSVT, 315–316

    SPV, 310

    SVV, 309–310

    Valsalva maneuver, 317–318

Pressure, EEO, 316–317

Pressure measurements, 296–301

  CVP, 296

  effects of cardiac cycle, 298

  effects of respiratory cycle, 297–298

  external reference landmark, 296–297

  physiologic and anatomic properties of heart, 298–301

  P_{pao}, 296

Propofol, lactic acidosis due to, 267–268

Pulmonary artery catheter, in cardiac output determination in ICU, 357–358

Pulmonary disease, NICO monitor in partial CO_2 rebreathing evaluation affected by, 387

Pulse contour waveform analysis, in cardiac output determination in ICU, 359

Pulse pressure variation (PPV), 310–313

Pyruvate dehydrogenase, inactivation of, cytopathic metabolic dysfunction in sepsis related to, 413

R

RBCs. See *Red blood cells (RBCs)*.

Rebreathing, partial CO_2, noninvasive monitoring cardiac output using, **383–392**. See also *Partial CO_2 rebreathing, noninvasive monitoring cardiac output using*.

Red blood cells (RBCs)

  physiology of, 340–341

  transfusion of, 329

Respiration, Cheyne-Stokes, 356

Respiratory cycle, effects of, 297–298

Respiratory systolic variation test (RSVT), 315–316

Right ventricular failure, acute, echocardiographic identification of, 374–376

RSVT. See *Respiratory systolic variation test (RSVT)*.

RVEDV, continuous, 301–303

S

Salicylates, lactic acidosis due to, 268

$SCVO_2$

    measurement of, 325–326

        SVO_2 measurement and, relationship between, 326–327

    monitoring of, bleeding indicated by, 329

SDF imaging. See *Sidestream dark-field (SDF) imaging.*

Sepsis

    cytopathic metabolic dysfunction in, mechanisms of, 413–414

    defined, 393

    hyperdynamic, cytopathic hypoxia and, 412–413

    hypodynamic, management of, 411–412

    incidence of, 393–394

    lactate in, 414–415

    microcirculation in, resuscitation of, 400–403

        drotrecogin alfa in, 402

        inotropes in, 400–401

        vasodilators in, 401–402

        vasopressors in, 400–401

    microcirculatory disturbances in, **393–408**

        correction of, 400–403

        measurement of, 395–398

            flowmetry in, 397

            fluorescence videomicroscopy in, 396

            indirect techniques in, 397–398

            microscopy/videomicroscopy in, 396

            OPS imaging in, 396–397

            prognostic value of, 398–400

            SDF imaging in, 397

            technical limitations in, 398

        mechanisms of, 394–395

    myocardial dysfunction related to, diagnosis of, echocardiography in, 372–374

    pharmacologic support of MAP in, 289–292

    physiology of, MAP and, 289

    tamponade vs., in acute hemodynamic instability of unknown cause, 376

Septic shock

    hemodynamic assessment of, echocardiography in, **365–382.** See also *Echocardiography, in hemodynamic assessment of septic shock.*

    hemodynamic support in, optimization of, central and mixed venous oxygen saturation in, **323–333**

        bleeding, 329

        clinical uses of, 327

        monitoring of, 327–329

        SVO_2 and $SCVO_2$ measurements, 325–327

        venous-to-arterial CO_2 difference, 329–330

Shock, septic. See *Septic shock.*

Sidestream dark-field (SDF) imaging, in microcirculatory dysfunction measurement, 397

SIRS. See *Systemic inflammatory response syndrome (SIRS).*

Sorbitol, lactic acidosis due to, 270

SPV. See *Systolic pressure variation (SPV).*

Storage lesion, 342–343
Storage medium, 343
Stroke volume variation (SVV), 309–310
Strychnine, lactic acidosis due to, 270
Sulfasalazine, lactic acidosis due to, 269
Superior vena cava, respiratory variability of, 312–313
Surviving Sepsis Campaign guidelines, 249–250
SVO$_2$ measurement, 325–326
    SCVO$_2$ measurement and, relationship between, 326–327
SVV. See *Stroke volume variation (SVV)*.
Systemic inflammatory response syndrome (SIRS), lactic acidosis and, 265
Systolic pressure variation (SPV), 310

T

Tamponade, sepsis vs., in acute hemodynamic instability of unknown cause, 376
TEB. See *Thoracic bioimpednace (TEB)*.
Thiamine deficiency, lactic acidosis due to, 269–270
Thoracic bioimpednace (TEB), in cardiac output determination in ICU, 360
Tissue hypoxia, causes of, 337
Tissue oxygenation
    effective, 410–411
    ineffective, 411
    measurement of, 337–338
Transfusion(s), immunomodulation related to, 343–346. See also
    Immunomodulation, transfusion-related.
Transgastric Doppler technique, in cardiac output determination in ICU, 363
Transpulmonary thermodilution, in cardiac output determination in ICU, 358

U

USCOM, in cardiac output determination in ICU, 363

V

Valproic acid, lactic acidosis due to, 270
Valsalva maneuver, 317–318
Vasodilators, in resuscitation of microcirculation in sepsis, 401–402
Vasopressin, in pharmacologic support of MAP in sepsis, 291
Vasopressors, in resuscitation of microcirculation in sepsis, 400–401
Vena cava
    inferior, respiratory variability of, 312–313
    superior, respiratory variability of, 312–313
Venous lactate, arterial lactate vs., 261–262
Venous oxygen saturation
    central, in optimizing hemodynamic support in septic shock, **323–333**. See also *Septic
    shock, hemodynamic support in.*
    mixed
        determinants of, 325

Venous oxygen (*continued*)
  in optimizing hemodynamic support in septic shock, **323–333.** See also
  Septic shock, hemodynamic support in.
  physiology of, 324–326
Venous-to-arterial CO_2 difference, 329–330
Videomicroscopy
  fluorescence, in microcirculatory dysfunction measurement, 396
  in microcirculatory dysfunction measurement, 396
Volume responsiveness, in hemodynamic assessment of septic shock, preload/prediction
  of, 370–372
Volumetric measurements, 301–303

  X

Xylitol, lactic acidosis due to, 270